Lael Wertenbaker

To Mend the Heart

Foreword by Dwight E. Harken, M.D.

The Viking Press | New York

Library of Congress Cataloging in Publication Data
Wertenbaker, Lael.
  To mend the heart.
  Includes index.
  1. Heart—Surgery—History.   I. Title.
RD598.W43   617'.412'009   79-3630
ISBN 0-670-47092-9

Printed in the United States of America
Set in VIP Caledonia

ACKNOWLEDGMENTS

American Heart Association: Diagram, "Your Heart and How It Works." Reprinted by permission of the American Heart Association.
Crown Publishers, Inc.: Selection from *The New American Medical Dictionary and Health Manual, New Revised Edition* by Robert E. Rothenberg, M.D., F.A.C.S. Copyright © 1975 by Robert E. Rothenberg.
E. P. Dutton, The Lantz Office, Incorporated, Michael Joseph Ltd.: Excerpts from *Hearts* by Thomas Thompson. Copyright © 1971 by Thomas Thompson. (A McCalls/Saturday Review Press Book).
Robert S. Litwak: Excerpts from "The Growth of Cardiac Surgery: Historical Notes" by Robert S. Litwak, *Cardiovascular Clinics Series: Cardiac Surgery 1,* Volume 3, Number 2. Copyright © 1971 by F. A. Davis Company.
Macmillan Publishing Co., Inc., and *Curtis Brown, Ltd.:* Excerpts from *One Life* by Christiaan Barnard and Curtis Bill Pepper. Copyright © 1969 by Christiaan Neethling Barnard.
Scottish Medical Journal: A selection from "At the Receiving End" by Ian Donald, *Scottish Medical Journal,* 1976, 21:49, pp. 323–28.

To wake the soul by tender strokes of art,
To raise the genius, and to mend the heart;
To make mankind in conscious virtue bold,
Live o'er each scene, and be what they behold:
For this the Tragic Muse first trod the stage.

—Alexander Pope, Prologue to Addison's *Cato*

To Mend the Heart

Fiction

Perilous Voyage
Unbidden Guests
The Afternoon Women
Eye of the Lion
Festival
Lament for Four Virgins

Nonfiction

The Magic of Light (with Jean Rosenthal)
The World of Pablo Picasso (with the editors of Time-Life Books)
You and the Armed Services
Portrait of Hotchkiss
Mister Junior
Death of a Man

Foreword

This story of cardiac surgery is timely. Recent decades have been a "golden age" for the development of surgical techniques and devices, and heart surgery is fortunate to have been initiated and to have flourished as the bellwether of that progress. Controls, costs, and consumerism may have ended such an age, and I have wanted to see documentation of heart surgery's evolution. Here it is.

I have lived to see the heart as the last organ to yield to surgical invasion; then to become the newest area of specialty. First there was a compelling dream; second a time when I knew every patient in the world who had had surgery within the heart. Third, as the field grew, I could only know every surgeon who performed heart surgery, then only every heart surgical center. Finally heart surgery has become worldwide. It is truly ubiquitous. Mine has been more than a unique observation point. I have enjoyed the ultimate privilege of participation.

Why did I want this book to be written, when public exposure to medicine in action has so often been counterproductive? Is it because of a compulsion to correct the tarnished image of Medicine? Possibly subconsciously; yes, even consciously. Could it have been born of jealousy or ego? Possibly, but I hope not. These and related questions have bedeviled me during this book's gestation and preparation, through its changing shape from a biography to a study with a broader scope. At times the purpose of my collaboration was as simple (and noble) as public education, given urgency by fear of time's erosion of memory. Occasionally motivation was as frivolous as lagniappe during bouts of insomnia.

My view of the pioneers and their contributions seemed important to set down. Inevitably it will be incomplete and even unkind in spite of being documented and tempered by Lael Wertenbaker with skill and integrity. That I've admired Lael for many years has proved to have advantages and disadvantages. Lael's fierce loyalty to her friends provides her with rose-tinted magnifying glasses. In the original biographical form she planned for the book I found she had perched me on a pedestal that was both uncomfortable and precarious. When she changed the book to a documentation of heart surgery, Lael generated many critical views of my colleagues in her tireless research. When possible, and in most of the unflattering material, she has mercifully spared me by revealing other sources. I respect her right to write *as* she chooses without necessarily endorsing *what* she chooses. There are still too many references to me, but here ego makes me permissive, while some modesty renders me uncomfortable.

If you are or know a distinguished cardiologist or heart surgeon who has been omitted from the text or from the Founders Group list (see Appendix), note, for example, that John J. Collins, Jr., Paul Ebert, Jack Matloff, Alden Harken, and Mortimer Buckley are also missing. That is very good company! Even to venture such a list, originally drawn up for the Second Ford Symposium in 1975, places me in a no-win position. On the other hand, it does indicate (painting with a broad brush) how various of the old and some not so old men have made cardiac surgery come about.

This book about heart surgery, incomplete as it is, provides an opportunity to salute some of those dedicated stalwarts whose competence, courage, and rugged physiques have transformed brave but disappointing adventures into consistent service to suffering children, women, and men. We salute the *doers* who have prevailed where *doubters* always have easy advantage. Also, an affectionate salute to Lael Wertenbaker who is per pound easily one of the greatest women of our time. Her search in interviews and libraries has turned up facts, embarrassing to some, interesting to more, and edifying to many. This defines the intended readership, with material too simple for some while too technical for others. We shall deem ourselves fortunate if there is something for most people.

Finally, Lael Wertenbaker has for Anne Harken and me changed what could have been lugubrious psychoanalysis into sparkling social interludes. We hope she can do as much for you.

Dwight Emary Harken, M.D.

Author's Note

This is a medical adventure story. The exploration of the heart has been as daring and rewarding as any penetration of little known areas that twentieth-century technology has made possible. I began this book as a biography of one extraordinary and leading pioneer in the terrain of the heart, surgeon Dwight Harken. Even after he persuaded me to broaden its scope, he remained the central figure because I felt he well deserved to be. I regret that there are many omissions in telling the story: so much happened and so many remarkable men were involved in so short a period of time.

In the Appendix of the book you will find a drawing and explanation of how the heart works, originally produced as a public service by the American Heart Association. I have also included a glossary of medical terms and definitions because I have discovered that it is necessary to use them in order to be exact; medical/lay equivalents are also included in the text in many instances. There is also a list compiled by Dwight Harken of those most prominent in developing the field of cardiac surgery and their major contributions, the Founders Group.

The generosity of those whom I interviewed or who wrote to me in the course of researching this book was overwhelming. I was permitted to tape record every interview I have used, with the understanding that these oral histories and informative comments were for inclusion in the book. I was also given tapes and some transcripts from "The Oral History of Twenty-five Years of American Cardiology," 1949–1974, which is available at the American College of Cardiology Extended Learning Library, to which some of the most prominent of the surgeons had contributed. The letters that came in answer to my requests or Dr. Harken's were carefully written to be helpful.

I relied to a great extent for anecdotal material on Dr. Harken's extraordinary memory and on the many historical notes he included in his lectures. For the most part he was confirmed by the memories of others, and where there were minor differences I have so indicated. Quotations not credited to others are from Harken.

In order to express my gratitude to the individuals who contributed so much so freely, and to credit published sources they gave me for reference or from which I derived information, a list is appended.

May I add that the medical profession is the most eager of all professions I have encountered in my journalistic lifetime to provide accurate information when it is honestly sought.

Contents

To Mend the Heart

1.

"To Pull Together
All We Know"

Nearly every surgeon who has actually entered a living human heart is still alive. Before the mid-twentieth century few surgeons had the temerity to tamper with the heart, and then only in life-and-death emergencies. It was the last sacred temple within the human body, the center and symbol of life.

The heart does lift with joy, flutter with fear, surge with love, pound with excitement, expand with wonder. How can any human being fail to react emotionally and unreasonably to his heart, which reacts so sensitively to him? How could even the most egocentric of surgeons assume the right to enter another man's heart? These emotional questions go beyond superstition or cowardice. They still cannot be answered entirely by statistics.

Scientific investigation stripped the heart of its poetry and mystery as long ago as the sixteenth century. Leonardo da Vinci made accurate drawings of its valves and William Harvey wrote of its sole function as a pump, a powerful, four-chambered mechanical pump. But not until 1944 did a surgeon, Dwight Harken, enter the chambers of the heart electively—by choice—to remove foreign bodies lodged within the hearts of wounded soldiers. There were no mortalities from his series, but as more complex procedures were pioneered in peacetime, risks ran high. Only in the past two decades has mortality from surgical intervention within the heart area dropped to levels consistent with other major procedures.

Now hundreds of thousands of people crippled by cardiac malfunction have been surgically restored to normal or near-normal lives. Unnumbered hearts beat on rhythmically with the aid of transistorized electronic control. Artificial valves are readily substituted for faulty ones, and some few individuals are alive with substitute hearts in place of their own. Institutions where cardiovascular (relating to the heart and blood vessels) surgery is performed are now within reach of almost everyone on earth. Diagnostic techniques, pre- and postoperative care, and surgical procedures are revised and improved almost daily.

Still, the tension in an operating room when the heart is the operative terrain is like that during a lively battle in a shooting war. There, no man, with no matter how much experience, escapes the feeling that he is wrestling with the angel of death. It is an awesome sight to see the human heart lolloping in the open chest of a preternaturally still body. At the slightest touch it quivers, shrinks, and surges. To watch it go quiet, stop—its function taken over by machines—is to feel inescapably the presence and reality of death. When it begins to beat again, that is resurrection.

For the surgeons and their teams, years of training have honed their skills, reinforced their courage. But what of the layman, the patient, who submits himself to them? His is the terrifying terrain they invade. It is his heart, harboring both the disease and the hope of cure. Some surgeons and medical men tell their patients as little as possible in the belief that ignorance is less disquieting. Others try to put their arcane knowledge into understandable terms, informing patients as thoroughly as possible.

It was in the interest of informing the public that Dwight Harken and his colleagues in cardiac care have given their time to aid in writing this history. Right now the layman can encompass a great deal. Reviewing history is a sound basis for acquiring knowledge, and the history of cardiac surgery is short. Knowledge may help one to make informed decisions, reduce awe and dependence on the experts, and knowing what has gone before can help in coping with what may come for anyone. As surgeon and epidemiologist George Blackburn said to Dwight Harken in one discussion, "Who is the great therapist and long-term help-me? It's each one of us! We are our own best physicians, benefiting from education by professional people in the field."

In 1975 the Henry Ford Second International Symposium on Cardiac Surgery took place in Detroit, Michigan. Invited were over seven hundred specialists in the medical treatment of the heart, physicians and engineers as well as surgeons. The panels of speakers were drawn from the most authoritative people in the world. Nearly all the surgeons present were still practicing their skills in the operating room. The few who had retired were still active as consultants; among them were Charles Philomore Bailey of Philadelphia and Lord Russell Brock of London, their names linked with that of Dwight Harken as pioneers who had operated blind within the heart, "seeing" only with their fingers, before it could be laid open.

Active as ever, Denton Cooley and Michael DeBakey had come up from Texas. DeBakey's early work on arterial disease had paved the way for coronary artery surgery. Cooley had outstripped his former chief in the speed and number of his cardiac surgeries. They kept far apart. Their feud was almost as famous as they were.

Japan's two leading cardiac surgeons were also personal antagonists. Juro Wada, chunky, aggressive, speaking machine-gun English, had first oxygenated venous blood by bubbling and de-bubbling it and had developed the tilting-disc hingeless heart valve. Shigeru Sakakibara, dignified, slim, and soft-spoken, founder of the Heart Institute of Japan in Tokyo, had vied with Dwight Harken, before Cooley and DeBakey set the records, for having performed more operations within the heart than anyone else. "We were both afraid to count," Sakakibara admitted, "for fear that he who counted might come in second!"

Among the speakers and panelists were Wilfred Bigelow from Canada, pioneer investigator in microcirculation, hypothermia, and pacemakers; Viking Björk of Sweden, innovator extraordinary of techniques and devices; Ake Senning of Switzerland, implanter of the first total pacemaker; Charles DuBost from

France, whose contributions include collaborating with Alain Carpentier on tissue valve replacement; René Favaloro from Argentina, leader in aortocoronary bypass surgery; Norman Shumway from California and Richard Lower, now in Virginia, pioneers in transplants. They were also among the distinguished names on the Founders Group list distributed at the symposium. This roster had been carefully assembled by Harken from the doctors themselves. Some omissions would be corrected later (see Appendix for the revised list). The one woman on the list, Helen Taussig, pioneer cardiologist, shared the podium with her colleagues. Of the seventy-four men listed, two were included as infamous because they had so authoritatively condemned the dream of cardiac surgery.

Another list accompanied that of the Founders Group. It was of the Turning Points—the thirteen creative quantum leaps that had ushered in each new era and vista in cardiac surgery:

Eras of Change in the Evolution of Cardiac Surgery

Turning Points	
	1
1896	REHN in Frankfurt—First successful suture of a heart wound
1925	SOUTTAR in London—First successful dilation of stenotic mitral valve
	2
1938	GROSS in Boston—Closure of patent ductus arteriosus
1944–45	HARKEN in World War II—Removal of intracardiac foreign bodies with no deaths, the first consistently successful intracardiac surgery
1944–45	BLALOCK and TAUSSIG in Baltimore—Development of the "blue baby" operation
1944–45	CRAFOORD in Stockholm and GROSS with HUFNAGEL in Boston (independently)—Correction of coarctation of the aorta
1948	BAILEY in Philadelphia, HARKEN in Boston, and BROCK in London—First, second, and third modern operation inside the heart—to relieve mitral stenosis

3

1953	GIBBON in Philadelphia, DENNIS in Minneapolis, and DODRILL in Detroit—First successful use of heart-lung machines

4

1952	HUFNAGEL of Washington, then in Boston—First caged-ball artificial valve installed (in descending thoracic aorta)
1960	HARKEN in Boston—First caged-ball heart valve in anatomic (aortic subcommen) position
1961	STARR in Portland—First caged-ball mitral valve
1967	FAVALORO in Cleveland—Made practical clinical use of coronary bypass, using saphenous vein grafts
1967–68	BARNARD in Cape Town, then KANTROWITZ in New York and SHUMWAY in Palo Alto using Shumway technique—Human cardiac transplantation

No one in that jealous and proud profession objected to the choice of Dwight Harken as the symposium's keynote speaker. He had perhaps made more separate contributions than anyone on the Founders Group list and had taken part in three of the Turning Points. His views, which inform this book more than any other's, were often controversial, but no one denied his right to hold them. His credentials were impeccable and his knowledge of the field encyclopedic.

Harken presented an hour-long review of cardiac surgical history. His professional audience listened intently. Even the uninformed layman could follow with comprehension and excitement the astounding progress that had been made between 1945 and 1975, the thirty years he called the "golden age" of heart surgery. His warning that the golden age was ending in a climate where caution, restriction, litigation, and suspicion were overwhelming innovation was echoed by almost every subsequent speaker.

In lauding the other golden age heroes, Harken differentiated "noble pioneering efforts" from "simple risk taking" and drew "the fine line between bold, aggressive, heroic surgery and just plain damned foolishness." It took bold surgeons to open all four of the major developments in heart surgery: extracardiac surgery, closed intracardiac surgery, open-heart surgery, and the replacement of parts and then of hearts entire.

The historic event that ushered in the thirty-year golden age was Dwight Harken's consistently successful elective invasions into the chambers of the heart during World War II.

In 1946 two documentary films were released concerning two of the most important developments of World War II affecting the postwar future of mankind. The first had been filmed in 1945 near the pretty green village of Cirencester in England, the second on Bikini, an uninhabited Pacific atoll. Honorable mention was awarded to the one of an operation in which Harken and his team invaded the sacred citadel of a man's heart and successfully removed a foreign body from an inner chamber. An Oscar went to the film that recorded the explosion of an atom bomb, the destructive power of which had already been demonstrated in the war.

By 1975, when the symposium was held, atomic weapons had proliferated and atomic annihilation threatened the future of all life on earth. Intracardiac surgery had given more years of healthy life to human beings than had been cut short by the bombs that fell on Hiroshima and Nagasaki. But when the documentaries were shown to successive audiences, nobody fainted while viewing the awesome emergence of the mushroom cloud; quite a few did so as they watched a metal fragment lifted from a living, bleeding human heart.

The night before the filming of that particular operation Dwight Harken sat in a Nissen hut and wrote in a letter to his wife, Anne: "If I kill this man, I shall be regarded as foolhardy rather than bold, and heart surgery could be set back by decades. If I succeed, heart surgery may well be on its way."

2.

Foreign Bodies and Purple Hearts

A man and his moment are never isolated. It was necessary for Harken's that there *be* a war, with its toll of young, strong wounded men. Scientific advances had to have included recently developed antibiotics, blood banks, and endotracheal anesthesia. Dwight Harken had to be the man he was, to have trained as he had, and to possess, as well as his surgical skill, the charisma, logic, and enthusiasm to persuade the Allied medical command in England to permit him to operate at his discretion around and within the hearts of soldiers. (In the Mediterranean theatre of the war Edward Delos Churchill, preeminent American surgeon, had decided the risks were too great and too little was known to permit any such attempts.)

In 1944 Harken was just thirty-four. He was one of the youngest men in the medical corps who was qualified as a thoracic surgeon, that is, in chest surgery. His dream that thoracic surgery should include the heart went back to his days as a brash, ambitious intern at Bellevue Hospital in New York. While participating in thoracic operations, it had seemed to him illogical to use the knife to correct infections and cancer of the pleural spaces in the lungs and in the esophagus. Those, he reasoned, might well yield to chemical or physical means, "while right there was the heart, untouched, a pump, a mechanical structure that should yield to mechanical [surgical] means!"

In 1938, the year he completed his residency at Bellevue, young Harken went to his most admired professor at Harvard to ask for advice. He wanted to specialize in thoracic surgery, although exclusive specialization in any area of the body was rare for a surgeon in those days. Dr. Edward Delos Churchill, chief of General Surgical Services at the Massachusetts General Hospital in Boston and John Homans Professor of Surgery at Harvard, had pioneered in complex thoracic surgical procedures. Where, asked Harken, should he himself go for the best training? Dr. Churchill suggested that his former pupil try for an appointment at the Brompton Hospital in London with surgeon A. Tudor Edwards. Mr. Tudor Edwards (surgeons are "mister" in England, physicians "doctor," and Tudor Edwards was always accorded his second and third names, without a hyphen) was considered by much of the English-speaking world to be the father of thoracic surgery. (Germany's Ernst Ferdinand Sauerbruch held that title on the Continent.) The Brompton claimed the distinction of being the first institution in the world devoted exclusively to chest diseases and one of the first to recognize the need for surgeons who had concentrated on thoracic surgery.

Harken applied for the appointment, although he was not sure how he would get to England if he received it. It was the time of the Great Depression. As an intern at Bellevue he had made $15 a month, and as a resident surgeon there in 1937 he was making not very much more. He had married his childhood sweetheart from Osceola, Iowa, Anne Hood, and the young couple were surviving on her salary as employment manager of Stern's Department Store. He could go from Bellevue to Harvard's distinguished Fifth Surgical Service at the Boston City Hospital when he finished his residency, with the promise of advancement and security and the charm of living in Cambridge.

No help would be forthcoming from home. Dr. Conreid Rex Harken, Dwight's father, had refused to help the couple unless they returned home and Dwight agreed to practice in the senior Harken's hospital in Osceola. Nevertheless, the sturdy young couple, both of pioneering stock, did not hesitate when Dwight Harken simultaneously won an appointment at the Brompton as junior clerk to Tudor Edwards and the New York Academy of Medicine's Alexander Cochrane Bowen Traveling Fellowship, offered each year to one graduate surgical intern in New York. In 1938 they left for London, to parlay that $1,800 fellowship into a year's living. Fortunately the clinical clerkship with Tudor Edwards was promptly upgraded to senior resident officer after the chief met his American clerk.

Dwight Harken was Senior Resident Surgeon on the famous Tudor Edwards team when Great Britain entered the war in September 1939. He was offered a commission in the British medical corps, but he decided to go back home. He expected to return with the American army in a few months. Because of isolationist sentiment in the United States, his return took three years longer than he had anticipated, and it was these three years that gave him vital laboratory and clinical experience.

A residency on the legendary Fifth (Harvard) Surgical Service at Boston City Hospital had been held open for him. Boston had appropriated $100,000 to build a hospital in 1861, and the Boston City opened its doors in 1864. Since then it had grown until its vast medical complex and resources were more extensive than those of its Boston sisters. And the master surgeon, Irving Walker, chief of the Fifth Surgical Service, was retiring. The acting chief was a general surgeon whose claim to fame rested on the superb care he lavished on the Harvard football team. Instead of relegating his new resident to routine surgery, this acting chief was happy to turn over the more exacting cases to Harken, or D.E.H., as he initialed his reports.

D.E.H. immediately sought out the patients on the medical services who needed major gastrointestinal surgery and rapidly became proficient in performing such surgery. When he learned that Edward Delos Churchill and Richard Sweet at the Massachusetts General Hospital were developing a transthoracic (through the chest) approach to remove cancerous portions of the upper part of the stomach and lower esophagus, he promptly adopted this procedure. By the time the two leading surgeons had reported two successes with this then stunning surgical tour de force, Harken had already amassed a series of sixteen, with a survival rate of fourteen.

Harken's local reputation grew, and while still a resident on the Fifth (Harvard) Surgical Service at Boston City, he became a "visit" or staff surgeon on the Second (Harvard) Service as well, and on the thoracic visiting staffs of Massachusetts Memorial and the Cambridge (later Mount Auburn) hospitals. He also taught Harvard medical students who were assigned to "the City" for their surgical training. Cornell Professor Lawrence Hinkle, from the height of his later eminence in preventive medicine, would describe being a student of Harken's in 1940:

> We all thought there would be a war for us and surgery was the best thing in a war. We were only allowed to hold a retractor or something, but when Dwight was operating, his enthusiasm was infectious. All that enthusiasm! We students trailed him everywhere. He was always out in front with that red hair, dashing up and down stairs or banging on the elevator doors, and he'd show us this patient and that patient, yelling for the X-rays if they weren't right there, doing workups, tearing down to pathology, on to the clinic, into the operating room. . . . It was like being caught in the tail of a whirlwind!

Harken seemed to move within his own field of extraordinary energy. Clinical experience alone did not satisfy his insatiable curiosity. Only animal experimentation could lead to cardiac surgery. He chose to study a disease of the heart that was completely, perfectly diagnosable and inevitably, routinely fatal: subacute bacterial endocarditis, or SBE, infections on the valves of the heart with resulting growths called vegetations. At the Mallory Institute of Pathology, close by the Boston City Hospital, he began to study the growths and the distribution patterns of those vegetations in the hearts of patients who had died of SBE. Then, by a complex procedure, he produced the same disease in live dogs and improved an instrument for looking around and locating the vegetations in their hearts. The first nineteen animals on which he operated to remove the vegetations died. By the time he reached his third experimental group of nineteen dogs, sixteen of which survived his surgery, penicillin had been discovered. This antibiotic chemically cured bacterial endocarditis.

Concurrently the United States had declared war on Japan and Germany. D.E.H. was offered a majority if he would join the army in July 1942, as soon as he had completed his Boston City Harvard residency. The surgeon who, by seniority, was slated to be the next chief of the Fifth (Harvard) Surgical Service, urged him not to enlist. Dr. Hominy was a pleasant gentleman, a veteran of World War I, and an adequate surgeon. He devoutly wished to be made chief, but there were procedures he knew himself inadequate to perform. "Dwight, you have the experience! If you will become my assistant, I'll be conveniently called out of town when a gastrectomy or an esophagogastrectomy comes up," he told Harken in Harken's living room. "I'll jump you right over the tour of duty in the outpatient clinic required of junior visits. You can skip several years on your way. Please! This can and should be done by declaring you essential here."

It was a tempting offer. Years gained. Unlimited clinical experience and the chance to continue his experimental work. Furthermore his sense of adventure was fully satisfied within his profession. He was a family man, devoted to his wife and their son, Alden, who had been born in 1941. A second child was on the way. Dr. Harken, his father, would be delighted to support and harbor his son's wife and his grandchildren if they would live in Osceola while he was at war, but otherwise proffered no help. Anne had no more desire to go back home than her husband, so he accepted Dr. Hominy's offer and a military exemption as "essential to the hospital and school."

That decision would not hold. Essential because his chief was afraid or unable to do certain surgery? Essential because as the younger men left, a lot of older doctors were unwilling to get out of bed for night work? Because it would further his career and he would be ahead of his contemporaries when they came back from the war? He had himself reclassified and volunteered, accepting a captaincy, and he and Anne borrowed the money to buy his uniform.

Harken's military career opened with orders to circumvent the privileges of rank, by which the army set such store. An old friend of his, Bryan Blades, a superb thoracic surgeon, had the civilian experience to be appointed chief of the thoracic service at Walter Reed Hospital near Washington, but he had been a captain in the reserves, so a captain he remained. He had to deal with majors and colonels on his service whom he considered rank incompetents. To Captain Harken he said, "Dwight, you just follow the so-and-sos around, especially so-and-so. As a junior officer, you can't countermand his orders, but just keep shouting *No!* Hold him back physically if necessary. He thinks the way to treat bronchiectitis is by radiation and he wants to close empyemas [the presence of pus in a cavity, as in the chest cavity] with blow bottles!" ("I did follow Bryan's instructions," said Harken, "and saved a lot of lives.")

The next opportunity that might have led him away from the front lines and field hospitals came with an offer to become chief of thoracic service at White Sulphur Springs in West Virginia. The luxurious accommodations there, intended for the rich and pampered in peacetime, had been commandeered as a general hospital for the U.S. Army Zone of the Interior. Dr. Daniel Elkin was chief of the whole surgical service. The former chairman of the Department of Surgery at Emory University in Georgia, he was considered an authority on what was then heart surgery—repairing stab wounds, provided the victim had not already bled to death.

Harken was pleased. At the time it seemed a wonderful way to fight a war. Chest surgery and postsurgical rehabilitation were areas of passionate interest to him, and both would be of prime importance to soldiers with chest wounds evacuated from the battle areas to the Zone of the Interior. Anne could join him there, with Alden, and their forthcoming child could be born in White Sulphur Springs. He was walking outside Walter Reed Hospital, contemplating this rosy picture, when he spotted a man in uniform who seemed unable to extricate himself from the bordering rhododenron bushes. After going to his aid, Harken recognized the man. "Heavens, Dr. Churchill, what are you doing?"

"Trying to get out of this confounded place," the distinguished Edward Delos Churchill replied testily, his face red with exertion. "I took a fire exit and landed in these confounded bushes. And what are you doing here, Dwight?"

Harken confessed that he was about to leave for White Sulphur Springs.

"Oh, my. Oh, no. No," said Colonel Churchill emphatically, once again deciding Harken's fate. "That's no place for a dynamic, aggressive, physically fit young man. You should be in the forward areas making contributions to the future of surgery. I'll see about it. Immediately."

Within forty-eight hours Harken had orders to report to Dodd Field near San Antonio, Texas, where the First Auxiliary Surgical Unit was staging. They were destined for the European Theatre of Operations.

The story of any hero, including one in the surgical war against heart disease, inevitably includes survival of boredom and discomfort and discouragement before and between heroic accomplishments. Dodd Field was a muddy expanse of flatland on the outskirts of Fort Sam Houston. There was nothing sensible for the medical men to do. They were obliged to participate in war-simulated training, often very hard on the older doctors as well as irrelevant, and to attend classes in compass interpretation and sextant reading. Harken's tent mate was a "tiresome old maid whiz kid who seemed preoccupied with combing his hair." The commanding officer was an army regular, "a braying jackass who was openly contemptuous of men with 'elegant training' who, in his opinion, thought they were superior." To humiliate any such presumption on Harken's part, he assigned him as assistant to a general practitioner with the rank of major and said they were to lead a thoracic team.

Harken was indignant. Abject with frustration, he was pacing the rutted roads between tents one night when an older doctor, also a captain, Kenneth Burton from Providence, Rhode Island, opened the flap of his tent and invited him in at 4 A.M. The big, furious redhead found Burton a companion in misery, but one who had accepted it with more philosophy.

"You know I'm an orthopedic surgeon and an editor of the orthopedic journal, Dwight," Burton said. "I've been put on a team to assist a second-rate GP and we're being called an orthopedic team! The difference between you and me is that I am able to sleep. I have learned to cooperate with the inevitable and you haven't learned that yet."

Harken learned to cooperate with as much of the inevitable as he could not manage to circumvent. As an outlet for his frantic energy, he organized a series of lectures on aspects of medicine, delivering the ones on thoracic surgery himself. Soon he was in demand as a speaker at nonmilitary medical meetings all over south Texas, adding an important skill to his surgical skill, that of speaking well in front of audiences.

In 1943, when his daughter Anne Louise was born in Cambridge, he could not get leave to go north and make her acquaintance. Later, when his unit was finally ordered to New York for embarkation, he managed to convey to his wife, despite tight security, when and where to meet him in Manhattan, and suggested she bring their new daughter. Anne Harken prudently considered that his tolerance for baby care was limited and that his second child, darling as she was, might spoil their reunion. The time they had together was brief and poignant, and by the time he saw his children, the baby was nearly three years old.

His unit sailed on the *Queen Mary*, stripped for troop transport. His Majesty's former luxury liner did not dally in order to go in convoy. As the ship pursued a choppy course across the Atlantic at top speed, depth charges were often dropped to discourage enemy submarines. The First Auxiliary Surgical Unit, debilitated by seasickness, debarked at Southampton, quickmarched to waiting trucks, and were rushed to Waterford, north of London. There they were to live in tents on another muddy field during the slow, monumental buildup of American troops in England. The second front the Allies hoped to open was still a long while off.

Harken had acquired no gift whatever for inaction. His mind buzzed with schemes and he quickly managed to procure a one-day pass to London. London had become "his" city in 1938, as much as New York and Boston were. Now, in 1943, her war-battered dynamism filled him with excitement. Debris had been cleaned away from empty spaces left by buildings destroyed in the blitz, and wild flowers were springing up in the rubble. Barrage balloons, silvery and elephantine, floated above the streets crowded with pedestrians moving with cheery confidence. V was for Victory.

A. Tudor Edwards, active advisor on thoracic surgery to wartime Britain's Ministry of Health despite a second coronary, was delighted to see his American former trainee. Yes, of course, Tudor Edwards would arrange for Harken to study the all too extensive British experience with chest wounds. Colonel Elliott Cutler, from Harvard's Peter Bent Brigham Hospital, was American chief of all surgery in the European Theatre of Operations. He welcomed Harken, who had been a pupil of his in medical school. Yes, he could order detached service for Harken. Cutler would assign him to update a manual for the Army Medical Corps on the management of chest injuries.

Harken moved into the ancient Bailey Hotel, whose other residents seemed to be about the same age as the building, and was given office space at 9 North Audley Street, the American ETO (European Theatre of Operations) Surgeon General's Headquarters. He did his evening drinking and socializing with the group of consultants serving with Surgeon General Hawley in the "Embassy Club" located in the basement of the embassy on Grosvenor (now Roosevelt) Square.

General Paul Hawley very much wanted Mr. Tudor Edwards to repeat his popular course of lectures on thoracic surgery for the benefit of the American surgeons. He sent Colonel Cutler to make the request of the great man and to suggest that if he himself were too ill, "one of our young men could do all the work." Tudor Edwards peremptorily refused. He was unable to take on the burden of giving the course himself, and he would not risk his prestige at the hands of any young American. As an afterthought to his refusal, he asked if Cutler and Hawley had any particular young man in mind.

"Well, yes," said Cutler. "Dwight Harken . . ."

"He's not *your* young man," said Tudor Edwards. "He's *mine!*"

So Harken was permitted to deliver the famous lectures. He began the program by inviting twelve American surgeons from

Waterford to London for two weeks. In addition to ingesting the accumulated wisdom of A. Tudor Edwards, they would visit British hospitals and meet their Allied confreres, which became the basis for considerable future cooperation on both sides. The detail was very popular. In relays of a dozen the American surgeons came from wherever they were stationed. London was an inexhaustibly enjoyable city, and to sleep in real beds an appreciated privilege. Harken also began traveling all over England, to clearing stations, field hospitals, and general hospitals, delivering copies of his updated manual and briefing the staffs on the care of chest injuries.

In the active Mediterranean Theatre of Operations Churchill, as chief of surgery, had already set up separate centers for the chest wounded. In the ETO Cutler wanted only general hospitals, under general surgical command.

"Cutler was," Harken would say, "a forthright man, of high standards, integrity, and skill. He thought of himself as the complete surgeon—general, thoracic, neuro—and he probably was as near to being one as was humanly possible that late in the evolution of surgery. A veritable Roger Bacon of surgery, 'the last man to know everything.' "

However, Harken thought Churchill was right and that separate chest centers with surgeons experienced in thoracic surgery in control were far preferable. If his awesome former chief, Mr. Tudor Edwards, could persuade General Hawley, Hawley could override Cutler, or perhaps even Cutler could be convinced. He enlisted Mrs. Tudor Edwards, who was very fond of her husband's American, as his ally. Together they connived to plan dinner parties at her house, with Hawley and Cutler as guests, A. Tudor Edwards as host, and Harken included (below the salt). Harken was in Mrs. Tudor Edwards' sewing room one day before the first dinner when Cutler himself burst into the room. "Where's the great man?" he demanded with his habitual lack of patience, ignoring Harken.

"Do sit down, Dr. Cutler," Eve Tudor Edwards said, knowing how much her husband enjoyed Cutler's sporadic visits. "I expect him any minute."

Cutler was still prancing around the sewing room when

Tudor Edwards arrived. "Now, Elliott," said the only man Harken ever knew who could talk down to Cutler, "you take fifteen grains of bromides, breathe through your mouth, and when you've settled down, we'll find out what you want."

The invitations were readily accepted, a welcome change from the officers' mess. Before each dinner party Harken briefed Tudor Edwards with fresh arguments in favor of chest centers, and then stayed on, uncharacteristically quiet in the background unless called upon for factual summaries or charts. General Hawley listened genially, Cutler politely, on these social occasions.

The general had a way of making subordinates forget rank when he talked to them privately. After summoning Captain Harken one day, he presented a problem for, he said, the captain's consideration. The Royal Masonic Hospital at Ravenscourt Park in London had asked Hawley for help. They had been very good to American soldiers injured in the blackout or in bombing raids. Most of their regular surgeons were serving elsewhere in the British army; only two medical students were there at night, with just one surgeon, the very senior Duncan Fitzwilliam, well past seventy, and occasionally Sir Victor Bonney, a famed but aging gynecologist, on call. The students had opened an abdomen one night in a case of acute appendicitis and had had great difficulty locating the appendix in order to remove it. "I suggested to them," Hawley told Harken, "that I had a young surgeon named Dwight Harken who might be willing to stay there at night, and who could certainly find appendices."

"Thank you, sir," said Harken, who immediately decided to recommend somebody else. He was busy enough and enjoyed his . free evenings. "May I think it over?"

"You may think it over," said General Hawley, "until exactly one o'clock today, at which time I am taking you to the Royal Masonic."

Harken would enjoy reminiscing about this interval in the war when only the American air force in England was engaged in active combat. The frequent German air raids on London occurred with Prussian precision on the dot of 4 A.M. Old Fitzwilliam, brave as a lion, was always the first one out of bed when the sirens sounded. He would march to Harken's room and stand in the doorway with his helmet askew on his white hair. "Dwight! Get up, put on your iron hat, look fierce, and come help me fight the Jerries!" Harken, Fitzwilliam, and Bonney, when he was there, would first help the staff at the Royal Masonic to shepherd patients who wanted to go down to the air raid shelters. Then Bonney, a timorous man, was left with nurses and patients in the shelter while Harken and Fitzwilliam headed for the roof to fire watch. One night two incendiary bombs fell on their sand-covered roof. Harken immediately scooped them up in a long-handled shovel and buried them in the ready sand-filled buckets. On another night Harken, who had been operating until 2:30 and was at last sound asleep, refused to get out of bed. Ten minutes later a bomb exploded nearby, shattering his window, and sent him in a flying leap onto broken glass. He rushed outside and joined Fitzwilliam, who was on his way to the Queen Elizabeth Lying-in Hospital, close by, which was on fire. They pulled patients out of the building and cared for them by the light of the blaze.

During the day Harken also took care of occasional emergency calls that came in to the surgeon general's office at North Audley. One was from a staging area outside London; an American soldier was bleeding to death in a British cottage hospital—one of the small local institutions, often made up of several small houses, or cottages, and without resident staffs. No anesthetist was on hand at headquarters. Harken telephoned Dr. Arthur Levin, an internist at the Royal Masonic with that broad competence he had so often admired in British physicians. "Come along, Arthur. A guy shot himself in the chest when he was caught by the MPs cheating in a crap game and I'm told the damn fool is exsanguinating and we'd better hurry."

An army pool car with a British driver was commandeered for Harken and they swung by the hospital to pick up Levin. The young soldier had mercifully missed his heart and great vessels, but had exploded the upper lobe of his right lung. Harken hastily inserted the endotracheal tube for Levin, who then took over the anesthesia. After opening the chest, Harken grabbed the pulmonary artery with his left hand, stemming the outflow of blood.

There were no suitable instruments on hand with which to control the hemorrhage, much less do a proper resection of a lobe of the lung. He called for a 14 French catheter. A flustered nurse found him one. Wrapping the catheter around the pedicle of the upper lobe of the lung, he pulled it tight and put a clamp on it, and closed the chest with tube and clamp protruding. Friends of the injured soldier gathered to volunteer blood for transfusion. After a gross cross-match and multiple transfusions had stabilized their patient, Harken and Levin transferred him to an American medical installation and went back to London.

"Well," Harken would say, "that was a nice example of emergency cottage kitchen table surgery. We went out there and saved that boy's life, for whatever public service that might or might not represent."

Harken was always ambivalent about attempted suicides. The surgeon's greatest ally is a patient's love of life. It had been his experience at Bellevue and Boston City that most would-be suicides would try and try again. He understood the suicidal impulse, would even feel it at moments when he lost a life that wanted to live, but was intolerant of people who succumbed to it. (In the future Harken would refuse to operate on heart patients who were unwilling to help themselves to live by quitting smoking.)

Another venture he referred to as "when the cow jumped over the moon." A British surgeon asked him to come north of London and help with the first pneumonectomy (surgical removal of an entire lung) to be performed in an Emergency Medical Service regional hospital. Harken took with him an expert anesthetist, Major Everett from Syracuse. While Everett diplomatically helped the less experienced British anesthetist, doing, said Harken, a particularly brilliant job, Harken with his British contemporary did the pneumonectomy, an operation that A. Tudor Edwards had pioneered. "That operation was completed with a certain amount of éclat," Harken admitted. Afterward they had an Anglo-American celebration.

On their way back in the blackout in a motor pool car, the exhausted Harken and Everett went sound asleep. Their British driver, a charming female, braked abruptly as an approaching car hit a large obstacle. Her passengers awakened to see a cow flying upward. Split seconds later, the cow, on its way back to the ground, came down on the hood of their car. Futile efforts by the doctors failed to resuscitate the badly disabled animal and it expired. They dragged the carcass to the roadside. Beef had to be salvaged, and they also felt they should compensate the owner, so they roused the occupants of the nearest farmhouse, who denied ownership. They left their names and address and continued on to London.

"All this was by way of dramatic contrast," Harken would say, "to most of our medical officers, who didn't have much to do. Some British hospitals were as desperately short staffed as the Royal Masonic had been. I worked out a program in which competent American surgeons could be secunded to British domestic institutions. For instance, Ronald Belsey, one of the truly great thoracic surgeons, took Walter Bugden, who would later do such good work in Syracuse, with him to Frenchy Park in Bristol. Edward Durno, later a congressman, worked with Rodney Mangot. Others went to places such as Birmingham, Southampton, Liverpool, and Newcastle. Our men were a godsend to the British, and working was a godsend for the Americans."

In the spring of 1944 Harken was summoned again to General Hawley's office. The call was not unexpected. Hawley was genial. "You may be pleased to know, Dwight, that we have decided to have designated chest centers."

"Yes, sir," said Harken. "That pleases me—a lot!"

Hawley made it perfectly clear that he had been well aware of Harken's machinations. "Colonel Cutler has agreed. Now, will you suggest logical men to head these centers?"

"Yes, sir," said Harken readily and reeled off his choices. Arthur Touroff, the senior surgeon experienced in chest surgery in the ETO, was from Mount Sinai Hospital in New York. Did the general know that Touroff had been the first man to tie off an infected patent ductus arteriosus following Robert Gross's successful ligation in Boston? George Somers was a colonel who had had fine thoracic training under John Alexander in Ann Arbor. Another good man, Robert Shaw, was also an Alexander trainee. "Each of them ought to head chest centers. Which one gets the first one is up to you and Colonel Cutler, and whether you appoint by seniority or merit is up to you."

"Of course it is," said Hawley. "And we have decided. You'll be in charge of the first one."

"Wouldn't it be awkward," asked Harken, giving the general advice, "for me, one of the most junior surgeons qualified in thoracic surgery in the ETO, to be head of the first center? Let me think about it."

"You may think about it," said Hawley, "until noon this Friday, when I am taking you to the 160th General to set up the first chest center. Your commanding officer, Colonel Leonard Heaton, will be receptive to change."

The 160th General was a vast huddle of empty Quonset huts installed outside the village of Cirencester in the low Cotswold hills. It had been designated as a thoracic and neurosurgical center. To combine the two was logical, since many chest wounds involved paraplegia (paralysis of the lower limbs). Stewart Rowe, an excellent neurosurgeon, was in charge of the neurosurgical area and became a consultant in his field for the area hospitals, as Harken did in thoracic surgery.

Over acres of once-verdant fields asphalt had been poured to accommodate future fleets of ambulances. One patient lay on a cot in one of the huts. He had a badly managed empyema that needed repair and was tended by Margot Evans, the chief and, so far, only nurse. Harken thought Nurse Evans looked far too fragile and elderly for what would come.

She had been chosen by Colonel Heaton, who was already in residence. Harken took immediately to Heaton, who was, he said, "dynamic, cooperative, helpful, wonderful" and who would, in his turn, become Surgeon General. They discussed the table of organization at the 160th. The TO precluded appropriate rank and offered little chance of promotion. In fact, there was no place on it for a consultant in thoracic surgery. Nevertheless they were both determined to have the best possible staff and the best possible equipment. Heaton gave Harken unspoken permission to beg, borrow, or steal both if necessary, and then sent him immediately back to London in a munitions carrier to buy the best British surgical instruments.

For his team, Harken combed the Army Medical Corps. At a casualty clearing station he found Paul Zoll, who had been transferred there from the Aleutians where he had nearly died of pneumonia. Zoll was an exceptionally promising cardiologist from Boston, a former classmate of Harken's. He was more interested in patient care than in army rank, and instantly agreed to go to the 160th.

Ashbel Williams, who had been a resident with Harken at Boston City and was a superb surgeon, was willing to trade his chances of promotion for matrimony. "I'm in love with Kay and she's a Wren," he explained. That meant she was subject to orders in the British services and there was a lot of red tape involved before she could marry an American officer. Heaton cut the tape. They were married. Wren Lieutenant Kay Williams was assigned on detached service with a British unit nearby and Captain and Mrs. Williams moved into a small cottage in Cirencester.

Harken propositioned William Stanton from San Antonio, a somewhat older man, to be his general surgical assistant. Stanton liked the way things were shaping up at the 160th, and agreed. So did William Sandusky, who had also trained at Boston City. He was an authority on chemotherapy, such as it was then, and the control of infections. Penicillin had just been released to add to his pharmacopoeia. Sandusky was tremendously excited by this breakthrough in antibiotics.

Chief Nurse Margot Evans, about whom Harken had already revised his first impression—the lady was indomitable—produced two crack scrub nurses. They were Lieutenants Shirley van Brackle and Addie Shirley. One was blond and one brunette, and Harken promptly nicknamed them "White Shirley" and "Black Shirley."

Central to a chest center's success was the anesthesiologist. Harken spoke to Cutler in London. "Name your man," said Cutler expansively. Harken named Charles Burstein, who had trained under the great Emery A. Rovenstein and had been a resident at Bellevue. Cutler protested. "He's not even in the army."

"That's not what you asked me!" said Harken.

It turned out that Burstein had just been inducted. Cutler arranged to have him sent on priority to the 160th. Burstein was able to collect excellent equipment when he got to England, where the art and science of anesthesia had been greatly advanced by pioneer Ivan Magill (later knighted), inventor of the endotracheal tube, with whom Harken had worked at the Brompton.

Among the maintenance troops coming to the 160th, Harken uncovered a remarkable artist. Good medical artists were rare. Sergeant Felix Weinstein had the necessary first qualification—he could reproduce with uncanny accuracy anything he looked at. In an operating room for the first time in his life, he drew what the layman saw—people in gowns and masks around a table, a draped patient with a dark hole in his body on the table. Harken gave him a cram course in anatomy and taught him to look at what was inside the hole. (Weinstein would go to Johns Hopkins after the war, where he became famous as a medical illustrator.)

On his various trips to London Harken besieged the highest authorities in the Allied medical command for permission to remove foreign bodies from the heart area. He argued that Edward Delos Churchill's prohibition of such attempts in the Mediterranean area was doubtless based on the prevalent assumption that the heart could not tolerate much manipulation, let alone invasion. There was the danger of ventricular fibrillation, that disorganized beating that resulted in circulatory arrest. Four minutes of ventricular fibrillation did cause brain death. But Harken had proved to his satisfaction that ventricular fibrillation could be avoided during his experiments producing bacterial endocarditis in dogs. On too many occasions he had hooked a safety pin onto the mitral valve leaflet margins of canine hearts with only a few extra systoles. Furthermore he had demonstrated during these operations that if he observed basic rules, such as not dislocating the heart, and if he did not apply electric currents of the wrong frequency, their hearts did not go awry.

While reviewing the British experience, he had come across many instances of fragments having been removed from the chest wall and lungs. Certainly men had survived with such fragments, over 1.5 by 1.5 centimeters, that had been driven directly into the heart or had migrated there through the venous return into the right auricle or ventricle. (In the future Harken would see for himself all types of migratory fragments, some of which had continued on through the heart and out into the lungs.) If such fragments were left embedded, he was sure the danger of infection, embolism, and insidious damage to the heart was greater than that of careful surgical removal.

Final decision rested with A. Tudor Edwards, Admiral Gordon Taylor, and Grey Turner, president of the Royal College of Surgeons, for the British, Hawley and Cutler for the Americans. Cutler, reconciled to chest centers, agreed with Harken, although he had abandoned his own attempts at clinical cardiac surgery in the 1920s.

Grey Turner told Harken that during World War I he had decided to remove a shell fragment that he thought was lodged in the pericardium, the sac around the heart. When he opened the wounded man's chest, he found that the fragment lay within the right ventricle. "As I looked at that wriggling, contorting structure, the heart, I concluded that to take that foreign body out of the right ventricle was beyond human and surgical capacity. But . . . you go ahead, young man. I agree with you for all the reasons you have given for attempting to remove foreign bodies from the heart. However, you have neglected an additional and important consideration: namely, the knowledge of an individual that he harbors an unwelcome visitor in the citadel of his well-being."

"That," said Harken, "was the British way of saying that it would scare the hell out of you to have a missile in your heart!"

Permission was granted.

On June 6, 1944, the people who stood in readiness at the 160th were distracted from their radios where they were listening to the first reports of the invasion of Europe by a crescendo of sound outside. They rushed to doors and windows to see ambulances arriving and short-legged stretchers being debouched onto the asphalt area. Soon the entire area was covered with them. At first Harken was sure that wounded of all kinds had been sent there and that triage officers would sort the chest wounded from among them. It was not so. Orderlies began bringing wounded into the huts at the chest center.

Margot Evans was already there. On her hands and knees she crawled among the stretchers, speaking to frightened and pain-racked young men. She was assuring them, as she would assure the waves of wounded men who arrived from that time on, that they were *lucky*. Each had fought his brave war and now, by the best of good fortune, had arrived at *the best center in the world for chest care*. She believed it and they believed her, taking comfort for their wounds. And, Harken would add, it was true.

The well-prepared chest center went into round-the-clock action as the battle for a foothold on the Continent was still in doubt on Omaha Beach. Wounded men were being evacuated to England across the Channel in swift, receding waves as incoming waves of men swept ashore. New arrivals were immediately given primary treatment. Chestfuls of blood were drained. At once Harken began a program of operations in his surgical theatre, half of a Quonset hut, scheduling two procedures at a time on the two tables and snatching naps when he could on a cot in the corner. When he noticed that Black and White Shirley were getting no rest at all, he insisted that they take turns. White Shirley, Lieutenant van Brackle, would say that thoracic surgery was different from ordinary or general surgery. "It's more nerve-racking for everybody."

Most of Harken's operations involved the lungs, pleural space, or chest wall. As soon as he learned of it, a procedure called decortication was adopted at the 160th. It had been developed in the Mediterranean theatre by Drs. Brewer, Samson, Burford, and Sheffs. A zone of peel or cortex, like the skin of an orange, formed on the lung and could be removed, without disturbing the pulp or fruit. Loose blood, clots, pus, and infected material often encapsulated and incarcerated the collapsed lung. Infection might be partially controlled by rib resection drainage, but the patient, chronically ill from infection, with a deformed body and lost lung function, would become a respiratory cripple. By decortication, the chest could be opened (thoracotomy) and the pleural space evacuated of all debris; stripped of its imprisoning cortex, the lung expanded like a flower from its bud to fill the pleural space and emancipate the chest cripple.

Missiles in the chest were located by X-ray. Some of them seemed to be within the shadow cast by the heart, the cardiac shadow. In a few it looked as if the missiles—common wartime word for foreign bodies—were actually within the heart chambers, but when the chest was opened, the missiles proved to have been only within the X-ray silhouette, the shadow cast by the heart. Surgery in all these cases required great skill and had rarely been attempted before, but, as anesthetist Burstein would say, "We approached every operation with the expectation of success—and we did succeed."

To get a better fix on the location of missiles, Harken began to use the fluoroscopic screen. This required direct inspection because it was simply a transient moving picture, using radiation X-rays to penetrate the patient's body. The pictures could not be examined later. Carefully rotating the patient under direct-inspection fluoroscopy, Harken found that missiles appearing to lie within the heart often "jumped" beyond the heart shadow, a very different surgical challenge.

In one case the fragment did seem to be clearly in the pericardial sac, but when the chest was opened and the ribs spread, he saw that the large foreign body lay within the right ventricle. The moment of cardiac invasion had come. The team was well rehearsed: White Shirley was alert and ready; Sandusky was prepared to assist. His cheerful optimism and certainty that everything would come out fine were undimmed by the tension of the moment.

Harken and Sandusky carefully placed the guy sutures around the site. Harken incised the epicardium covering the heart muscle, then the myocardium, the heart muscle itself. All eyes focused on the endocardium, the membrane lining of the chambers, which was pouting out over the fragment. Prayerfully, holding his breath, Harken put a Kocker clamp through the last layer of heart wall, grasped the missile, and pulled it to the edge of the site, where it stuck. As it stuck in the incision, it obstructed the blood loss.

"Thus, for a moment, I stood with my clamp on the fragment that was inside the heart, and the heart was not bleeding. Then, suddenly, with a pop as if a champagne cork had been drawn, the fragment jumped out of the ventricle, forced by the pressure within the chamber, and the tension I was keeping on the clamp engaged the foreign body. Blood poured out in a torrent! Sandusky grasped the sutures and crossed them, only partially stemming that spectacular hemorrhage. I threw the clamp and the missile toward White Shirley. It missed her and went onto the floor beyond the operating table. I tried to cross the sutures to complete stemming the flood. It wasn't enough. I told the first and second assistants to cross the sutures and I put my finger over the awful leak. The torrent slowed, stopped, and with my finger *in situ*, I took large needles swedged with silk and began passing them through the heart muscle wall, under my finger and out the other side. With four of these in, I slowly removed my finger as one after the other was tied. Paul Zoll was monitoring the electrocardiogram. About a liter of blood had been lost, but twelve hundred cubic centimeters were returned by the pressure technique in a minute and a few seconds. Blood pressure did drop, but the only instant of panic was when we discovered that one suture had gone through the glove on the finger that had stemmed the flood. I was sutured to the wall of the heart! We cut the glove and I got loose. Blood pressure returned. By the time we closed his chest, the patient was well on the way to recovery, and aside from some signs indicating slight and transient myocardial damage, we found nothing to worry about. The next day the patient felt very well indeed."

Harken wrote to Anne that night about this long-prepared-for and anticipated first. She knew then that her husband was beginning to realize his dream of surgery within the heart.

The irrepressible Sandusky opined the next day that an alternative resolution to the crisis might have been to cut off Harken's finger and leave it behind.

The stream of casualties was unending. Harken's heroine of the war became the elderly Margot Evans, whose calm confidence expressed in her alto voice was contagious. He had no doubt about the positive metabolic effect of a patient's morale and motivation when the margin was narrow. "She was a unique life support system," said Harken.

Each procedure that involved the heart area was a dangerous venture into *terra incognita,* with the distances in millimeters and the timing in milliseconds. Harken had learned from his experimentation on dogs that minimal dislocation of the heart from its normal position (optimum position of function) was a major consideration, which meant that the surgeon's versatility of approach was taxed.

The missiles in that area were located by palpation and stabilized with the fingers. Double sutures were placed delicately over the foreign body while the exposed heart was kept moist with a 1 percent procaine solution "to reduce irritability." ("Everybody believed that worked," said Harken, "but we learned years later that we might as well have used warm water!") Paul Zoll checked continuously to see if any manipulation was being badly tolerated. The unprecedented series built up, slowly, until it included thirteen missiles removed from within the right chambers of the heart.

At one time Harken and Zoll thought that perhaps a giant electric magnet could be used to transfix the metal fragments instead of clamps. A special model was ordered and sent over from the States. When it was turned on in the operating room, the results were disastrous. The regular electric equipment in the operating room went immediately awry and, worse still, every metal instrument in the magnetic vicinity migrated at top speed toward the magnet. The magnet was turned off, the shambles cleaned up, and that idea was retired to the files under "another good notion gone wrong."

It was now obvious that direct entry into the right ventricle did not necessarily cause death. Nor did migration into that chamber by way of the veins kill a man. In fact, having survived thus far, most patients could survive without surgical intervention, but these previously untried elective operations meant that they would live without potential time bombs within the "citadel of their well-being." There were no deaths in the series, and

Harken ardently believed he was proving that intracardiac surgery had a future.

No fragments had been found in the left ventricle so far. It was logical to conclude that direct entry into the left ventricle, which pumped blood into the body under much greater pressure than that exerted through the right ventricle, must be almost immediately fatal. Men thus wounded on the battlefield would have suffered exsanguinating hemorrhage and died.

Most of the operations at the 160th still came under the heading of thoracic rather than cardiac surgery. Word spread quickly through the ETO that some very interesting and exciting procedures in chest surgery were going on at the 160th. Surgeons on leave or detached service began to come in from all over the area. Men from other teams were sent to work with Harken for two or three weeks at a time. Showman and teacher, Harken never minded a crowd.

The patients, he warned, were no ordinary mix. The extraordinary recovery record was partly credited to their youth, resilience, and confidence in their personal invulnerability to death. They were physically and psychologically fit. That made rehabilitation techniques all the more important. But even such patients could easily end up chest cripples. The side of the chest that was cut lost its natural connection with the motor cortex control from the brain. For a time the patient had no control, voluntary or involuntary, of the area. As the middle motor convolution in the brain on the opposite side of the head became paralyzed from disuse, fused lung syndrome could result. The British had developed Specific Remedial Breathing Exercises to reorient the alienated or divorced motor connection. By touching the part of the chest that needed moving, while breathing forcibly, the patient sent an impulse to the brain that the brain recognized. Then, by concentrating, the patient could reestablish the connection and begin to use that side of his chest both voluntarily and involuntarily.

Expatiating on the anatomical reasons for the forceful expirations that reinforced activity in the lungs, Harken often stripped off his shirt and demonstrated with his own splendidly expandable torso. It was a crusade, and he would later carry it home to the States and consider it one of the most important contributions of his life to the healing arts. At the 160th, he trained a drill sergeant who had recovered from a chest wound himself. Daily the sergeant, a master of discipline, routed postoperative patients out of bed to *breathe in, breathe out*—no matter how painful they found it.

So many visitors came that Colonel Heaton and Harken (promoted by then to major) worked out a system of tours. The "A" tour, for VIP tourists who were not medical men, was short and dramatic. "B," a longer tour, was offered to the physicians and medical technicians. "C," for surgeons, had everything, including instruction.

Russell Brock, a British surgeon who had been at the Brompton on the service of Mr. J. E. H. Roberts, the hated rival of Mr. Tudor Edwards, while Harken was there before the war, was entitled to "C." Brock, who would later be knighted and then given a life peerage for his pioneer cardiac surgery, was interested but skeptical when he watched Harken remove a missile from a soldier's right ventricle.

"I really don't see what useful purpose we can put this to after the war, Dwight," he said. "We won't see such fragments in hearts then."

Harken emphatically disagreed. "Russell, if you'd read the manuscript of your own marvelous Lawrence O'Shaughnessy, you'd know he already had the idea of doing something very like what I'm doing! With this same technique, I could probably open up a congenital pulmonic valvular stenosis. If he hadn't died at Dunkirk, O'Shaughnessy would probably have come back and done it. I'll show you."

Brock looked at Harken's copy of the unfinished manuscript O'Shaughnessy had written before war intervened. Harken had studied the draft, which was to have been the Hunterion lecture O'Shaughnessy had been invited to deliver. Included was a picture of an obstructed valve and a description of a projected operation to open the stenosis (constriction of a passageway) by inserting a cutting valvulotome by way of the ventricle. Brock read it carefully, but remained skeptical. In 1946 Russell Brock would perform the first successful operation on a congenital pulmonary stenosis by the method suggested in O'Shaughnessy's paper and demonstrated by Harken's procedure. He did not then nor thereafter mention Harken or his own compatriot O'Shaughnessy in connection with that triumph. "Perhaps he had really forgotten what I showed him at the 160th," Harken would say with some charity.

When a three-star general notified the 160th that he was arriving on an inspection tour, Heaton conferred with Harken on how to save their showplace from the officer's famous sadism; he prided himself on the black marks he handed out for waste or dirt. Rumor had it that after inspecting one post, he had forced its commanding officer to eat the scraps he had found in the post's garbage pails which he considered edible and which therefore should not have been wasted. He also ran his white-gloved fingers over door and window sills.

"Well, after all, medically he's just another layman," Harken said to Heaton. "You greet him with your usual charm and give me a signal. Delay him six or seven minutes and then offer to show him some important, unique, exciting things that are making surgical history here. Put him in surgical garb and bring him in."

Harken was normally as bad as the general about his operating theatre. "Keep it tidy! Keep it clean!" he would bark. This time he gleefully ordered the staff to pick up nothing, to leave everything *in situ*. Bloody towels and sponges littered the floor by the time Heaton's signal came. Harken prepared an open chest, making a foot-long incision exposing the lungs and the heart, doing its frantic flipflop. Heaton, the general, and two attendant officers, gowned and masked, came in. "Bring the general over here where he can see this," Harken invited enthusiastically.

The general advanced, looked, burst into perspiration, staggered slightly, backed away—and was escorted outside by his officers. Heaton followed and inquired whether he might care now to inspect the food service, kitchens, and garbage disposal.

The general said that he had concluded that the 160th warranted a superior rating and that he was in a hurry to leave for his next inspection.

General Ossopof of the Soviet Union, destined to become surgeon general of the Red Army, arrived to stay several days. Young, blond, handsome, and polite, he assiduously observed everything, but of each case Harken showed him, he remarked, through his interpreter, "We do just the same in Russia."

Watching Zoll and Harken conduct a session to locate fragments and visualize them by fluoroscopy, Ossopof said again, "Just the same in Russia!" Harken grinned. He knew perfectly well that the best equipment in the U.S.S.R., manufactured by General Electric and Westinghouse, was quite incapable of visualizing foreign bodies such as they were showing him.

On the third day Major Harken accompanied General Ossopof through his wards. The boys who could do so came to attention, stood beside their beds, and exposed their incisions. In some cases they displayed in their hands the metal fragments that Harken had removed from lungs, great vessels, or hearts.

"Tell the major," said Ossopof to his interpreter, "that his incisions are too long!"

Harken believed in six-, ten-, or twelve-inch incisions for good exposure. He lost his temper. "Tell the general that when he has done a hundred and fifty such operations with shorter incisions and equally fast recovery, I'll change. But I want him to know that incisions in Americans heal from the *sides* not from the *ends*, and when *length* affords better exposure, it is the *method of choice*."

Ossopof put his big hands on Harken's shoulders. "To the bar," he said *basso profundo*. "We drink. No more rounds today! To the bar."

The Queen Mother of England came in her Daimler, and red carpet was rolled out over the asphalt. She demanded of Harken, "Tell me what *we* have done for you." Harken had not recovered from the bruising battles he had had with the British to get equipment, but nevertheless diplomatically replied, "Why, Your Majesty, you have contributed everything, from the ground on which we walk to the surgical methods taught by your great pioneer

Mr. Tudor Edwards—the very where and how of our success."
Harken thought he was laying it on a bit thick, but Her Majesty
merely nodded, satisfied.

In the spring of 1945 *New York Times* reporter Kathleen
McLaughlin trailed the VIPs to the 160th, following up intel-
ligence that medical miracles were occurring daily in the lovely
Cotswold valley. "Generalissimo and pivotal personality is
Dwight E. Harken, chief surgeon," wrote the correspondent,
describing him as a sandy-red-haired six-foot Bostonian who looked
only slightly older than the age of his average case.

When Harken had word that Elliott Cutler, now a general,
was coming with British Surgeon General Hood, he staged their
reception with care. As if it were a random choice, he led them
first to a particular ward where he had arranged for a handsome
young corporal to call the patients to attention. The visiting party
came to a halt as the corporal shouted "Ten*shun!*" and saluted
stiffly.

"By the way," said Harken, "this soldier had a problem that
might interest you gentlemen. I took a shell fragment from his
heart."

Cutler, wide-eyed and pleased, said, "General Hood, well,
here's a boy out of whose heart Dwight has actually taken a
foreign body. Isn't that interesting? Corporal, when was your
operation?"

"Fixty-six hours ago, sir!"

Hood was astounded and Cutler expressed his pleasure, embarrassment, or disbelief with a gesture characteristic of him. He
leaned over sharply, covered his smiling face with his hand, and
then righted himself. "Well, what do you think of that, General
Hood?"

Hood said, "I always thought I was a bit of a liar myself!"

Harken's strongly held theories about early ambulation at a
time when healthy women were kept in bed weeks after normal
childbirth were not normally carried this far. "It was a bit rough
on the youngster," he later admitted. "But the kid was willing to
make quite an effort, was glad to do it. The missile had been in
the solid wall of his left ventricle and I was certain it wouldn't
damage him to get up so soon. He was plucky and showed no sign

of pain. The boys were all so glad to be there. They knew it was a showplace, the best place, where they got the best treatment, so the boys always tossed the ball back."

The stream of casualties flowing into the 160th slowed down. A British general had once remarked that Americans fought their wars by making an incredible quantity of lethal objects and then tossing them wholesale at the enemy. The things to throw were now sent barreling through France along the Red Ball Highway and the army was pitching them at a rapidly retreating enemy.

Harken often went elsewhere at night to act as consultant on difficult thoracic problems, taking with him a nurse and anesthetist and sometimes an assistant surgeon. "We were young and vigorous and didn't worry about sleeping. The next morning after these trips, we'd just go back to work."

Another additional activity was Harken's participation in the selection of chest-injured German prisoners to exchange for American prisoners. Germany's Sauerbruch was involved in selecting the Americans. He was Tudor Edwards' rival in fame and had been called to England to treat His British Majesty's empyema in 1935. For this Tudor Edwards would never forgive either his sovereign or Sauerbruch, and he maintained that the royal empyema had been badly mismanaged. Sauerbruch "cheated" in choosing the Americans, Harken claimed, sending over irreparable paraplegics or amputees with chest wounds that could never be repaired, ignoring the humane principle of selecting those who were ready to go home. Also ignored, the Americans learned, was the Geneva covenant, which forbade the return to combat of exchanged prisoners. The Germans, well cared for by the Americans, said Harken, often seemed reluctant to be repatriated.

Examination indicated that one particularly attractive young American artillery officer who came in to the 160th had a fragment in the pericardium, slightly posterior to the left ventricle. He was prepared for operation. Harken dissected a thinly damaged zone of heart muscle stuck to the pericardium. Then he and his team saw what they had not seen before. The missile site lay within the left ventricle. There had been a laceration of the ventricle.

The thickened left ventricular wall had, because of missile damage, developed an out-pouching or "blowout area." Scar tissue had formed under the heart, in the heart wall, and outside the heart, but was limited by the sac around the heart. The missile lay within this blowout area, imbedded in its own cocoon, as if it had built a little igloo and the lining of the heart had grown over it. The aneurysm (dilatation of the wall) acted as an idle cylinder in a motor does. When the wall of the heart contracted to expel blood into the aorta, the zone of aneurysm moved paradoxically in the wrong direction, sapping the strength of the contraction.

Harken put purse string and guy sutures around the left ventricular aneurysm. He found that old blood and clot were sequestered in the depths of the cocoon. He incised it. The anticipated sudden and powerful rush of blood occurred as the cocoon burst and extruded out through the cardiotomy site. The bleeding was barely sufficiently controlled by crossing the guy sutures, tightening the purse string sutures, and then oversewing to reinforce. Each time the heart was lifted from the pericardium, it grew irritable. Harken replaced it to rest. Lift it out . . . work . . . replace . . . lift . . . work. Circulation was repeatedly restored—a wonderful demonstration of the principle that the heart should not be dislocated from the position of optimum function, thought Harken.

In a strenuously tense and brief time the operation was completed. Surgically a left ventricle had been invaded, an abscess excised in a pumping heart under the enormous systemic pressure. Cloth as well as the missile had been removed. The patient recovered extraordinarily well, and when the foreign materials taken from his heart were cultured in the laboratory they were found to grow pathogenic organisms. This was Harken's twelfth operation within a heart, and the first and only one within a left ventricle.

By early December 1944 almost everyone in England thought the war would soon be over. "Home for Christmas,"

Margot Evans told those of her boys nearly well enough to travel.

A few days before Christmas Harken was flabbergasted to see stretchers once again covering the entire asphalt loading and unloading area. He went out and asked several of the young men whether they had come in from the forward areas because the army had begun a program of redeployment. "Oh, no," they told him. "We're here because we are losing the war."

These were the chest wounded from the last desperate German push, from Bastogne and the Battle of the Bulge. The thinly stretched Allied lines had been breached. In Paris there was panic, even at SHAEF, the Allied high command post outside the city. "Nothing between the German army and Paris in a direct line but one MP and two short-order cooks," quipped an officer at SHAEF. German soldiers who spoke perfect English were infiltrating the area in American uniforms, their objective to capture SHAEF. Checkpoints were set up everywhere and infiltrators were trapped by questions about American baseball heroes and by their lack of familiarity with current American slang.

American casualties from the German push were high. The air force was immobilized by bad weather. Then, when a small flight of German jets flew over one battlefield at a speed against which the Americans had no defense, there was further panic. If jets, the first ever seen, were in mass production in Germany, the enemy could still win the war. The jet airplanes were not in mass production, but before the tide of Allied victory swept once more toward Berlin, chest wounded soldiers were pouring into the 160th.

In order to promote Major Harken and get around the fixed table of organization for the 160th, HQ in London found a medical officer due for promotion who would exchange it for a chance to work with Harken. The night Major William Cassebaum arrived to join Lieutenant Colonel Harken, Harken had to do an emergency operation on a young man emaciated from multiple, long-standing injuries. The patient had developed a secondary hemorrhage from the spleen which required an immediate splenectomy. There must be no delay. Harken had been forty-eight hours without sleep and could scarcely stand. Using a transthoracic approach, with the patient left side up, his incision went through the lower intercostal (between ribs) space, beginning over the eighth interspace in the mid-auxiliary line. Then Harken's knife slipped off the rib and cut through the interspace and underlying diaphragm. Instantly as the ribs were spread the spleen popped out, tethered only by an unusually long pedicle. Without indicating that this was fortuitous, Harken simply and quickly tied off the splenic artery and vein and cut off the spleen. Mission accomplished. Emergency over. Cassebaum, a fine general surgeon himself, was dazzled. "My God," he said to the man for whom he had forfeited his promotion, "I heard you were fast, but I didn't think anybody could do it that fast!"

The Allies could no longer lose the war and peace was delayed only by Hitler's intransigence. It had to come soon.

Harken's series of extraordinary heart and great vessel operations had grown to well over a hundred. Wartime reputations faded very quickly in peacetime, and in spite of the record, he might not be able to continue experiments in heart surgery. He would return to the States one of a huge number of discharged surgeons looking for appointments. What he needed was solid, objective proof and documentation of those wartime cardiac interventions.

Colonel Heaton had been promoted and replaced as commanding officer by a pleasant, unimaginative officer who always went through channels and by the book. He was inclined to say "Impossible" or "No" to any irregular request. When Harken asked him if he could arrange for some of his operations to be filmed, he was told that the commanding officer would petition through channels but that it was probably impossible to arrange. So Harken himself asked Elliott Roosevelt of the Signal Corps to loan him a camera crew. Roosevelt agreed and Harken decided to risk criticism by filming the operation he contemplated on patient Private First Class Leroy Rohrbach. He would choose as the date the one set for a visit by his former colleagues at the Brompton, including his old chief A. Tudor Edwards.

Rohrbach lay in Harken's special ward. He had a piece of metal in his right ventricle. Harken originally had attempted to remove the missile when it was still in the right ventricle, but it had wriggled from his forceps and migrated to the right auricle Weeks later Harken had exposed the fragment again, but lost it as it moved back to the right ventricle. He had tried to send Rohrbach home to the United States so someone else could challenge the elusive missile.

Rohrbach might not die because the fragment was still in his heart, but he wanted the damn thing out. He was afraid nobody else would even try to remove it. "Sir," he said, "you've been kicking around in my heart quite a lot. Why don't you take one more crack?"

To operate on a man's heart for the third time was to add risk to risk to risk. Harken was sure that if he failed, he would be regarded as an irresponsible fool. But if he succeeded, he would have dramatic proof of his contention that the heart was capable of withstanding a good deal of trauma. He wrote to Anne Harken the night before the operation: "If I succeed, heart surgery may well be on its way."

3.

"Wonderful, Healthy American Soldiers!"

Thirty years later Mr. Norman R. Barrett, F.R.C.S. (Fellow of the Royal College of Surgeons), would write in reminiscence:

> The news had come to us in London that Dwight had successfully operated upon a series of wounded men who had foreign bodies in the heart, the pericardium, the large vessels, and the mediastinum. No surgeon had had such an experience and few thought it was possible to tackle these cases. It is true that various individuals had made isolated attempts—"smash and grab raids"—but there were no guiding lines regarding techniques; and the problem of control of hemorrhage seemed almost insuperable to most of us. Moreover there were other problems: even supposing the bleeding could be controlled, would the heart continue to beat when open and would it heal well afterwards?
>
> You can understand that, under these circumstances, Dwight had not only the responsibility of demonstrating a new and dangerous technique, but he was about to do so before the critical eyes of his former chief.
>
> In the event Mr. Tudor Edwards and the rest of the old Brompton team went on a visit to Dwight's unit. The patient was a soldier who had a piece of metal about the size of a lump of sugar in the right ventricle. Two other attempts had been made to get this foreign body out of his heart. Both had failed because the foreign body moved.

That morning Harken strode from his quarters at his usual pace, rapid as a hiker's descent down a mountain. Within the ugly Quonset huts the busy hospital routine went on, but the beautiful valley was quiet. The blue sky overhead was empty except for feathery clouds. Not so long before the daylight bomber flights from British bases had domed the valley with sound. One day soon the Americans would fulfill their promise to remove all traces of their war, carting away the huts, uprooting the asphalt paving, replanting the grass. By odd coincidence, the land on which the 160th was installed belonged to the Hood family, one of whose ancestors had been killed in the Battle of Bunker Hill and another of whom had gone west in the States. One of the American Hoods was Harken's wife, Anne Hood Harken.

Harken dashed through the ward to which he had taken Cutler and British Surgeon General Hood (who might have been a distant relation of his wife's), perhaps for luck. He paused by the bed where a sergeant from Iowa lay as the ward came to attention; he had been under artillery fire, leading his men against enemy pillboxes east of Metz, near the German border, when a shell fragment entered his heart. The wound had festered and his fever prevented Harken from operating. Convinced that his heart would stand the strain now, Harken had scheduled the Iowan for the following day. Perhaps that operation to remove the fragment and drain the abscess could also be filmed. "See you tomorrow, Sergeant," said Harken. "And when you get home to Iowa, be sure to give the folks my regards."

On his feet, at attention, was a nineteen-year-old from Brooklyn. Hit by a splinter of a shell from a German eighty-eight inside the enemy's country, he had walked more than half a mile to a forward field hospital. He was evacuated to the 160th, and the two-inch slug that had pierced his pericardium was in Harken's collection of war trophies.

A young corporal saluted as Harken passed him, permitting his fingers to vibrate, the ghost of a grin on his immobile countenance. Harken grinned back. The plucky kid was the one who had done him proud. The boys always tossed the ball back and now Private First Class Rohrbach had entrusted his heart to surgeon Harken. The surgeon's British peers and his great chief would be watching while he made that third attempt to remove the fragment that had migrated back into Rohrbach's right ventricle. Elliott Roosevelt had sent over Sergeant Cissna from the Signal Corps to record the procedure on film. Cissna had been chief cameraman at a major movie studio in Hollywood before the war. The course of postwar intracardiac surgery, with its life-saving, life-prolonging potential, was up to Harken that day.

Cissna had set up his equipment in the operating room. Cables for the cameras and lights snaked over the floor. Cissna had never filmed anything like this. Even fake scenes of operations were rare in motion pictures in those days, and there was no popular television, which would make such scenes a staple of public entertainment. Cissna sprawled with his assistant on scaffolding erected above the operating table.

Patient Rohrbach was brought in, still quite conscious. Harken scrubbed in with his surgical team. They were a great team, he thought, cossetted, argued, chivvied, and scolded into a near-perfect unit. His first assistant today was Joe Lynch, affectionately described by artist Weinstein as "a telephone pole with an Adam's apple." An outstanding man. Hank, the second assistant, was the only newcomer, and he was superb. He had requested the assignment as "secunded" to Harken at the 160th, and walked in a short time before. They had never met, but Harken recognized him instantly. Six foot five, with very short cropped white hair despite his youth, a shaggy brow, and a remarkable lack of occiput above his neck. "You've got to be a Saltonstall," Harken had exclaimed. He was Dr. Henry Saltonstall.

Anesthetist Charles Burstein was certainly the very best there was, thought Harken. He had already inserted two large-caliber cannulae (instruments devised to fit various body channels) into Rohrbach's anticubital veins (those in front of the elbow) so that the rapid blood transfusions could be given under pressure, transfusions of hitherto unprecedented magnitude.

Under the table, in which cramped space he could on this occasion best monitor the electrocardiograms, was Paul Zoll. Zoll had helped to fluoroscope Rohrbach all three times.

Both Shirleys scrubbed in. They were alert, ferociously well trained, rugged, efficient.

Masks already hid the faces of the visitors from the famous London hospital. Colleagues from his own days at the Brompton, Russell Brock, who had come down again, and Norman Barrett, were there. Barrett, a generous fellow and a close friend, wished him well. Was Brock, dour, solid, and circumspect, as generous?

The greatly revered A. Tudor Edwards was too ill and fragile to stand, much less to scrub. He was seated on a stool, his head above the ether shield, with drapes drawn around his neck tying him into the field with towel clips. His bright beady black eyes peered over his metal-framed half-spectacles. Ill or not, Harken's former chief would miss nothing.

Conversation was mush-mouthed through the masks, but far from murmurous. Harken, always a talkative man in the operating room, kept oral track of every detail, and his was a carrying baritone. Casual medical chatter belied the tension. Rohrbach no longer heard anything. His anesthetized body was tilted left side down, right shoulder up, so that the apex of his heart was down and to the left. Harken hoped by this position to keep and trap the missile where it had eluded him in the first operation. The missile had returned to the place where it had been after its frustrating escape from the right auricle in the second operation.

The chest was opened with a semicircular incision over the fifth interspace below Rohrbach's left nipple. Overhead the camera began to whirr. The team began bathing and sucking away the tranquilizing procaine to reduce the irritability of Rohrbach's exposed heart. As expected, there were massive adhesions fusing the chest wall to the pericardium and the pericardium to the epicardium and the heart wall, which made exposure difficult.

Harken gingerly put his hand on the heart. He could palpate the missile—about two centimeters by one centimeter by one centimeter in size—under the very thin wall of the right ventricle. Carefully he placed a series of sutures around an area of about three square centimeters, so that when he went through the clear zone within the circle of adhesions he could cross them to stop bleeding.

The tension grew almost unbearable. The surgeons suffered what they called "dry-mouth syndrome." From the platform over the table a film box fell into the sterile operating field. The possible contamination had to be ignored. Color film continued to move through the camera, which was focused on the surgeon's hands and the patient's heart. As in all the previous intracardiac operations, the knife carefully divided the epicardium and its covering adhesions, then the muscular wall, until the lining endocardium pouted into the incision with its underlying contained shell fragment.

Harken plunged a heavy Kocher clamp into Rohrbach's heart and the clamp grasped the missile. The heart wriggled in protest and wrested the missile from the forceps. Blood spurted in a column the diameter of a man's middle finger and rose to a height of eight inches before sweeping down, from left to right, across Harken's left hand. Lynch pulled the sutures across the incision to control the flow of blood. Two medical corpsmen pumped blood to replace the loss into the cannulae in Rohrbach's arm veins, replacing slightly more than was lost through the geyser from his heart. Burstein relayed what soft-voiced Paul Zoll was reporting. Private Rohrbach's blood pressure was not dropping and the electrocardiogram was not alarming.

Harken plunged the forceps in again. The missile was torn loose again. Harken could still feel it and he made a third try, calling out, *"Joe, grab it from your side!"*

Deftly Joe Lynch placed his clamp at a ninety-degree angle from Harken's. With four-point fixation, the two men lifted the missile out, up, and across the left side of the table. According to accurate film measurements, this took sixteen seconds. They crossed and tied the guide sutures, controlling the blood spout with the sutures and with their fingers. Thirty seconds. Then they carefully reinforced the whole area with a free covering of pericardium.

During this brief, vital time the two orderlies used upside down double-stoppered glass bottles (Dr. Carl Walter had not yet invented plastic transfusion receptacles). They pumped air into the tops of the bottles. Blood was thus forced well into the veins. Throughout, Rohrbach's heart behaved quite well, with very little ventricular irritability.

Heartbeats, including Rohrbach's, steadied. The rib spreader was removed and the ribs were approximated (pulled together) and heavy catgut sutures were placed with care around the rib cage protecting the heart. Subcutaneous tissues and skin were aligned and sewn over the cage to create a firm, normal chest wall. That done, the members of the surgical team and the visitors moved away casually. Beyond the sterile field, masks were removed and surgical gloves pulled off.

Dwight Harken, in his stained operating clothes, went straight to Tudor Edwards. "Did I do well by you, my great chief?"

"Rawther! Rawther! Rawther!" said Tudor Edwards.

Before returning to the Signal Corps, cameraman Cissna filmed Private First Class Rohrbach the next day. Rohrbach was comfortable and responsive. He managed to sit up in bed and smile for the camera. (Harken was still receiving loquacious letters from civilian Leroy Rohrbach in 1975.)

On their second day there, Cissna and his assistant also filmed the operation on the sergeant who was Harken's fellow Iowan. The unwelcome invader in this patient's pericardium was a jagged piece of iron, surrounded by a gas gangrene abscess. His heart had to be lifted from the sac in order to get at the iron and cleanse the abscess. Dislocated, the heart dilated, and its beat became very irregular. Harken would say, "I knew what was happening, of course, from watching animal hearts in the laboratory dilate and then go through fibrillation, and then stop. When it misbehaved too badly, I just put the heart back for a rest."

Paul Zoll documented the electrocardiographic changes on his long cardiographic strips. "Oh, they were *very* interesting," he would comment. The sergeant recovered well.

Some months later, after VJ day ended World War II, Lieutenant Colonel Harken left for home. On the wallowing troopship he spent most of his time energetically participating in and combating an epidemic of seasickness. In his locker was the film, the Legion of Merit medal, and his collection of trophies—foreign bodies, mostly shell fragments he had removed from the forbidden territory in and around the heart.

In Dr. Frank Brown Berry's *Surgery in World War II: Thoracic Surgery*, Volume II (1965), this first "consistently successful series of operations in this area"—seventy-eight within or

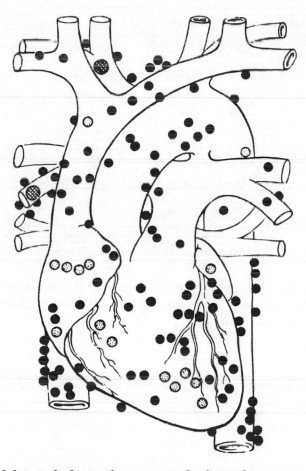

Position of foreign bodies within or near the heart that were removed by Lieutenant Colonel Harken's thoracic team at the 160th General Hospital in England.

in relation to the great vessels, fifty-six in or in relation to the heart—was noted:

> The series of 134 operations performed by Lt. Colonel Dwight E. Harken, M.D., in which foreign bodies were removed from the heart and great vessels constituted a remarkable achievement. There were no deaths in the series and all the patients left the chest center with normally functioning hearts.

In the future Dr. Harken would often be asked to testify at legislative hearings necessitated by groups opposed to animal experimentation.

"Think of four groups of nineteen patients each," he would open, regarding his audience solemnly through his spectacles. "In the first group of nineteen I opened the heart, dealt with a foreign body in the heart, closed the heart, and they all died. In the second group of nineteen I opened the heart, dealt with the foreign body in the heart, closed the heart, and nine died. In the third group of nineteen only three died. Dismal, but getting better?"

Here he would pause and regard his often horrified listeners owlishly. "In the fourth group I opened the heart, dealt with the foreign bodies in the heart, closed the heart, and they all lived." Another pause. "There was an important difference. The first three groups of patients were all experimental laboratory animals on whom I learned how. The fourth group were all *wonderful, healthy American soldiers!*"

4.

A Long, Long Road

"The road to the heart is only two or three centimeters in a direct line, but it has taken twenty-four hundred years to travel it!" remarked surgeon B. F. Sherman in 1896 after Ludwig Rehn in Germany successfully repaired a stab wound that had penetrated the heart; it is a quotation that would often be repeated. Rehn's suturing of the heart was the first recorded instance of cardiac surgery.

Suturing of chest wounds had been mentioned by Homer in the *Iliad*. A papyrus, not discovered and translated until the twentieth century, contained earlier references to two successfully treated chest wounds, one of them sutured, and both bound with fresh meat, grease, honey, and lint. This stretched, as it were, the date of the earliest crude thoracic surgery to about 3000 B.C., making that road to the heart some five thousand years long.

The great second-century A.D. Greek physician and philosopher, Galen, had been the first man to report that he had seen a living heart beating within an open chest. His medical writings were extensive, and until the sixteenth century he was considered the greatest of all medical authorities. He wrote that he had watched a heart continuing to function when he removed part of a war-wounded man's sternum and a piece of the pericardium to cure an abscess.

Chest wounds have always been common in wars because the chest, caging the vulnerable heart, is the prime target of those with intent to kill. Until the mid-twentieth century penetration of the chest wall to any depth, by knife, ax, sword, spear, arrow, bullet, or bayonet, was seldom amenable to the crude surgery available. Those warriors who did not bleed to death most often died of subsequent infection.

The recovery rate might have improved in the thirteenth century if his medical contemporaries had heeded an Italian physician named Theodoric. He was a remarkably modern-minded man and wrote feelingly about the need for medical men to be less rash and violent. "Let physicians be foresighted, gentle, and circumspect around the sensitive parts and ticklish places," he begged. About chest wounds, he insisted that they healed more readily "if the stitches are placed in accordance with the size of the wound so that the natural heat cannot escape in any way or the air outside be able to enter." Accepted medical theory was adamant that leaving the chest open so that infection could be better treated was preferable. Arguments against Theodoric's idea that chest wounds should be closed to keep air out continued until the influenza epidemic of 1917.

Firearms were first used in the battle over Crécy in the Hundred Years War between England and France. Gunshot wounds in the chest were routinely fatal, but in 1676 British physician Richard Wiseman wrote that in spite of the overwhelming incidence of mortality from them, "It is not consistent with Religion or Humanity to leave such people without help: for sometimes we happily prolong the life of some, and now and then cure one."

The mortality rate for men with penetrating chest wounds in the Crimean War (1853–56) was staggering, 91.6 percent in the French army, 97.2 percent in the British. As time went on, treatment improved, and such wounds were more often quickly closed, but not until the latter part of World War I did more than half, 53.3 percent, of the chest wounded survive. This was the record of military surgery during combat years and of no ordinary mix. From battlefield surgery have come many radical revisions of hitherto accepted practices, but it often takes years before the revisions are accepted in peacetime. Peacetime pioneers, in theory or deed, are subject to suspicious supervision, criticism, and conventional rejection by their peers.

It takes time to displace what is widely assumed to be right. William Harvey's new and radical conception of the circulation of the blood, which would lead down the long road to heart surgery, was fiercely disputed for over two centuries. Harvey's lectures on the subject, delivered in 1616, and the paper, *De Motu Cordis*, in which he expanded this conception, published in 1628, are a joy to review for the simple elegance of his deductive reasoning. Harvey was a British physiologist and amateur naturalist. He made three major discoveries: first, that the heart had unidirectional valves and was a pump; second, that arterial blood was forcibly pumped away from the heart as the stream from cut arteries clearly attested; third, that the venous blood clearly returned in the direction of the heart, as obstructing the venous blood on the surface of the arm clearly showed. And he irascibly defended these discoveries.

That new ideas are clearly more likely to be wrong than right gives the nihilists a distinct advantage. If they say "No," they may well prove to be justified; if they are wrong, they incur no blame—they merely followed accepted and hallowed methods. Pioneers, on the other hand, face every disadvantage. If they are right, it may be a long, controversial time before their rightness is admitted. If they are wrong, they are scathingly denounced. And even correct theories confirmed in the laboratory may have to wait many years before they are clinically applicable.

For instance, in France Julien Cesar Legallois demonstrated that his new concept of resuscitating hearts after ischemic arrest (caused when the blood supply is cut off) was correct by injecting arterial blood directly into the circulatory system in animals. This concept was later validated under certain conditions in open-heart surgery. At the time, the objection to human trial of the method was understandable. In order to inject the blood, Legallois decapitated his experimental animals.

It takes courage to maintain a heretical stand in the hierarchical world of physicians and surgeons.

In the late nineteenth century two men in the medical capitals of Europe, Vienna and London, laid down the law about surgery in the heart. Professor Christian Albert Theodor Billroth, whose own extensive abdominal operations were called by the irreverent "autopsies *in vivo*," declared that even to consider suturing a heart wound was out of the question. "Any surgeon who would attempt an operation on the heart should lose the respect of his colleagues." In the spring of 1896 Sir Stephen Paget made his pronouncement: "The heart alone of all viscera has reached the limits set by nature to surgery. No new method and no new technique can overcome the natural obstacles surrounding a wound of the heart." Both men are included in the Founders Group list along with their pronouncements. Thus, Billroth's and Paget's places in surgical history are assured not by their accomplishments but by these dicta, which were remarkably badly timed.

On September 8, 1896, a young German soldier was stabbed in a beer hall brawl in Frankfurt, Germany. He was picked up by the police on the sidewalk at 3 A.M. and taken to the Frankfurt hospital. Probing by the house surgeon on duty indicated that the knife had reached into his heart. The soldier, William Justus, was given a shot of morphine and an ice pack was placed over the wound. He was then left in his bed to die.

Dr. Ludwig Rehn, visiting surgeon at the hospital, arrived there on the evening of the 9th. William Justus, by some miracle, was still alive. Rehn observed his own golden rule: "If we see a case which may be saved only by operation, then it is our duty to operate!" A courageous man who had done some unusual work on lung wounds, Rehn had already saved many lives with a new and widely disputed operation for appendicitis. At 7:30 on September 9 he decided to risk his reputation and had patient Justus prepared for surgery.

Ether dropped on gauze was used to anesthetize the patient. His weak pulse did not falter. Rehn went in between the fourth and fifth ribs, exposed the fifth rib and divided it with bone scissors, then bent it outward to expose the pericardium, which was distended. When he opened this, he saw that blood from the penetration had drained into the sac, threatening to choke the heart. Rehn snipped a window to drain the pericardial sac and saw behind his incision the heart's chambers. From the right ventricle blood was flowing. Holding the heart in his hand, the surgeon put two stitches in the lacerated heart and a third stitch in the pericardium which drew the protective sac together. The heart stopped beating for an instant, and then began to beat again. Within two weeks Justus was up and walking around the wards.

In subsequent lectures, exhibiting Justus, who would willingly bare his incision, Rehn admitted that they had been lucky. After the operation he discovered that his patient had recently been dismissed from the army because he had heart trouble, giving him a slow pulse. Paradoxically, it was possible that the slow loss of blood from his wound had helped him to survive until the surgery. His heartbeat, further weakened, meant that less blood leaked into the pleural space. The cold night had helped the blood around the wound to congeal. The slow pulse gave the surgeon fewer problems in placing the sutures.

It is also possible, Harken suggests, that the pressure of the collection of blood in the surrounding pericardial sac had stopped the leak from the heart. If Justus had not suffered tamponade (obstruction of the heart's ability to accept and eject blood) in the more than forty hours that elapsed before Rehn operated, he might well have survived without Rehn's aggressive surgical intervention.

That does not diminish the immense importance of the operation. It was listed first as the Turning Point that led from chest to heart surgery because it proved that tampering with a man's heart would not kill him.

Rehn kept track of the suturing of heart wounds thereafter, recording 134 in the next ten years, with 40 percent survival. This was, of course, the simplest *extra*cardiac surgery. Before the chambers of the heart could be entered and *intra*cardiac surgery become feasible, a number of things would have to happen in the laboratory, in men's minds, and in the operating room.

Thoracic surgery was already developing its modern heroes in the early 1900s. Radical lung surgery was pioneered before World War II by Tudor Edwards in England, Sauerbruch in Germany, and Evarts Graham and Churchill in the United States. A major problem was that opening the chest often led to fatal collapse of the lungs. To reduce pressure, Sauerbruch experimented with an operating chamber in which the bodies of the patient and the surgical team were inside a negative pressure chamber while their heads remained outside. This technique was discarded as too cumbersome even before Ivan Magill in England designed his apparatus for administering oxygen and anesthetic gases through an endotracheal tube.

Magill's tube was inserted into the windpipe (trachea) and made airtight by packing the throat or by fitting the tube with a balloon cuff. Anesthetic agents and oxygen were administered directly. A bag like a football bladder on the anesthetist's end of the tube allowed him to inflate and deflate (ventilate) the lungs at will while administering any gaseous agents he elected. Magill's invention, together with the development of techniques for blood transfusion, permitted thoracic surgery's radical extensions.

A few men began to call themselves specialists in thoracic surgery and even the heart was less than sacrosanct. Sauerbruch, a few years after Rehn's publicized first, found he could starve a heart of blood for a minute at a time without significant damage to the patient. In 1901 Norwegian surgeon Kristian Igelsrud took a stopped heart in his hand and pumped it until it beat again voluntarily. This was the precursor of open-chest cardiac massage—a bastard term for what should be called "manual systole." (The manipulation is a rhythmic propulsive substitution of circulating force bearing only a misleading relationship to "massage.")

The first American Nobel Laureate in Medicine and Physiology (1912), Alexis Carrel, was a prophet of the future, changing more thinking than fact. He predicted and plotted heart valve surgery and even artificial hearts on the basis of animal experimentation.

World War I, absorbing the energy, money, and manpower of the Western nations, slowed experimentation and the careful accumulation of knowledge, but galvanized surgery. After the war, *Lancet*, England's prestigious medical journal, published a record of two soldiers from whose right ventricles foreign bodies had been successfully removed. Transfusions had compensated for blood loss. One of them died of sepsis, a grave problem at the time for all wounded. At autopsy his heart was found to have already firmly healed. These two cases were dismissed as instances of life-or-death wartime surgical chance taking and chance survival, and no one appears to have accorded them any significance.

The war did lead to the realization that thoracic surgery should be a recognized specialty. In London A. Tudor Edwards and J. E. H. Roberts were appointed to the Brompton Hospital as staff surgeons. The hospital had been originally established by the Fowles family when one of their parlor maids coughed up blood in the 1850s. Lord Fowles wanted the local physician to send her to a sanatorium for consumptives, but was told there were no such institutions. Whereupon the charitably minded nobleman vacated his manor house to make it into a hospital for consumptives. The original manor house remained in use as a vast medical complex grew up around it. Meanwhile, victims of tuberculosis began to be segregated in sanatoria rather than in hospitals. In 1920 Tudor Edwards and J. E. H. Roberts were appointed surgeons at the Brompton, mostly to treat surgically tuberculosis of the gastrointestinal tract, including the rectum. They both saw things that should be done in the chest, including surgery by which the tuberculus cavities were collapsed to rest and heal, and in time the Brompton became a great center for chest surgery, including resection (removal) of diseased lungs.

In 1920 the three men who would open the area of blind (closed) intracardiac valvular surgery were still schoolboys: the slightly older Russell Brock in England, Charles Bailey in New Jersey, and Dwight Harken in Iowa. If any of the three as children and youths dreamed of different careers, they scarcely remembered them. They would bring to surgery the total absorption, concentration, and natural talent that made them daring innovators as well as superior technicians.

If ever a boy was set willy-nilly upon a single path to his career, it was young Dwight. His father, Dr. C. R. Harken, began taking him along as "anesthetist" when he was seven. Cornelia Rex Harken was doctor to most of Clark County, Iowa. Farms were often too isolated on the vast rolling fields and pastureland for "city care." The two of them would set forth, by horse and carriage before Dr. Harken acquired one of the first automobiles seen in Osceola, to outlying farmhouses for the home delivery of babies. Obstetrical anesthesia consisted of a cloth soaked in chloroform, which the laboring woman held above her face. She would drift to sleep, and her hand and the cloth would fall. Young Dwight's responsibility was to snatch it off if it fell on her face, which could cause excessive anesthesia, or to pick it up and restore it to her hand when she needed it again. Through the natural combination of Dr. Harken's obstetrical skill, the ruggedness of the Iowan farm folk, and a paucity of pathogenic bacteria in the environment, there was a fine crop of healthy babies in that area.

Following a delivery, there was often immediate consideration given to a name for the newborn. If Dr. Harken had liked his baptismal names, there would have been a plethora of Conreids and Rexes in the region. Since he did not, so many male children were named for his two sons that in one year there were three Dwights and three Aldens, none of them Harkens, on the Osceola high school football team.

Dr. Harken's consuming ambition was to emulate the already famous Mayo Clinic in Rochester, Minnesota, dominated by Dr. Mayo's two sons. C. R. Harken had already established the first hospital in Osceola. When Dwight and his younger brother, Alden, grew up, it was to become the Harken Clinic, with Dwight, he had decided, as the surgeon, and Alden the physician. More autocratic than fatherly, Dr. Harken assumed he would remain the undisputed head man at his clinic.

C. R. Harken kept himself medically up to date and in no way resembled a comfortable, old-fashioned general practitioner. Dignified, always impeccably tailored, handsome, and authoritative, he ran his extensive practice as he did his family, brooking neither criticism nor opposition. The Bible Belt townspeople and country folk accepted his authority and respected the medical care he lavished on them, although he was known to be irreligious. However, if they had realized that he was performing the devil's work—animal experimentation—in their midst, he might well have been run out of the county.

His laboratory was in the attic of his hospital garage, the entrance hidden behind the top-floor laundry tubs. It was accessible through a trap door. Only four people knew about it besides his wife and two sons: the hospital superintendent, his chief nurse, the sheriff of Osceola, and the Reverend Mr. Tice who lived next door. Harken swore to Tice that no animal would suffer pain while it was contributing to knowledge that might save human lives. The sheriff, one of whose duties was to dispose of unwanted animals or strays at $2 each, profited by selling them instead to Dr. Harken for another $2. Young Dwight was his father's laboratory anesthetist. He would place the animal in a large tile bin with a sponge soaked in chloroform or ether, cap the bin, and when the scratching stopped, haul the anethetized animal to the operating table. Beside the table, he ran a steam gauge ether drip that controlled a vaporizing tube to maintain ether delivery.

Dr. Harken went by train to Chicago every Sunday night and spent Monday observing new surgical techniques in that city. He arrived back in Osceola at 4 A.M. on Tuesdays. By the time he was twelve years old, Dwight was driving his father to and from the railroad station in Dr. Harken's Dodge touring car. One pre-dawn Tuesday Dr. Harken leapt from the train in unusual excitement. As they drove home, tall man and big son, he told the boy about a brand-new operation with which he could help people. When they arrived at the house, he rushed in and awakened his wife. Edna Harken came downstairs in a dressing gown and the three of them sat in the kitchen by the stove while Dr. Harken talked on.

"You've seen women around here with those big unsightly growths on their necks. It's caused by the thyroid gland. It's even more interesting because they get thyrotoxic sometimes and their · eyes pop out and they eat too much and can't stand hot weather. They're like—like—automobiles at full throttle with the clutch in. Those glands can come out! We'll work on dogs and then we'll take them out of people. You know, we've called a lot of folks crazy when they weren't crazy. It's their glands. The endocrine glands."

In the 1950s, when C. R. Harken's son Dwight was performing the then dramatic valvuloplasty for mitral stenosis, which became the surgery for heart disease resulting from rheumatic fever, he learned of a paper C. R. Harken, M.D., had published in

1914. It contained observations connecting heart disease with tonsular infection by a streptococcus that grew green on cultures. The country doctor was actually describing rheumatic fever and commented astutely that "Rheumatism is not a father to, but a member of the flock. Endocarditis, myocarditis, and pericarditis do not so often trace their ancestry to rheumatism, they trace their ancestry to a strain of micro-organisms whose Adam found his Eden in the tonsular crypt."

"My God, Dad," said Dwight Harken, by then internationally famous for his achievements in surgery, "you were the first to make this connection. You should have been famous!"

Dr. Harken never forgave Dwight for not returning to Osceola, especially after his other son, Alden, was stricken with multiple sclerosis and had to give up his ambition to go to medical school and came home to die. He repeated bitterly, "Dwight, you scrubbed for me in my operating room from eleven to sixteen, and then you left me!"

Dwight Harken had left Osceola for Harvard, and did not return again except as a visitor, but he never lost his sense of identity with his birthplace. For one thing, he appreciated the training his father had given him, and for another he carried with him his love for the hometown girl who would become his partner for life. In 1976, at one dinner given in Canada to honor his achievements, the speaker enumerated the number of remarkably right decisions Harken had made in his career at each crossroad in cardiac surgery. Another doctor rose to protest the speech: "You have left out the most important decision Dwight ever made! And that was to marry Anne Hood Harken!" The entire company rose and applauded.

Hoods and Harkens were both first families in the Midwest, descended from pioneering British stock. The Hoods had moved to Osceola from Creston, Iowa, when Anne Louise was twelve. Dwight, the same age, committed himself at first sight of the big-eyed, dark-haired girl who had a strange, enchanting way of smiling. Both were strong-willed and intelligent and at fifteen announced their intent to marry when they graduated from high school. Their parents thought it was much too soon for an engagement and the Hoods sent Anne Louise west to college while Dr.

Harken decreed Harvard for Dwight, vetoing their plan to go together to the University of Iowa.

At Harvard Dwight was a good enough student. The fact that he had a sex-linked reading disability, which his father had inherited and passed on, went unnoticed until his second year in Harvard Medical School, when there were excessive demands for rapid fine-print reading of material he found distinctly uninteresting. Before the end of that year, rather than fail, student Harken decided to relinquish a medical career and transferred to the Massachusetts School of Art. That really suited no one, least of all his father, and the next year he returned to repeat second-year medical training. Toward the end of it, medical students were sent to hospitals to learn by observation and participation as well as from textbooks. Contact with live patients so stimulated Harken that he shot to the top of the class.

After his third year in medical school he married Anne Hood, who was easily able to find work in Cambridge. Then Dwight Harken won his choice of an internship at Bellevue. The couple moved to New York. He won first place in the house officer examinations given to candidates for Bellevue, which gave him first choice among the open programs, and elected the one that offered six months in pathology, six in medicine, and then surgery, leading to a position as house surgeon. "That exciting mishmash set me on fire!"

Laboratory work in pathology so excited him that he decided to become a pathologist. He would haunt pathology laboratories for the rest of his life, although he turned out to have an allergy to formalin rather than the much more common intolerance to scrubbing. Being with or near formalin caused painful swelling of his hands and difficulty in breathing.

Medicine, in turn, tempted him, and he also would remain intensely interested in all of its aspects. But when he got into surgery the only question that remained was how to get ahead in a hurry. Established surgeons did not readily make room for newcomers and it was a long, arduous way to the top. Every branch of surgery, including the latest specialty, thoracic surgery, had monumental figures in dominant positions. The great and kindly Dr. Evarts Graham was already president of the American Association for Thoracic Surgery and founding editor of its journal. Graham was credited with the first resection of the lungs for cancer, although Dr. Isaac Bigger preceded him. (Dr. Graham's patient would outlive him. Graham was addicted to cigarettes and intractably refused to admit that heavy smoking contributed to lung cancer. He would die of it in 1957.) While Harken was at Harvard his mentor-professor, Dr. Edward Delos Churchill, a quiet man, surgical philosopher, and thinker, had stressed thoracic surgery, but did not think that a surgeon specializing in it exclusively could yet earn a decent living. The mercurial and dramatic Elliott Cutler, for his part, had insisted that all surgeons continue to do all surgery.

During his medical student days Harken had watched Churchill perform an operation for constrictive pericarditis, removing the scar tissue that incarcerated the heart and severely embarrassed its function so that it could neither accept nor eject blood properly. When the surgeon emancipated the heart from its constricting calcific sarcophagus, it fairly danced in its new freedom, becoming immediately larger, fuller of blood, freer to function. This extracardiac procedure, which would become Cutler's favorite operation, had intrigued Harken beyond measure. One could fairly see dysfunction and function in the living heart.

Just before Harken moved on from medicine to surgery at Bellevue, a patient came into his ward with fluid in the abdomen, massive swelling of the legs, and massive enlargement of the liver. His name was Cancerini and he was serving a long sentence in the Tombs, New York's famous prison, but had been released to Bellevue for treatment.

Cancerini was correctly diagnosed. His constrictive pericarditis had reached the point where he had no comfort and little life left. Harken began to convey his enthusiasm for Churchill's surgery to his seniors at Bellevue, who had the skill to do the pericardiectomy. If they decided to attempt the procedure, the timing would coincide with his own transfer onto the surgical service.

The operation was scheduled, the first pericardiectomy in New York, and Harken was allowed to join the surgical team. An unusual number of visitors dropped in to watch. Harken, permitted to remove quite a lot of the dense scar tissue himself, noticed that some of the spectators were sneezing and coughing, but it was too late to control the crowd. When Cancerini's heart did its "lovely" liberation dance, the excited visitors pressed close for a better view.

Cancerini, a former prizefighter, was a tough man with a strong will to live, even if in the Tombs. He recovered well—until infection set in. There was little to be done about that at the time. Harken fought to keep his patient alive. "He almost crawled into the oxygen tent with the fellow, *willing* him to survive," said one of his associates.

The incision broke down completely, laying Cancerini's chest open. Harken put a petri dish, a glass plate about an inch deep and five inches in diameter, over the opening, fused the plate on the chest with the kind of adhesive used to patch inner tubes, creating a window through which he could watch Cancerini's heart in action. During his long vigil Harken talked to his courageous patient while he observed his heart beating, the moment-to-moment wonders of blood circulation.

Dr. Marjorie Davis, chief surgeon at the Toronto Women's Hospital, and one of the first women who had been accepted at Bellevue, would talk about the days when she interned with Harken. "We all wanted autopsies," she said, "but it was very difficult and emotional in those days to get permission from relatives. Dwight was fantastic. He would promise them anything in the world—and deliver what he promised. Arrange the funeral, get the embalming done, send his wife out to beg clothes for the corpse."

When Cancerini died, Harken traced down his patient's estranged wife and got her permission to perform an autopsy. After it, he devised a noble funeral for the ex-prizefighter. He enlisted the hospital chaplain, borrowed a purple blanket to cover the body, collected flowers from the wards, and persuaded nurses and other interns to attend Cancerini's send-off to a pauper's grave.

In 1938 Harken became Dr. Fenwick Beekman's resident on the Children's Surgical Service at Bellevue. He nearly died himself of streptococcal septicemia (bloodstream infection) when he pricked his finger with a scalpel during an operation. The accident was not uncommon, nor was rapid death from the resulting infection. A year earlier he probably would have succumbed to streptococcus hemolyticus septicemia, but Prontalyn, early among the sulfonamides, had come into experimental use. It was a major medical breakthrough. Harken was Case Number 61 in the Rockefeller Institute's program to study the drug.

Late in 1938 he was on his way to England with Anne on the New York Academy's Bowen Traveling Fellowship. He and Norman Barrett, who would become a famous thoracic surgeon in England, were colleagues as clinical clerks on the A. Tudor Edwards team at the Brompton. Barrett and his wife, Betty, became close, helpful friends of the young Harkens and Barrett later wrote of their earlier days together.

The Brompton Hospital had always been devoted to the study of chest diseases. The patients were cared for by visiting surgeons and physicians who had a number of resident young doctors, who lived in the Hospital. The two senior surgeons each had a team composed of an "assistant surgeon" and a number of residents and juniors of various grades. The "firm" to which Dwight Harken was assigned was run by Mr. Tudor Edwards and Mr. Price Thomas. Dwight and I were colleagues and we occupied rather humble positions. These were still the days when the leaders of the surgical world were great men whom few would dare to challenge. They were days when pneumonectomy was still a most hazardous procedure even in the hands of the elite.

At that time thoracic surgery was largely concerned with the management of pulmonary tuberculosis, and for this disease relaxation therapy (by various types of pneumothorax or thoracoplasty) combined with long bed-rest in a sanitarium was the most advanced form of therapy. It was true that, at the Brompton, various operations upon the lung itself were being tentatively assayed, and upon some occasions a pneumonectomy for carcinoma would be done. There were of course many who suffered from empyema and this was often so serious as to be a fatal condition. Indeed no real advances had been made in the management of pleural sepsis since the great work of Evarts Graham done during the influenza epidemic after the first World War. It is against this background of limited enterprise that Dwight got his early training and there was nothing upon the horizon to suggest the beginning of cardiac, mediastinal or diaphragmatic surgery.

A. Tudor Edwards, born in 1890, was a remarkably handsome man, with smooth, center-parted black hair and an exquisitely trimmed mustache. When his American junior clerk reported for duty, Tudor Edwards made it peremptorily clear that he expected Harken to qualify for practice in England. There was no reciprocity across the Atlantic. Conjoint board examinations would be offered in about three months, those by the Royal College of Surgeons in about six. Harken had best begin studying immediately, since medical customs in England differed considerably from those in America.

Harken could not abide the wait. He discovered that there was another set of qualifying examinations he could take in three weeks, offered by the Society of Apothecaries in London. He began "swotting up" for them at night in the furnished flat he shared with Anne.

The ultimate was not expected of licentiates of the Ancient, Royal, Worshipful, and Honorable Guild, the Society of Apothecaries, but they were legally licensed to practice medicine and surgery in England as well as to write prescriptions and "commit a lunatic." Their examiners were chosen for their distinction. Harken's recall of the ordeal remained vivid. "Oh, those first day's written examinations were *awful*. What did I know about British forensic medicine anyway? I'd had only three weeks to prepare. Anne hung around outside, in her devoted fashion, and when I emerged, I told her I had failed miserably. I was not going back next day for my vivers—the oral examinations involving anatomy and live patients. It was no use. I wanted to stick my head in the shilling grate in our little digs, disgraced, but Anne insisted we go back inside and talk to somebody first."

The honorable secretary of the society, one Mr. Carpenter, was kind. He was not permitted to reveal his grades to a candidate, but he would allow himself to assure this candidate that he had done very well.

On his second day Harken was examined by Mr. Duncan Fitzwilliam, later to fire watch with him at the Royal Masonic during the war. The towering Fitzwilliam crouched on a chair at one side of a small table. Behind the table were tiers of oaken shelves on which lay rows of very dusty skeletal specimens.

"I understand that you are to be examined in anatomy, sir," said Fitzwilliam, clipping the words.

"Yes, sir."

Fitzwilliam unfolded himself from his chair to his full height of six feet five, reached up to a top shelf, and removed a skull, which he turned upside down, exposing the base.

"Oh, no," protested Harken, thrusting his fists against his own skull. "Oh, no!"

"What do you mean, 'Oh, no,' sir?" asked Fitzwilliam, looking at the skull in his hand as if about to recite "Alas, poor Yorick."

"You'll take a pencil, won't you, and poke the tip into various foramina, and if I'm lucky enough to guess the names of these little holes, you'll ask me what nerves go through them. I've been away from anatomy and neurology so long the chances of my answering correctly about twelve nerves going through twelve holes are so small I'd rather you asked me something else."

"And what do I do about a grade?" asked the tall gentleman, caressing the cranium.

"I assume you'd give me zero so far."

Fitzwilliam nodded and restored the skull to the shelf. "Fair enough." His back to Harken, he selected a dinosaur-sized human bone from another shelf.

Both men sat down across from each other at the small table and Harken took the bone. "This is a large tibia and fibula with cross union where there was a fracture and osteomyelitis, sir," said Harken with confidence. He had done plenty of orthopedic surgery at Bellevue.

"You've failed. Again," Fitzwilliam said.

"Sir!" said Harken. "That's exactly what it is!"

"Your answer was unromantic, colorless, and uninteresting," said Fitzwilliam. "What is the story behind that tibia?"

Harken was as unfamiliar with British humor as he was with British medical practice and he failed to see the frosty twinkle in his examiner's blue eyes. "I beg your pardon," he said indignantly. "I didn't know I was here to romance! All right. Many years ago along Fleet Street a large Zulu prince visiting England stepped off a curb and was run over by a taxicab. He lay in the gutter and got dirt in the compound comminuted fracture of his right leg. He was a very tall man and this is a very large bone. He developed osteomyelitis and that accounts for the cross union!"

"You have failed again," said Mr. Duncan Fitzwilliam. Before Harken could protest in astonishment, he went on, "Don't you recognize that when the Worshipful Society of Apothecaries got this collection of bones together there were no taxicabs? He was run over by a *hansom* cab."

Harken realized that he was being teased and befriended, not persecuted, by this great surgeon, and went more jauntily with him into the big guild hall where a number of patients were waiting. Among them, one little boy sat with his mother. Harken was told to examine the child and suggest treatment for the swollen area below the boy's right knee.

"Sir," said Harken, temerity returning with his certainty and his interest in a live patient, "I know you British think we jump to X-rays and the laboratory pretty hastily in the United States, but having determined immediately that this swelling has been weeks growing, that it is not tender and is cold, I would be afraid of a bone tumor such as osteogenic sarcoma, tuberculosis or Brodie's abscess, and I would have X-rays taken *at once*!"

"That's all right. That's exactly what I did. Here are the X-rays."

Harken looked carefully at the films. They were difficult to read. There was no clean-cut giant cell tumor with punched-out appearance. There was no clean-cut osteomyelitis with destruction of the bone. There was no clear onion skinning suggesting periosteal proliferation characteristic of osteogenic sarcoma. He said so. "It has some of the characteristics of all the three principal lesions that concern me, but I can't tell which one—sir—but it makes a lot of difference to this little boy, so I would take the X-rays to an expert bone roentgenologist who could make this distinction!"

"Exactly what I did," said Fitzwilliam. "It is osteogenic sarcoma."

"Sir!" Harken's face turned brick red. "Then how can you justify the fact that this little boy is sitting here instead of in a hospital undergoing final confirmation prior to having his leg amputated?"

"A valid criticism," said his examiner thoughtfully. "But it takes supreme skill in the face of a perfectly good differential diagnosis to decide on amputation. I was about to make a decision."

Harken was certain the case was urgent; the leg should come off at once. Fitzwilliam nodded, accepted Harken's opinion, and sent the American doctor on his way while he took care of the boy.

The next examination was in midwifery, a skill by which the apothecaries set special store. In order to return to A. Tudor Edwards with a license to practice, Harken supposed he could deliver a baby, but his experience in that area had been minimal. During his twelve required days on district obstetrics in medical school, only one baby had been born in all East Boston so far as he knew. Babies galore before and babies afterward, but only one birth at which he had officiated.

In the room where the examinations in midwifery were conducted, a formidable panel of obstetricians, Fellows of the Royal College of Surgeons, sat behind a table on which there was an equally formidable display of forceps, ranging from ancient iron ones to nickel-plated, chrome, and stainless steel ones. On another table lay a manikin with a wooden pelvis and a rubber vagina. A doll had been inserted into "her" birth canal and Harken was asked to determine the position of the "baby" and to recommend a method of delivery.

The panelists could not see the hand he inserted, so instead of gently using the tip of his finger to check the identifying points for its position, Harken reached up and grabbed for the nose and back of the head, which told him what he needed to know—that the occiput was "midposition and posterior" and it would be most impractical to deliver the "baby" without mutilating its face. He announced a midposition occiput posterior and said that he would use the "Scanzoni maneuver" for delivery.

"The *what?*" demanded one of the examiners.

"The Scanzoni maneuver of double application of forceps rotating the baby and delivering it in the appropriate fashion," said the candidate, who had only read about the procedure.

The examiner looked incredulous and apprehensive. "Well, sir, let's see you demonstrate that remarkable maneuver!"

Harken assumed that the maneuver must have been invented somewhere between the rusty iron and the latest stainless steel forceps so he chose a reasonable-looking chrome-plated instrument along the line. Rotating the doll's head within the manikin, ninety degrees one way, removing, replacing the forceps and rotating the head another ninety degrees, he delivered the doll "uneventfully," occiput forward. He managed to conceal the force he used and to palm a four-by-four-centimeter piece of the manikin's rubber vagina—in a live patient that would have resulted in considerable hemorrhage—and presented the doll in perfect condition.

"Now where on earth," inquired another member of the panel testily, "did you learn to do a thing like that?"

"Gentlemen," said Harken, "that is unfair. I make no pretense to being a midwife. I studied at a good school under a respectable group of obstetricians and what I've done today should not reflect on them."

One of the examiners looked at the others. "That's the young fellow who's going to work with Tudor Edwards and he came from Harvard and that means he would have been trained by Fritz Irving and we all know that Fritz might well have done a damn fool thing like that!"

Harken was given an L.M.S.S.A. (Licentiate in Medicine and Surgery of the Society of Apothecaries) "with distinction," which qualified him for practice in England. Tudor Edwards never let him forget that no L.M.S.S.A. had ever before been— or would ever again become—senior resident officer at the Brompton.

According to one of the society's officers it had been considered "outside of enough" when in June 1945 it was decided to ask an American to deliver the Joseph Strickland Goodall Lecture, the society's triannual high honor offered to the man they considered outstanding. When they learned that Harken was an L.M.S.S.A., and one of their own, they were incredulous and overjoyed. This had never happened before, either.

Among the guests were Lord Horder, the king's physician, Duncan Fitzwilliam, past president of the Royal College of Surgeons, American Surgeon General Hawley, Clement Price Thomas, later to be knighted after removing the king's lung successfully, Russell Brock, and A. Tudor Edwards.

Although he grumbled at the L.M.S.S.A. in 1938, Tudor Edwards had immediately offered Harken his residency at the Brompton. This would carry a badly needed stipend if his resident could get permission to accept it. One condition of the Alexander Bowen Fellowship was that the fellow devote himself exclusively to study and earn no additional income. Harken wrote to the Academy of Medicine in New York and suggested that his unusual opportunity would enhance the advantages of the year. The academy, without sacrificing the principle involved, invited Tudor Edwards to become an honorary member. He accepted and was appointed an ad hoc committee of one to decide the question. Harken was made a resident and assigned a pleasant bedroom in the "new building," constructed in 1896, and a sitting room with a fireplace in the former Fowles Manor House.

His American resident admired Tudor Edwards immensely, but, without it diminishing his respect, he came to the conclusion that his chief, a consummate technician and a bold adventurer in surgery, was neither a solid investigator nor a natural teacher. He began slipping away when he could to watch Tudor Edwards' arch rival, J. E. H. Roberts, who carefully answered all Harken's eager questions.

"When you were with Tudor Edwards," Harken would say, "you became excited about the patient or subject, learned and worked without fatigue. You *saw* the answers—the results, not the method—as if they had come from a computer. To learn from

Roberts was to be taken logically, segmentally, through the rationale of the operation." Harken began to consider how the teaching/learning techniques of these two men could be combined. The question of how knowledge could best be transferred from one mind to another was one that would never cease to preoccupy him.

Tudor Edwards had performed the first elective lobectomy (removal of a lobe of the lung) at the Brompton in 1931 and was popularizing the procedure. The removal of an entire lung, pneumonectomy, when justified, especially for lung cancers, gave the surgeon license to take long chances. After a pneumonectomy Tudor Edwards carefully oversewed the bronchial stump to prevent leakage. If the stump did open, fluid in the chest cavity left by lung removal would dump into the trachea, the other lung's bronchial tree, and drown the patient.

Nothing eased Tudor Edwards' distress when a patient died. So distraught he could not talk, he would turn white and shrink, literally holding himself up on the side of a scrub sink or bed. Sometimes he clutched his chest in agony, which came from what he would not admit were anginal attacks provoked by exhaustion and his emotions of humiliation and despair.

Resident Harken took a bed next to the patient after such operations. He had learned to move in fast with an intercostal tube, draining off fluid as an emergency measure. He also instituted regular transfusions for patients, by no means standard practice then. Bellevue at the time maintained the first blood bank in the world. At the Brompton blood had to be procured from suitable donors in the mornings before surgery. Mortality dropped, and Tudor Edwards grew increasingly benign toward his American trainee, grateful for these improvements and for Harken's evident dedication to patient care.

With her husband working day and night at the hospital, Anne Harken, in "digs" nearby, suffered from loneliness and bad weather. It seemed to both their advantages that she move to Paris, where she could live more cheaply and learn the French language. In the late spring of 1939 Dwight was able to take a weekend off to join her. While he was gone, Tudor Edwards suffered a severe heart attack. Harken rushed back to rejoin the team operating without its chief and to perform some of the major operations.

As war grew imminent, the Brompton was emptied of its civilian patients. It was to be "Clearing Station Number II" for casualties, expected to number ten thousand in the first week of conflict. Harken was appointed "second surgeon" with nothing to do except play chess and listen to the wireless or to a player piano for which there was only one roll of music, "The Carey Dancers." Citizens of neutral countries were urged to depart at once and, refusing a majority in the British medical corps, Dwight Harken left with Anne. That brought to an end what they would both call "one of the greatest experiences of our lives."

Before Harken went to work on his dogs in the Boston laboratory, evidence was already accumulating that heart surgery was not an impossible dream.

5.

Milestones

During the 1920s in the United States, Drs. Duff Allen and Evarts Graham had developed a cardioscope, which made it possible to see something of the heart's mitral valve. So-called because it was shaped like a bishop's miter, the valve opened to permit blood to exit into the left ventricle (pumping chamber) and closed to prevent the blood from leaking back into the atrium (reservoir). Mitral stenosis was a common and crippling heart problem, which afflicted more women than men (the reason for the sex differentiation remains a mystery). When the orifice was too narrow, the normal healthy flow was inhibited. The condition was readily diagnosable and surgeons Elliott Cutler and Claude Beck collaborated with cardiologist Samuel Levine at the Peter Bent Brigham Hospital in Boston to attempt relieving it surgically. Cutler and Beck devised a valvulotome, an instrument designed to cut the obstructing tissue.

Cutler failed to recognize that he could not successfully substitute incompetence—failure of the valve to close tightly after the orifice was enlarged—for stenosis. Very little was known at the time about the individual function of the valve leaflets. Leakage followed the Cutler operations and blood regurgitated into the atrium, increasing the pressure in the lungs. After one miraculous success, the rest of the operations were failures and he called a halt to the series in 1928. (He would later bequeath his valvulotome to D.E.H., who succeeded in relieving mitral stenosis with a different approach to the valve and with due regard for the nature of incompetence resulting from leaflet damage.)

In 1929, in Germany, a new approach to gaining knowledge of blood flow was tried by a youthful fanatic. Dr. Werner Forssmann reached into his own heart with a catheter threaded through his veins. He was too daring and too far ahead of his time. That achievement, presaging angiography and pressure measurements now routinely in use for determining obstructions and flow, would not be recognized for decades.

Dr. Forssmann, twenty-five years old, got the idea from an illustration in a veterinary journal. If the veterinary surgeon could pass a long, slim catheter into the vein of a horse for the purpose of taking blood samples, Forssmann argued with his colleagues, it should be feasible to reach the human heart by this means. He envisioned the possibility of feeding in emergency drugs during an operation instead of injecting them into peripheral veins. Forssmann tried the procedure on a cadaver. It worked. He did not dare risk an attempt on a live fellow human, so he induced another doctor to help him try it on himself. An incision was made in the crook of his elbow, a wide-bore needle inserted, and the oiled rubber tube slipped down the needle along the vein. After sixteen inches of tube had been inserted, the other doctor balked and refused to continue the experiment.

A week later Forssmann dragooned an unwilling nurse to aid him, prepared his own vein, slid the tube along, and placed himself behind a fluoroscope screen while the nurse held a mirror. He felt a tingling pain, then a burning sensation as the tube slid toward the right atrium. He manipulated it to enter the chamber. His heart maintained its steady rhythm. The screen monitored but did not fix the image. Who would believe him? With the catheter in his heart, Forssmann walked out of the room, along a corridor, and up two flights of stairs to an X-ray room where he could take fixed pictures of his heart with the tube in place. A colleague, Dr. Joseph Fischman, recalled the incident in a letter written to Dr. Harken:

It happened on a hot summer afternoon on a Sunday in 1929. I was at that time resident in general surgery in the Berlin City Hospital, Berlin-Neukolln, in which same hospital Forssmann was—I think—a surgical intern. I and a few others of the resident staff were alarmed by the news that Dr. Forssmann had committed suicide. Upon arrival in his room we found Dr. F. lying on his bed silent and pale, staring at the ceiling, his clothes and the bed linen spotted with blood. He refused to give any information. The idea of suicide appeared to be not too remote as Dr. F. was a rather queer, peculiar person, lone and desolate, hardly ever mingling with his co-workers socially. One never knew whether he was thinking or mentally deficient. On closer investigation of the situation one found his condition medically satisfactory. There were a few surgical instruments lying around and also a ureter catheter— possibly still inserted into his anticubital vein (whether left or right, I do not remember). This latter was removed and a dressing applied to the wound. Whether he inserted the catheter in order to quench his scientific thirst or else, I never was able to find out. What I still remember vividly [is] that the catheter was in the vein at a length of at least two and half feet.

That much to the scenery. An interesting addition as an aftermath to the above, that shortly after the episode, Dr. Ferdinand Sauerbruch—whose mental integrity, with all merits granted to his medical ingenuity, also sometimes appeared to be questionable—claimed Dr. F. for his Department at the University Hospital Charite as his co-worker and that Dr. F.'s "silly" acting initiated a splendid career for him.

The "splendid career" did not, in fact, last long. Forssmann's report of the experiment, in which he gave meticulous credit to another German doctor who he discovered had inserted tubes into the thigh veins of patients, caused a brief flurry, but Sauerbruch soon dismissed him as a crank. According to reporter and writer Hugh McLeave in his book *The Risk Takers,* Forssmann then went to Eberswalde, fifty miles north of Berlin, where he established himself as a general practitioner. His practice dwindled and for a time he left medicine, earning his living for a year by felling trees. McLeave records that in 1944 he was working obscurely in a Berlin hospital. Recognition did not come to him until almost thirty years after his self-experiment, in 1956, when Werner Forssmann shared the Nobel Prize in Medicine and Physiology with Drs. Dickinson W. Richards, Jr., and André F. Cournand, who had followed up his work in catheterization of the heart.

Before World War II, in 1938, another Turning Point in heart surgical history was achieved in Boston. This was the treatment of patent ductus arteriosus by surgery. The duct, open in newborn infants, had been described by the Greek physician Galen in the second century A.D. It lay between the aorta, or main artery to the body, and the pulmonary arteries, which carry blood from the heart to the lungs. Normally it closed within three days after birth. When it remained open, or patent, the shunting of blood damaged the lungs and overworked the heart. Failure of the duct to close was responsible for seventeen out of every hundred cases of congenital heart disease. The chances that a child born with this defect would survive to maturity were very poor indeed.

In Boston surgeon John Strieder made one dramatic, courageous attempt to save a thirty-two-year-old woman with the fatal ductus complications of SBE (subacute bacterial endocarditis) but it was unsuccessful. The "first" credit went to surgeon Robert Gross. Favorably located in the large, busy Boston Children's Hospital, Gross was small, indefatigable, ruthless, brilliant, and good-looking, characteristics not unsuited to a pioneer. He studied congenital anomalies in autopsies and worked in well-equipped research laboratories experimenting with techniques for closing patent ducti.

On the 26th of August, 1938, Robert Gross tried his own procedure on a seven-year-old girl. She was scrawny and undersized. Her mother, able to hear the constant buzzing in her chest, brought her to Children's Hospital. Through the stethoscope Gross heard the rough machinery murmur, punctuated by sounds like pistol shots. By X-ray he documented the ballooning of her pulmonary artery. The defect was very likely to cause her demise at any time.

He opened the child's chest, packed away her left lung to

obtain exposure of the mediastinum (the space beneath the breastbone containing the heart, aorta, vena cava, trachea, and other vessels and nerves), and slit the pericardium to expose the pulmonary artery and aorta where they lay side by side. Running above the pulmonary artery, which should no longer have the communication with the adjacent aorta, lay the unclosed duct. It was about a third of an inch wide and a fifth of an inch long. Blood pounded from the high-pressure aorta to the low-pressure lung vessels. He touched the outside of the duct and felt a vibration or thrill over the entire region. Listening with a sterile stethoscope, he heard an almost deafening roar, a sound very much like a large volume of escaping steam.

Gross passed silk ligature around the duct and with it obstructed the ductus for three minutes to see how the heart and lungs would behave. Satisfied, he tightened and tied the ligature permanently, closing off the channel. The lung was expanded and the chest wall closed. Two days later the little girl was sitting up. And the operation was curative, not palliative. By the time she grew up, married, and had her own child, Gross and his Boston team alone had closed fifteen hundred patent ducti with an incredibly low mortality rate.

The earliest case of an operation by which mitral stenosis was corrected in a procedure not too far removed from the dramatic operations performed by Charles Bailey and Harken in 1948 was only very belatedly recognized. The report of it had been buried in a conspiracy of silence. Harken did not hear of it until 1961, by which time he was perhaps the most famous heart surgeon in the world and people were coming from everywhere to Boston for his operations to correct mitral stenosis. He wrote to the surgeon who had achieved this unsung Turning Point to ask why he had failed to follow up that brilliant initial success.

The surgeon was Henry Souttar, later knighted for his other contributions to surgery and medicine. In the early 1920s he was consultant at the London Hospital and already well known for his invention of many devices including the eyeless surgical needle. Working on cadavers and animals, Souttar had concluded that replacing the valves of the heart with artificial ones was out of the question, but that it should be possible to divide a stenosed, constricted, or obstructed mitral valve with a scalpel or his finger. He presented a lecture on this potential mitral valve surgery, but it was skeptically, even indignantly, received. Sir James Mackenzie, the king's physician and the acknowledged authority in England on heart disease, commented testily, "Indeed! The only heart disease I know of is that of the muscle, and *no* operation will correct it."

In 1925 London cardiologist T. B. Layton was at his wit's end over one patient, a dark-haired, bright-eyed endearing little girl named Lily Hine. Lily was a slum child from London's East End, skinny and miserable. She had the classic physical signs of mitral stenosis: a long, rumbling murmur in her chest as the left ventricle, the main pumping chamber, relaxed; a soft blowing sound when it tensed. Her valve disease induced severe breathlessness, a rasping, hacking cough, and her rheumatic fever caused pain throughout her limbs. She had been coming to the hospital for four years, since 1921, and only the use of digitalis, a stimulant derived from foxglove that was already in common use for weak hearts, kept her alive. Dr. Layton was certain in 1925 that she could live no longer than six more months.

"Natural causes"—or an identifiable disease—on death certificates aroused no interest and offered no risk to the doctor. Death in the operating room was subject to scrutiny and possible reprimand by the formidable British coroner, who could break medical reputations. Nevertheless Layton took Lily to Souttar and the two men agreed that his untried operation was the little girl's only chance for survival.

Her parents consented. Lily, trusting her cardiologist and the soft-spoken surgeon, willingly agreed. John Challis, one of the best anesthetists, or "gas men," at the time, risked his own reputation to assist. Anesthesia caused as many deaths as surgery in those days, and ether or chloroform were all he had to use on a child with a very weak heart. "Challis did a very brave thing," Souttar would say.

Souttar made careful sketches for the surgery, devising his method of entering the heart without massive blood loss. Then, on May 6, 1925, Lily Hine was anesthetized by Challis, who slipped the marvelous new tube invented by Ivan Magill into her windpipe. The hollow tube fitted exactly through the throat into the trachea. Through a rubber bag attached to his end of the tube he could deliver the gases of his choice. He could, by squeezing and releasing the bag, effect inflation or deflation of her lungs, preventing collapse and aiding the breathing function. Souttar made a C-shaped incision over the heart area, resected the ribs, and exposed the heart. Lily's pulse accelerated; they had to wait five minutes until her heartbeat steadied and pulse slowed.

With a clamp Souttar isolated the end of the arterial appendage (a tiny "ear" of the reservoir) and made the crucial half-inch incision through which he could thrust his forefinger while stay stitches held the wall of the heart's appendage tight against his finger to hold back the blood. For perhaps two minutes he explored the mitral valve, tension on the circumscribing sutures preventing much blood loss. Lily Hine's blood pressure fell to zero, but there was no change in the cardiac rhythm. As Souttar explored the interior of the heart with his finger, the jet of blood coming back from the left ventricle told him the valve was leaking. The chordae tendineae (heart strings), which tied the valve to the wall of the ventricle, prevented the blood pressure from pushing some of the flood back into the atrium. With each beat of Lily's heart Souttar could feel the valve leaflets partially opening and partially closing. They had not fused as much as he and Layton had thought. He did not have to use a knife to separate the fused leaflets because he thought he could break down the adhesions between them with his finger.

He thought he had succeeded. The worst danger seemed past. Souttar gently withdrew his finger from the auricular appendage. Then the unforeseen and unfortunate happened: the silk that should have closed the incision snapped. Blood spurted. With inspired controlled haste, Souttar pressed the leaking atrium against the heart wall, while an assistant tied off the appendage. This stopped the blood issuing with great force from the incision and the torn appendage. Lily's blood pressure climbed again, and her chest could be closed.

The operation had taken just sixty minutes, rapid by any standard. Souttar felt that he had broken the adhesions that stuck the leaflets together, causing stenosis. The next day Lily Hine told him that she felt "ever so much better!" Souttar concluded that the heart was as amenable to surgical treatment as any other organ.

In 1961 Sir Henry Souttar replied to Dwight Harken's inquiry as to why he had failed to follow up such a dramatic and important success. His answer was succinct:

Dear Dr. Harken,

Thank you so much for your very kind letter. I did not repeat the operation because I could not get another case. Although my patient made an uninterrupted recovery the Physicians declared that it was all nonsense and in fact the operation was unjustifiable. In fact it is of no use to be ahead of one's time!

The tear of the appendage had no real bearing on the case but I thought I ought to mention it as it was a detail to avoid. It is wonderful to think of the immense series you have built up and it is a pleasure to think that my little attempt should have opened the way. Cardiac surgery has reached levels of which we never dreamt, and it is a privilege to have contact with one who has done so much toward it as yourself.

> With very kind regards,
> Sincerely yours,
> Henry Souttar

Before he died, at the age of eighty-six, Sir Henry Souttar gave his own ironic epitaph to British writer Hugh McLeave. "I am," he said, "the only surgeon in the world who has operated on the heart with *no* mortality!"

6.

One First, Two Firsts, and Three Firsts

"Blue babies" lived short, breathless lives. They had a syndrome described by a Marseilles doctor, Etienne Fallot, in 1888, and dubbed "*la maladie bleue*" for the summer-sky color of their complexions. The medical designation would be "tetralogy of Fallot" in honor of the man who discovered that four separate defects in-the heart made up the congenital syndrome. The valve leading from the right ventricle is narrow and thick, which causes the lower chamber to balloon and hyperatrophy (dilate and thicken). The septum (partition dividing the chambers) has a hole in it allowing blood to shunt from the left ventricle back into the right rather than going out to the rest of the body. The aorta is misplaced, overriding both chambers and the septal defect so as to steal blood from the right side of the heart. Venous blood, its oxygen used up and therefore blue, normally goes to the lungs for oxygenation before returning to the left ventricle and aorta to supply the body. When, as in these cases, it partially bypasses the lungs, the blue hue justifies the descriptive term. Babies with tetralogy of Fallot were born to die early.

An operation successfully palliating the syndrome was developed by surgeon Alfred Blalock and cardiologist Helen Taussig in Baltimore. It was an example of cooperation among medical and surgical as well as administrative and technical people. Taussig thought that recycling the blood through the lungs would add extra oxygen. She took her plan and concept to Gross, whose forte was closing ducti, but he was not interested. So she returned to Baltimore and approached Dr. Alfred Blalock.

Dr. Edward A. Park, chairman of the Department of Pediatrics at Johns Hopkins in Baltimore, encouraged surgeon Blalock to experiment. It was Park who suggested that techniques Blalock was developing for an operation on coarctation of the aorta (narrowing or closure of the walls of the vessel) might be used in rescuing cyanotic children, following up Helen Taussig's idea that if some additional blood could be detoured from the aorta to the lungs, it would save the little blue victims.

Park had appointed Helen Taussig to take charge of the Cardiac Clinic at Johns Hopkins in spite of opposition to female physicians. According to her, he "literally forced the staff to refer patients to me." She had observed that some of the children with tetralogy of Fallot had, in addition to the classic quartet of defects, a patent ductus. These fared better than their fellow sufferers unless and until the open duct was tied off by the method Boston's Gross had devised. She concluded that the blood shunted through this additional defect, in cyanotic babies bypassing the right chamber, actually helped to increase the blood supply to the lungs.

For a year Blalock and Taussig, with the help of Vivien Thomas, Blalock's technical assistant, worked on animals. Blalock was ready, on October 29, 1944, to take a dying fifteen-month-old blue baby to the operating room. There he delicately isolated and divided an arterial branch of the aorta and joined it to the pulmonary artery as it led to the lung on that side of the chest. He released the clamps, listened, and felt for the telltale thrill from the heart that would prove that the flow in the pulmonary artery had been boosted with blood from the aorta. The thrill came.

Postoperatively the little girl was watched by six doctors in turn. Her lungs collapsed repeatedly and not until the 25th of January was she well enough to be discharged from the hospital.

She was followed by two more cases. Said Dr. Taussig in a 1965 lecture cited by Robert S. Litwak:

The fact that the first three operations [for tetralogy of Fallot] were successful attests to the brilliancy of Dr. Blalock's skill. It was, however, only at the end of the third operation that we *saw* the value of the operation. It was on an utterly miserable small six-year-old boy who had a red blood cell count of 10 million [twice normal] and was no longer able to walk. When Dr. Blalock first removed the clamps the blood welled up in the child's chest. Dr. Blalock quickly controlled the hemorrhage. . . . Suddenly Dr. Merle Harmel [the anesthesiologist] cried, "He's a lovely color now," and I walked around to the head of the table and saw his lovely normal pink lips! The child woke up in the operating room and asked, "Is the operation over?" When Dr. Blalock said, "Yes," the child said, "May I get up now?" From that moment on he was a happy, active child.

The Blalock-Taussig procedure, not curative but a life-saving corrective operation, was reported in a model fifteen-thousand-word paper with classic illustrations. Their description was so exact that many chest surgeons were able to perform the operation. And the drama of "a cure for blue babies" was a sensation in the popular press.

The next Turning Point was a procedure for removing the constricted zone—or coarctation—of the aorta and rejoining the ends. The first man to succeed was surgeon Clarence Crafoord in Stockholm.

In 1935–36 Crafoord had demonstrated on laboratory dogs that the flow of blood to all organs except the brain could remain suspended for as long as twenty to twenty-five minutes without organ damage if an adequate flow to the brain was secured. He managed this by creating anastomoses (jointures) between the carotid (large arteries on either side of the neck) and jugular vessels on one side of the patient-animal and the corresponding vessels in a dog of the same size lying beside it. This led him to take the risk of placing clamp forceps on the aorta above and below the point of entry in certain human patients on whom he was performing an operation for patent ductus arteriosus. The clamps were left in place during the time it took to divide the duct and suture the aorta. In one patient this was twenty-seven minutes—with the aorta shut off below the point where the subclavian artery arose—and there were no noticeable disturbances then or later in the patient's internal organs.

Crafoord began to consider that it was possible to treat congenital coarctation of the aortic isthmus (the narrow part of the vessel) by surgical means. Coarctation of the aorta was easy enough to diagnose, once physicians thought of looking for it. The upper part of the body had a fierce pulse and high blood pressure, while the lower half had almost no pulse and low blood pressure. If the blocked part could be excised and the ends rejoined—a very delicate and untried procedure—the normal flow to the whole body would be restored.

Physician-in-Chief G. Nylin agreed enthusiastically to collaborate with surgeon Crafoord as soon as they found a patient who justified the experimental operation. In the fall of 1944 two such patients turned up at the same time. One of them, an undersized, pale schoolboy aged twelve, was sent to Nylin. The other, a middle-aged farmer, came to Crafoord. Both were suffering from heart failure and were incapable of exertion. Consent to try the untried was readily obtained from the families and the patients. Crafoord performed the two operations within twelve days of each other. For the anastomosis, he used a stitch he had devised, turning up the ends of the cut artery as a tailor would the bottoms of trousers. Five months later the boy was back in school and the farmer was again vigorously tilling his fields. The Crafoord-Nylin report was received for publication on June 1, 1945.

A little later in Boston Robert Gross and Charles Hufnagel, in their second attempt, successfully took a kink out of an aorta and rejoined the ends. They went on to work out methods of replacing excised portions of the artery by preserved arterial grafts when the ends could not be drawn together.

There was considerable controversy over who deserved the greater credit. Crafoord had visited Gross in Boston and met Hufnagel in the Harvard research laboratory before his operation. He had been shown the Hufnagel-Gross technique for rejoining the free ends of the aorta after removal of the constricted zone, but at the time no one had yet performed the operation on a human being. On the list of Turning Points, Crafoord and Gross in Boston were given equal credit for this one, independently.

VE Day in May 1945, ending the European war with the unconditional surrender of Germany, was followed by VJ Day in September when Japan formally surrendered. Seven million Americans in the armed forces began surging home at the rate of twenty-five thousand a day. Whatever their prewar professions, veterans were apt to find civilians entrenched in them. Surgeons who had taken over on the home front were understandably disinclined to step aside for long-absent heroes.

Even the distinguished Edward Delos Churchill, Harvard Homans Professor, found his place at Massachusetts General Hospital preempted by Richard Sweet. Sweet, a brilliant technician, did very well for his patients, and Churchill found himself practically a nonoperating surgeon, which did not suit him at all. In truth, the two men made a remarkable combination. Churchill, a surgical scholar, had the new ideas and devised the methods to implement them; Sweet, a technical genius, retained the heavy operating schedule. Neither man quite understood, appreciated, or enjoyed the situation.

Harken returned and was mustered out at his current rank of lieutenant colonel. Before he left England he completed the thoracic surgery still required at the 160th, and in addition to lecturing for the Society of Apothecaries, showed to the Royal College of Surgeons his film of the heart operation, his case of foreign bodies, and a dramatic drawing of the heart area with 134 black dots pinpointing all the locations from which he had removed the missiles. Soon after he reentered practice in Boston he was invited to lecture on the spectrum of army surgery, including his series, at the first postwar meeting of the American Association for Thoracic Surgery, sharing the podium with Alfred Blalock and Helen Taussig.

Anne Harken went to the meeting with her husband. She was in their hotel room there when a tall, round-headed, somewhat bellicose Philadelphia surgeon came to visit. His name was Charles Bailey and he was making a reputation as an extraordinarily skillful young surgeon. "Dwight," he said, "I know you're working toward mitral surgery, and I'm going to give you a hell of a run for your money! I'll outpace you." At the time both Harkens forgot the challenge.

In Boston Elliott Cutler talked to Harken about following him as Moseley Professor at Harvard. He declined to be interviewed for that coveted chair, although Robert Williams, outstanding internist at the Boston City Hospital's Thorndike Division, had begun a campaign for his appointment. No one, Harken thought, could remain a really active good general surgeon, a scholar, an administrator, a teacher, an investigator, and at the same time develop the new field of heart surgery. This was perhaps the only time he accepted limitations on the energy and abilities of one man: himself.

Instead he accepted a subordinate role with Dr. John Strieder and an assistant professorship at Tufts Medical School in Boston. Strieder had been asked to establish a thoracic service at the Boston City Hospital. He, Cutler, Sweet, Churchill, and Richard Overholt all served Greater Boston as thoracic consultants. Hitherto none of the hospitals had thought they needed full-time staff thoracic surgeons. The association with Strieder was not altogether happy for either man. Though their personalities were totally incompatible, Harken said he "accepted and appreciated the solid, understated, ethical conduct, leadership, and unique orderly teaching ability of John Strieder."

Harken could never help finding much more than his share of the work in any situation. He discovered that most community hospital staff physicians did not recognize which of their patients could benefit from esophageal, lung, diaphragmatic, and pleural surgery. Soon he was visiting many of the hospitals on Strieder's list that the senior man rarely attended. Educating staff men as he went along, Harken began operating in Cambridge, Winthrop, Malden, Melrose, Wakefield, Waltham, Newton, and Wellesley, which, plus Boston City, represented the northwest quadrant of Greater Boston. He began getting so many cases of his own that he had to almost literally kick in the doors of hospitals to find beds for them.

Once he tried to book a patient with lung cancer into the Massachusetts Memorial Hospital only to find the surgical beds glutted with Reginald Smithwick's patients who were having sympathectomies. This was Smithwick's operation for high blood pressure by removing lumbar sympathetic nerves. His patients almost invariably improved, their blood pressure did drop, and the operation had become socially popular—whole bridge clubs seemed to get sympathectomized. But blood pressure also dropped when other major operations were performed and the patients stayed in bed for comparable periods of time on the same miserable hospital starvation diet. Before the operation became outmoded, Harken articulated principles involving the delivery of health care. Smithwick's flood of operations had the positive effect of improving general care at the hospital because he insisted on better anesthesia, a blood bank, an improved X-ray department. Since sympathectomy was not dangerous, just expensive, Smithwick was never required to defend himself by proving that patients were really better off for having that specific procedure. "When we get excited about a new operation," Harken would reiterate after that, "we *must* compare the results with a medical regimen without the surgical procedure!"

In order to gain access to more beds and more operating days Harken began to use the Seventh Day Adventists Hospital on Sundays and agreed to help out at Chelsea Naval Hospital if they would schedule thoracic operations there at night. Driving like a maniac to cover his territory, he gained vast experience and lost sleep. Nevertheless when General Paul Hawley and a civilian consultant to the Veterans Administration, Bryan Blades, asked him to clean up a surgical situation at the Veterans Hospital, largely for tuberculosis patients, in Rutland, Massachusetts, some fifty miles from Boston, he agreed.

The situation at Rutland highlighted a problem that was threatening to become a national scandal in veterans' hospitals. In a dramatic sweep D.E.H. reformed procedures and brought in new surgeons. When General Rankin, General Hawley's successor as VA chief of surgery, visited Rutland later, he was presented with the human proof of what the change had meant to the veterans. Harken had developed a modification of thoracoplasty (an operation to remove ribs and collapse the lung) that did not leave the chest wall on one side so damaged that the patient could never stand straight again. His postoperative patients presented themselves with military bearing. General Rankin trumpeted this difference.

When streptomycin was released, Harken resorted to his high-level military support system to obtain large, early supplies of it for Rutland. This miracle drug so diminished the scourge of tuberculosis (and obviated most surgery for it) that in due course Rutland and many other TB sanatoriums would be closed or converted to other uses.

As soon as he had returned from the war Harken had resumed his laboratory work with a view to performing mitral surgery. Into his life had walked a "doctor with a hair ribbon," an M.D. with surgical training. Leona Norman, nicknamed "Missy," was a big, beautiful orthodox Jewish woman who was searching for a satisfactory medical niche. She did not need money, and accepted Harken's offer to become his assistant in the laboratory. Together they slipped out at every opportunity, day or night, to the Mallory Institute where they snipped the valves from the institute's array of preserved human hearts. On dogs Harken practiced what he would call "valvuloplasty," devising and revising instruments to make it work.

Previous investigators had studied valvulotomy, simple incision and opening of the stenotic mitral valve. Others had tried to excise valve segments—valvulectomy—to exchange stenosis for insufficiency, as Cutler had. Charles Bailey would call his own procedure by lateral incisions "commissurotomy"—a term that caught on, but Harken would always prefer "valvuloplasty"— making the best possible valve of the whole stenotic complex— because, he said, "it was first, it was better, and it was mine!"

He had learned that damage to the major mitral leaflet, at the base of the aortic valve, would send his dogs into congestive heart failure. That leaflet constituted a vital baffle, shunting blood out through the aorta to the body. To cut or tear it in correcting mitral stenosis could produce devastating mitral incompetence, or regurgitation. This probably accounted for Cutler's failures. Cutler intended to cut a piece from the major mitral leaflet. If he had succeeded every time, he would have lost all his patients instead of all but the first.

On the other hand, a piece could be taken out of the mural leaflet, the opposite and minor one, leaving the baffle effect of the major leaflet unaffected. When the heart contracted (systole), the major leaflet closed to occlude the minor leaflet's defect. The operation lessened the stenosis and permitted forward flow of blood in diastole and leakage did not occur.

Intracardiac surgery for mitral stenosis was practical, Harken was convinced. He was ready to try it clinically. With cardiologist Laurence Ellis and his associates at Boston City Hospital, D.E.H's group began to formulate principles that differed substantially from Cutler's: The heart must not be displaced from the position of optimum function; the stenotic mitral valve should be approached from the atrial side; selective insufficiency could be achieved by wedge-shaped resections of the mural leaflet, or fused commissural bridges could be broken or incised to restore leaflet action—"valvuloplasty." Above all, the integrity of the major leaflet must be preserved.

Meantime, Charles Bailey was very much in the race. Some colleagues at the Hahnemann Medical College and Hospital in Philadelphia deplored what they considered his ruthlessness, but no one denied his technical brilliance as a surgeon. He attempted a mitral valve operation in 1945, but his patient died of hemorrhage. The next year he tried again. He had accepted Cutler's concept that relief of mitral stenosis required excision of a portion of the valve, but this patient developed severe hypotension before Bailey's valvulotome could be positioned, so he inserted his finger into the atrium. The patient ultimately succumbed, but this operation was of importance because it established in Bailey's mind the basis for a sound operation and disabused him of the idea that incompetence must accompany relief of the stenosis. He could not try again at that time because physicians were adamant in refusing to refer patients with mitral stenosis to him.

Bailey was always something of a loner, whereas Harken was convivial even with those who thought him overenthusiastic and even abrasive. But one hospital to which he did not return after initial ventures was Boston's Beth Israel. Harken's explanation of this differs considerably and in great detail from Paul Zoll's, but both admitted that it did not work out. Their collaboration, which had been so successful and exciting at the 160th during the war, was terminated in peacetime.

Cardiologist Paul Zoll, who returned to Beth Israel in 1945, asked Harken to perform a couple of complex thoracic operations at Beth Israel with a view to having him there regularly in the future. He would say, "The people and the nurses and the setup were not exactly the way he wanted and Dwight got the hospital in an uproar. He was just a little bit too vigorous and they couldn't stand his style—stirring people up if they didn't meet his specifications got them all upset. I still feel the hospital missed a real chance to have an innovative new surgeon, and if he was a little too impatient and in a little too much of a hurry, I think that's tolerable and in some ways good. But it never came off there. Too bad. It was a long time before Beth Israel had very active cardiac surgery. Quite a long time."

When Joseph Brodeur came into Boston City Hospital he was coughing up so much blood that it seemed likely he would drown in his own blood any minute. His symptoms indicated mitral stenosis so advanced that the valve was reduced to an inadequate pinhole. Brodeur had nothing to lose by permitting Harken to try out his plan of inserting a valvulotome through the pulmonary vein into the right atrium and thence to the valve to relieve the stenosis.

Outside the operating room door Dr. Crawford Adams monitored the primitive electrocardiographic equipment, which began to spew its reams of paper. Brodeur suffered from tachycardia, an onomatopoetic word for rapid heartbeat. Not even such a superb cardiologist as Laurence Brewster Ellis, said Harken, who often added in a man's middle name when identifying him, or senior cardiologist James Faulkner, had realized that rapid heartbeat was a serious complication uniquely disadvantageous in patients with mitral stenosis.

"It's very simple once you think of it," Harken said. "After all, the dam between the left atrium and the left ventricle means the blood can only get through into the ventricle during diastole

[the rest period]. It is then pumped out to the body during systole. If the heartbeat is rapid, there is less time between beats
and total time for drainage from the atrium into the ventricle. If
there is any back leakage [regurgitation] of an incompetent as well
as stenotic valve, blood is not only given less time for forward
flow in diastole, but with more beats and any regurgitation there
is actual back flow every time the heart contracts. Thus in two
ways tachycardia interferes with forward circulation and builds up
blood in the lungs. With the lungs thus engorged, breathing inevitably becomes difficult and possibly the patient spits up blood.
This simple, obvious clinico-patho-physiologic fact was first articulated in relation to Brodeur, but it took a long time before this
was fully appreciated because *we see what we look for and we
look for what we know!"*

From the bushels of electrocardiographic tracking paper
Harken would follow the heartbeats in their course. Later his
conclusion that tachycardia was the enemy of mitral patients was
so taken for granted that everybody, said Harken, now thought that
he discovered it for himself. Perhaps many of them did. When
progress in a direction is in the air, discovery is a vague and dis-
persed matter. Whether it has come by grapevine or from simulta-
neous observation is often difficult to discern.

In Joseph Brodeur's case, Harken invaded the heart with his
valvulotome and withdrew it "probably sufficiently correcting his
stenosis so that he would have been substantially improved"—and
Brodeur survived. But not for long. His rapid heartbeat caused
more congestion, he coughed up more blood, and died the following day. Had the observation concerning rapid heartbeat preceded this experience rather than derived from it, Joseph
Brodeur might well have lived, "substantially improved." It was
failures like this that haunted Harken.

June 1948 was a remarkable month in the history of heart
surgery. Three men opened the era of closed or "blind" surgery
within the heart, which preceded the era of open-heart surgery.

On the morning of June 10 Charles Bailey operated on a patient with mitral stenosis at the Philadelphia General Hospital.
He was accompanied by cardiologist Thomas Durant, who had

agreed to accept the risk for his patient. The problems he encountered frustrated Bailey. The anesthesia did not work properly, the lungs adhered to all structures, cardiac arrythmias (irregularities in beat) occurred every time the heart was touched. When intravenous quinidine was administered, the heart stopped, as if poisoned, and all desperate efforts by Bailey and the team to restore the beat were futile.

There was an immediate necropsy, or autopsy. Bailey explained to Durant what he had been attempting. It should have been possible for him to split the fused mitral leaflets the way a plastic surgeon separated fused lips in a burn victim. In his article on the history of cardiac surgery, Dr. Robert Litwak recalls their exchange: Durant said, "Charlie, you mean you are trying to open the commissures [tissues binding together opposite but corresponding parts, in these cases deforming the heart valve]?" "That's right," exclaimed Bailey, "and we'll call the procedure commissurotomy!"

That afternoon, before news of his failure could precede him, Bailey took his assistant surgeon to the Episcopal Hospital where a patient and Dr. Robert Glover waited for him. Told the risk, the twenty-four-year-old patient insisted that Bailey go ahead. The operation this time went smoothly. A sharp, buttonhook-shaped tiny knife slid along Bailey's finger and was inserted through the valve orifice. The commissure was cut and Bailey broke up some fine remaining fibrous strands with his finger. The patient was well and active thereafter until she was killed in an automobile accident.

Six days later in Boston, unaware of Bailey's success, Dwight Harken introduced a cardiovalvulotome into the heart of a twenty-seven-year-old man with severe mitral stenosis. The cutting edge was directed at the lateral commissure. The hook engaged and the instrument was closed, eliciting the sensation and sound of a snip, although the segment was not recovered. The maneuver was repeated with the instrument directed at the commissure, and finally a segment of the stenotic tunnel was removed in a third maneuver. Valvuloplasty. The patient made what surgeons call, with profound satisfaction, "an uneventful recovery." Though D.E.H. published his report first, the question of who had been the first would be in dispute for many years. Eventually Bailey got credit, by that six days, but never without that credit extending to Harken for publishing first.

That same month, June 1948, Russell Brock in England performed a closed "pulmonary valvotomy," as he called it, and three months later joined Harken and Bailey in both credit and fact by performing an operation for mitral stenosis. In the annals of medicine the three are listed as triplets, the three great pioneers of modern intracardiac surgery.

The time had come. Souttar's concept and approach were validated after twenty-three years had gone by. The efforts of Cutler, Levine, and Beck in the 1920s had borne fruit. Bailey, Harken, and Brock would suffer, each according to his capacity for personal suffering, from "the pain of the pioneer," as Harken would describe it. Mortality was always high in the early days of a new and complex surgical procedure. An unproven operation was only justified if the patient was very ill, which increased the risk. It took time to smooth out techniques and solve the problems of anesthesia and pre- and postoperative care. There was inevitably devastating criticism of the men who persevered in risky clinical pioneering. "Such criticism," Harken would say bitterly, "is always the tool of men frustrated by their own inability to create."

All three of them—in Boston, Philadelphia, and London— would go on in spite of everything.

7.

Blind Surgery

Drama is defined as characters in action. The blind era of heart surgery is dramatically Shakespearean, and the three great protagonists lived in an unbearably intense atmosphere of triumph and tragedy. Desperately ill patients came to them, in Boston, Philadelphia, and London, pleading for miracles. Surgeons came from all over the world to observe the three pioneers pry into obstructed hearts with their fingers or delicate tiny knives, hoping against hope to save the lives entrusted to their skills.

They were literally groping in the dark, trying to cure what they could not see. Even with the tightly drawn sutures, which kept the point of entry into the heart from bleeding out, the disturbance to that vital organ must be brief. They literally raced against death, and death was often the winner. In 1949 only those three were attempting what had never been done before, and they had to withstand the strain not only of the operations but of the constant and severe criticism of most of the medical profession as well. It took extraordinary courage and resilience and confidence to continue.

In the first 1948 issue of *British Medical Journal* Russell Brock, a cool as well as a courageous man, wrote of the day after his fourth death in succession. "Despair stalked before us and everyone's morale was low. I said to my team that we could only do one of two things—give up or go on—and that it was impossible to give up as we were certainly in the right. The only thing, therefore, was to go on."

Dwight Harken, the most mercurial of the three, whose emotions were always involved with his patients, suffered extremes of elation and despair. He would later describe his worst crisis with recall so total that he relived the day. He had already lost five patients out of nine. After the sixth death, one at the Naval Hospital, he went home to give up. Nothing, he said to Anne, was worth the pain. Nothing could induce him to continue doing cardiac surgery. Then he went upstairs and went to bed as if despair were a disease.

Laurence Ellis, the Boston cardiologist and president of the New England Cardiovascular Society, who had sent his otherwise hopeless patients to Harken, came over, went up, and sat by his bedside. Both men would remember their conversation exactly.

Ellis was soft-spoken to the point of sounding inarticulate, as if he were muttering to himself. "Dwight," he said, "I understand you are going to quit heart surgery."

Harken spoke painfully. "I don't have to earn my living this way! I can't stand it! I can't live this awful way."

"Well," said Ellis, "seems to me rather a criminal thing for you to waste those people's lives."

This shocked Harken. "What do you mean, waste their lives?"

"You must have learned something."

"Of course I did! Christ almighty," said Harken.

"Don't you think you could do better in the future?" Ellis asked.

"What future? No respectable physician would send me a patient now, after a record like that!"

"I'm considered a respectable physician," replied Ellis. "Your patients were dying, so you haven't lost any lives. They were already lost. You've spared them some terminal suffering perhaps, and you have also given four of those ten a better chance to live. I think you might well do a lot better in the future."

Harken went back and did enough better so that in 1949 when he and Anne met Dr. John Gibbon, by this time professor of surgery at Jefferson Medical School, and his wife, Maly, on the boardwalk at Atlantic City during a medical convention, their conversation was quite different in tone. Gibbon told Harken that he should not "fiddle around" with mitral stenosis by closed techniques. Within a year, Gibbon said, he would have a machine to bypass the heart.

"Jack," Harken replied, "I wouldn't dream of waiting around and stopping my work. By the time you fellows make heart-lung machines safe enough for us to use routinely, I shall have taken care of over a thousand people!"

Later Charles Bailey came up from Philadelphia to plead with Harken. They should, he thought, both go all out to persuade better-risk patients, those who were not already sick unto death, to have the surgery. The figures would look better. High mortality rates were no way to gain acceptance for a new operation.

"I will only take people who have nothing to lose but a little longer life of misery and discomfort," Harken answered. "Charlie, if the operation is as good as we think it is, we don't have to sacrifice anyone who can wait a little longer! We'll learn to avoid errors in anesthesia, errors in getting into and out of the atrial appendage, errors in knocking off blood clots. If we lose anybody in a good-risk category, anyone who could wait for a better operation when we are better and who are still getting some happiness out of life, that's a *bad thing*. That's unacceptable to me!"

Bailey resented his rival's high moral tone. They were, he would say, "two tigers on the same hill and if Dwight was redheaded, I had a red-headed mother! I come from the City of Brotherly Love, but when Dwight attacked me, I attacked right back. I didn't think he had been anointed from on high to set limitations on what I should do or the patients I should try to help!"

Harken continued, during these experimental days, to accept only high-risk patients who were much more likely to die of invasion than those whose hearts were not already severely damaged. One of these was a remarkably good-looking young woman named Florence Mahoney. She was hopelessly limited by her mitral stenosis and had been cared for by a devoted husband. Harken booked her into the Chelsea Naval Hospital, where he was also booking Theresa Trelligan.

The consultant on anesthesia at the Chelsea Naval was a man who doubted the value of Harken's operations, Leo Hand. He was in the operating room when Harken went into Florence Mahoney's heart.

Harken was using at the time reverse scissors on a curved valvulotome, something like Bailey's instrument, he said, "but infinitely better." He had almost completed the delicate procedure when he tore her auricle. Blood poured out. He grasped the torn margins of the appendage and occluded them with his fingers. The bleeding stopped, but there seemed no way of getting around Harken's staying fingers to control the hemorrhage and free his hand. A senior assisting surgeon made a big loop of silk thread around Harken's wrist, lowered it to the fingers and slid it down toward the heart. It slipped off. Harken grasped the margins again and again until they finally successfully placed the loop and tied it. By that time Florence Mahoney's heart had stopped. Harken took the heart in his hand and pumped for it (manual systole). This was too much for Leo Hand. He left the operating room swearing that there would be no more heart operations in his bailiwick.

When her heart did finally take over for itself, Florence Mahoney had lost so much blood and had had low blood pressure for so long that it was some days before her brain fully regained normal function, even after she recovered and was much improved. Successful resuscitation by manual systole was rare in those days. The media heard about Florence Mahoney and could not wait to tell the story, with pictures of the beautiful girl. Her surgeon explained to her what the radio and newspaper commotion was about, how he had held her heart and pumped it for her until it beat for itself. It was now behaving quite normally.

"Well," she said, looking stunned, "thank you very much!"

Hand protested such experimentation to the commanding officers at the Chelsea Naval Hospital. A halt was called to cardiac surgery on the premises. Harken had to move Theresa Trelligan over to the Boston City Hospital. Her mitral valvuloplasty pro-

ceeded uneventfully and she would become, later on, an active
worker for Mended Hearts, an association for those who have undergone cardiac surgery.

Presenting patients was never an ordeal for Harken. He
approached this part of the medical routine with confidence and
always had ready and logical answers for questions from critical
peers. Two months after her surgery at Chelsea Naval Hospital he
presented the beautiful Mrs. Mahoney at Boston City Hospital.
His colleagues and a number of distinguished visitors were there.
Harken wanted to stress accurate assessment of results by such
objective means as catheterization. He told the large audience
that it would be possible by that technique to see how much she
had improved.

"I know how much I have improved," Florence Mahoney informed the assemblage. "Before I could not walk at all, let alone
climb stairs. Day before yesterday I climbed the Flume in the
Appalachians."

When handsome, able Francis Moore was made chief of
surgery at the Peter Bent Brigham Hospital, famous for the early
and brilliant neurosurgery performed there by Dr. Harvey Cushing, one of his first appointments was Dwight E. Harken as chief
thoracic surgeon. It was an ideal base for Harken. His letter to his
father in February 1950 gives a contemporary rather than retro-
spective picture of what was happening.

> After very trying times last summer when we had three deaths
> on the table and one shortly after surgery, we went into the dol-
> drums and even despaired of the future of true valvuloplasty. Fol-
> lowing the deaths on the table, before leaving the room, I placed
> my finger on the heart and found to my great surprise that I could
> fracture the site of the previous commissure and convert this fixed
> stenotic tunnel into leaflets that became a true valve again. Of
> course this was what I had been trying to do with powerful cutting
> instruments and it is what my only competitor, Bailey of Philadel-
> phia, has been trying to do with a knife on his finger. He has also
> tried to convince me that I could orient myself much more quickly
> with the finger, and I have tried to convince him that he couldn't
> cut anything with the tiny little knife he was using.

This was a very interesting phenomenon that with my finger I could fracture the fused commissure site with a blunt finger dissection better than I could open it with Bailey's knife or my own valvulotome.

On the strength of this serendipitous experience I sent letters out to the pathology departments of the major hospitals in Boston and asked that I be called in the event of any patient's dying from mitral stenosis. A number of pathologists cooperated and soon I had had experience with six more patients with mitral stenosis and had been able to work out a satisfactory "finger fracture valvuloplasty." The next step was to make satisfactory clamps, variations of those you have seen for holding the renal pedicle. We devised the clamps (shaped to conform to various atrial appendages and with shanks so softened that trauma to the heart was unlikely). This done, we were ready to proceed with human trial.

I have now performed the operation eight times, and only one of these patients has died. With the death of the patient, I changed my approach to a lateral one and four consecutive patients are doing well.

The improvement shown by these patients following *finger fracture valvuloplasty* is positively startling. Bedridden patients with pulmonary edema and right-sided heart failure, on Salyrgan twice a week and ammonium chloride [the most powerful depleting—diuretic—agent at the time] daily, are converted into patients who are able to be up and about, indulging in the most strenuous activities.

We are now accepting patients on a freer basis, and of course the number needing such surgery is tremendous. I am doing two or three next week.

A follow-up note on Florence Mahoney, whom I talked about on my Midwestern speaking trip a year ago, who had been bedridden for two years. She came into the office on the anniversary of her valvuloplasty and brought Jill [Harken's daughter] the loveliest sweater she had knitted on a trip through the mountains. She was an important patient because she represents the first patient in the surgery of mitral stenosis to have demonstrated objective improvement by cardiac output studies and pulmonary pressures.

Friday morning at the Brigham Hospital rounds for the Harvard third- and fourth-year students and outside visitors, the finger fracture valvuloplasty was the subject of discussion. We presented a number of our patients, and described the background for our surgery and our optimism for the future. Fran Moore, now Moseley Professor of Surgery and successor to Cushing and Cutler, closed the discussion by saying "This is a great day for the Brigham. I am sorry my predecessors, whose pictures are on the wall, could not be here." He then broke off because he became emotional and left the room. I regard this as the nicest compliment I have ever had. It was approached only by the clapping of the Royal College of Surgeons when I announced that the surgical removal of foreign bodies in or around the hearts and great vessels had been accomplished in 134 patients with no deaths. The Brigham audience similarly broke into applause when Fran stopped speaking, and I felt definitely that the dark days were over.

Such letters to his father were sent regularly by Dwight for many years. Their relationship was ambivalent and cut deep both ways. Dr. C. R. Harken not only never forgave his older son for refusing to return to Osceola, but would never accord him the final parental accolade for his work. When Dwight talked about his father, respect vied with other complex emotions, invariably upsetting him. Leona Norman would describe one visit to Boston made by Dr. C R. Harken during these exciting and tension-ridden days.

"Dr. Harken, Sr., scrubbed and joined us on the floor rather than in the gallery. What a handsome man he was! Very smooth, very impressive, very charming. Well, Dwight performed with incredible brilliance and things were very tense and all of us were very much occupied. The surgery was successful, the patient survived, and we all relaxed and looked around for Dr. Harken . . . but he was gone. He had left and gone to the doctors' room, for a nap. Dwight looked absolutely stricken, although he never said anything except, very softly, 'He slept through it!' I felt that it was so cruel and then I felt I understood a great deal about Dwight. That monumental effort he was putting out, hypertensive, aggressive, wild, erratic, was designed to succeed in his father's eyes. He was looking for that word of approval which he was *never* going to get!"

Harken's memory of the incident was less simplistic and even touched with humor. "I remember it vividly," he said. "When Dad came to visit me, I took him to Boston City to see me

wrap an aneurysm of the upper portion of the aorta. It was before
we could remove and reconstitute continuity with grafts; so we
wrapped aneurysms, hoping that the cellophane would produce a
scar tissue protective cocoon about the potential blowout area.
This aneurysm was stuck to all surrounding structures. Dad
seemed bored with the tedious dissection and went to the
surgeons' room for a nap. As I dissected the treacherously thin sac
under great pressure of blood, I tore a small hole in it. The bleeding was alarming and controlled only with great difficulty. I
thought Dad would be excited by such a nerve-shattering experience so I sent out for him, repeatedly, but my intern messengers
did not have the courage to wake him up. He was pretty formidable. At last the operation was successfully concluded and I
awakened him myself. I said, 'Dad, I tore a hole in that aneurysm.' 'I assumed you would,' he said, 'the way you were going
at it.' I said, 'Do you mean to tell me you thought your son would
be in that unbelievable crisis and you were not interested enough
to watch?' 'No,' he replied, 'I'd not be interested. I don't do that
sort of surgery and I'm not sure you should!' "

There is no record of the reply Dr. C. R. Harken may have
made when he received a letter from Robert Cutler, president of
the Peter Bent Brigham Hospital Board of Trustees. Cutler wrote:

> You probably know that it was my older brother, Dr. Elliott
> Cutler, who first attempted in 1923 the operation which Dwight has
> now so marvelously brought to perfection. It must fill you with great
> pride to have such an accomplished son who is doing so much for
> medical progress.

There was no ambivalence in the relationship between the
Philadelphia and Boston pioneers with their rival firsts. When
Charles Bailey and Dwight Harken spoke from the same plat-
forms, sober debates turned into donnybrooks. Often they were
scheduled together to provide the "fun." They argued over everything—patient selection, surgical approaches, instruments, and
morals and ethics. They were even embrangled over the structure
of the mitral valve. The living, working valve was very different
from the one in cadavers, which looked like a collapsed little para-
chute. Harken claimed that the mitral valve had four leaflets.

"I said it had two," Bailey would admit. "I had the authority of the great anatomists on that and I said Dwight must have figured from a bull's heart, which was different. That was understandable, I said, there was a lot of bull in Boston. Actually we were both wrong. The mitral valve is a skirtlike structure, but the way it closes in the normal state does give the impression of tetracuspid structure. He was more right than I was."

Robert Litwak, a member of the Founders Group for his own future innovations, trained under both men.

"There was no question in Bailey's mind," he would say, "that Harken was completely off base, but when I got to Boston from Philadelphia, Dwight was developing a beautiful series and you could see the evolution of his own surgical team. Bailey was much more of a loner. Both were superb surgeons and gentlemen, but me, I became a 'Harken student' and that's the way it was. I think there are many of us around the world who have been profoundly influenced by his personality, his superior intellect, his innovativeness. At conferences he always had new ideas and I don't think he ever got up in the morning without wondering why the sun rose in the east, he was so full of questions. And he was just plain fearless. If you are fearless because you don't feel, that's simply being insensitive. Dwight was sensitive."

Some of his trainees shivered when they recalled D.E.H. and his uncompromising demands for perfection, and more than one broke down and left. One of those who was grateful because he stuck it out said, "Dwight could be terribly cruel to us and to everybody except patients. But those of us who got close were aware that under all the trappings this warm, soft, quivering, loving, giving human being was so vulnerable he had to encase and protect it."

None denied his dramatic effectiveness as a teacher. "The obligation of a creative surgeon is to innovate, then perfect, simplify, and finally standardize any new technique so that it can be conducted safely as it is *handed on*," Harken would preach.

"Handing on" had to go on well before the perfection and standardization. In those days of early mitral valve surgery every procedure was a learning one for the surgeon as well as for the team, trainees, and visitors. Diagnostic techniques, though improving, were still relatively crude, and "incredible surprises" were apt to be uncovered when the surgeons got into a chest. They had to work their way through unforeseen adhesions, thromboses, calcified valves. Control of blood pressure was poorly understood and low blood pressure could spell death. One junior of his heard Harken remark as he approached the table, "Well, men, let's get into the chest before the blood pressure finds out we're there!"

Before the defibrillator—for the administration of shocks when a heart's ventricle fibrillated (that terrifying form of fatal quivering)—was improved, everyone in the operating theatre was endangered. The original alternating-current models were ungrounded, exposed, and unprotected. To add to the nervousness, the two electrodes intended to defibrillate the heart could easily ignite explosive gases in the operating room, although it never happened.

Teaching valvuloplasty was for D.E.H. a constant obligation and challenge. No one, including the surgeon, could see what was happening at the crucial valve level. Harken would assess the situation, then, to make the blind manipulation more comprehensible, would hold up his hand, cupped, showing how it should be done. He would then permit visiting surgeons or residents to feel the valve themselves before he corrected the stenosis. While he was working on the valve, he would do a shadow procedure with his other hand to show what his operating finger was doing. The assistants would then in turn check what he had accomplished. This best conceivable way of teaching his technique was employed whenever, and only, if it posed no risk to the patient.

Writing about the operation for the October 1951 issue of *The Annals of Surgery*, Harken explained that finger fracture had proved to be the best procedure, with an assortment of tiny knives or valvulotomes for backup use as needed:

> The great temptation is to force the fracture rather than to slip the knife along the finger or to withdraw the finger and then to reinsert it with the appropriate valvulotome. If a second or third maneuver, advancing the exploring fracture finger 2 or 3 centimeters

through the valve, fails, *the surgeon must not use force*, but rather gently retreat in order to resort to incisional valvuloplasty.

The 1951 annual report of the Peter Bent Brigham Hospital contained a paragraph by Francis Moore:

> Visitors from all over the world appear in a steady stream to learn the techniques in this new field of surgery. The rapidity with which such a field ceases to be "new" and becomes "accepted" is frightening. . . . Mitral stenosis operations are being done in so many hospitals in the country that the only cases now referred from elsewhere are the "tough ones" that the inexperienced man does not wish to undertake.

One example of the spread of the new techniques came from John Hayward, a distinguished surgeon in Melbourne, Australia.

> Dear Dwight [he wrote in June 1952],
> You will be interested to hear that I did my first mitral last Friday week. She had an auricular appendage too small for my finger, which split the atrial wall. You can imagine what happened when the finger was withdrawn. We got out of it by the skin of our teeth and many pints of blood, and she can now walk upstairs without difficulty. As she could only walk fifty yards on the flat before the operation, she is very pleased with herself, so your very able instruction has borne fruit already. I have a second one to do tomorrow, another next week and several others lined up for the future.
> I have never spent a happier or more instructive week than the one with you and your family. Also please thank Dr. Ellis for the catheters he gave us.

The operation did not "cure" mitral stenosis; that claim was not made. But the clinical improvement following the operation was generally spectacular, especially after Harken felt justified in taking less high-risk patients, those in whom terminal changes had not taken place.

Patients attested to this spectacular improvement, sometimes in humorous fashion. One of Harken's favorites was a former football player from South Boston, who had been known for his cheerful barroom bellicosity. The Irishman had grown weaker and weaker from his progressing mitral stenosis until his companions began calling him "sissy" to his face. Five weeks after Harken restored his mitral valve function, he rose from convalescence at home, went to his local bar, carefully beat up his old friends, broke all the bottles in the bar, and left in triumph. No one had the heart to sue him.

Harken asked the Irishman to return to the hospital for postoperative catheterization, which would confirm his improvement. Under the drapes, the patient heard the indiscreet operators and technicians talking among themselves. "Well," said one of them, "I can't see any change in these measurements since his surgery."

"Man," said the satisfied patient, "I don't know what the hell you're measuring, but I'm sure as hell a lot better! What counts with me is better."

Another patient, this one from Texas, was also asked to submit to right-sided catheter study while he was still in the hospital. When the orderlies went to get him, he was not there, although his crutches, wheelchair, and clothes were. It turned out that the large Texas roughneck had a mind of his own and had simply put on a bathrobe over his hospital "johnnie," walked to the nearest hospital exit, hailed a taxi, and taken a plane home to Austin. Harken saw his former patient when he was lecturing in Texas a year later. "That was a terrible thing you did to me!" Harken said. "Okay, Doc, but you were going to measure me to see if I was better and I already knew that. I tried the stairs and they was fine. I didn't need no catheter to tell me what I already knowed."

Among the criticisms Harken endured from colleagues, even as his mitral operations became more and more successful, was that he explained too much to patients. Telling the "truth" to patients was not a popular concept among many doctors. Harken believed in the patient's right to know, and some cardiologists felt that his careful explanations were often "frightening."

Another severe criticism was that he was getting too much publicity. The attitude of the medical profession toward media exposure was that it was self-seeking and unethical. This would change, even in Boston, as hospitals began to open public relations departments. At the time, attention by an eager press embarrassed Harken, particularly when it brought pitiful letters from many people whose conditions, the result of other types of heart disease, could not be improved by anything a surgeon could then do.

Nevertheless the press sniffed out dramatic cases and the patients were seldom loath to talk. One such was Helen Keith. Because it was thought she could not survive general anesthetic, she was operated on under epidural (local). When her heart went into ventricular fibrillation, Harken maintained its action with his hands for twelve minutes. This was a record at the time. Within half an hour after that prolonged cardiac arrest, Mrs. Keith had been able to answer questions and move her arms and legs. Discovering her, the reporters praised her extraordinary courage and her surgeon's daring.

One vivid report from a patient was published in the *American Weekly*, the Hearst newspaper Sunday supplement distributed all over the United States. In it, Cameron Dewar, who had been a regular dance critic for a Boston newspaper, carefully traced his own cardiac history. He had grown progressively more handicapped over the years, and had been variously diagnosed as having everything from pleurisy to stomach ulcers. After he moved to California two psychiatrists had pronounced him a "cardiac neurotic." When he reached the point where to see a dancer dance made him cringe and the effort of eating a bowl of soup left him breathless, he went to see cardiologist Laurence Ellis in Boston.

Ellis, Dewar reported, tested him with "fearsome gadgets" and ignored his protests. If Dewar could not withstand the tests, Ellis said, he would never get through an operation such as Ellis thought he needed. The operation was only a "slim hope" anyway, and Dewar nearly slunk back home to let nature take its inevitable course. Then he read of a Harken patient who had had the same operation and was back playing professional basketball.

The operation was explained to him by a "vigorous man in his early forties, Dr. Dwight E. Harken," who told him that 10 percent of all heart disease was caused by mitral stenosis, and that more than half a million Americans suffered from it.

Even in his postoperative pain Dewar's overriding thought was that he was breathing normally: "Air never tasted so good!" Before he left Boston, Harken showed him a motion picture of his own operation.

As the picture flashed on the screen [wrote Dewar] there I was in glorious Technicolor, lying on my right side with my left arm strapped over my head. For a moment I thought I could never take this and when I saw the doctor's scalpel advance on my own flesh I was sure of it.

I writhed as the knife cut into my chest wall, from the breastbone in a sweeping downward stroke and over to a point under the left arm. Muscles and tissues were being divided and intercostal nerves blocked. Cartilage and ribs were spread [with the recently developed Harken rib spreader] and the pericardium—the sac that surrounds the heart—lay exposed.

As the sac was cut open the surgeon told me to watch closely, for here was "the big scene." And there was my heart on the screen, pulsating to the rhythm of my own.

At the top of the heart was an appendage that looked like a little ear. The amputation of this "ear" is a vital job, for should it be filled with clot, Dr. Harken pointed out, results can be disastrous. I saw him grasp it lightly with a clamp, while another surgeon drew stitches around it like a purse string. The "ear" was then cut off and saved for observation. [Actually, Harken would say in comment, the opened ear was allowed to open and out popped a clot that could have caused a stroke.]

The four surgeons necessary to effect this operation were now working at an increased tempo, for the sooner the heart is sewn up the better. While one held the clamps and another the purse strings, Dr. Harken slowly inserted the tip of his right index finger into the opening. Slow, gentle motions, he said, were imperative if the deadly clots were to be left undisturbed and if the heart wall was not to be torn.

The miracle was already happening. I could see my putty-like skin take on color as the first real surge of blood in years rushed through my heart.

The doctor's finger was now going deeper and he was, he said, determining the position of the funnel of the valve. His finger came out and he explained that every three or four seconds this was necessary, to allow the blood to return to the valve. Finally he withdrew his finger and the surgeon pulled the purse strings tight. The worst, said Dr. Harken, was over.

On the screen I saw blood flowing freely, but Dr. Harken assured me that it was all to the good since the bleeding would permit blood containing clots to get out.

Through all this split-second timing was vital. The four surgeons were like a backfield team. Dr. Harken drew my attention to the anesthetist. Here, he said, more than in any other operation, was the final key. It was the development of a technique of anesthesia for chest work that brought surgery of the heart within range.

My life was now in the hands of this skilled technician as he hung on every movement of the busy surgeons. The wound was swathed, the stitches set in place, the flesh smoothed and bandaged and the job was done.

The curtain closed on the screen and I staggered from the room. "Surely," Dr. Harken said, "this proves that the sanctity of the heart can be violated without dire results." I heartily agreed, for here I was, living proof. And my heart beat only slightly faster than normal.

It was 1953 before John Gibbon, who had hoped to have one in 1949, as he told Harken, successfully used his heart-lung machine, and it was nearly the end of the decade before Drs. Kirklin, Lillehei, and Dewall, among others, improved it acceptably. Much of the best and most complicated surgery had to wait for open-heart techniques, but in many cases of mitral stenosis, those without severe valve stone formation or rigid scarring, the closed-heart finger fracture would remain the safest and best means of treatment. Unfortunately a new generation of open-heart surgeons would have far too little experience with closed techniques to take advantage of its superiority.

Meantime Harken was one of the busiest as well as the most famous of cardiac surgeons and, with Laurence Ellis, was establishing guidelines and collecting data for the proper selection of patients. Ellis had located an ideal control group in Denmark, since no cardiac surgery was done there. Copenhagen's Dr. Olleson offered medical care roughly equivalent to that in the United States and classified his patients in roughly the same way. Group I patients were those with benign mitral stenosis. Group IIs were

handicapped to some extent but stable. Group IIIs were struggling along on medical treatment with progressive symptoms and
a poor prognosis for the future. Group IVs were prone to chronic
failure, and often had irreversible damage to the heart muscle,
the liver, or the lungs.

In their report for the October 1951 issue of *The Annals of
Surgery* Harken, Ellis, and cardiologist Lewis Dexter dismissed
consideration of surgery for Group I patients until appearance of
symptoms shifted them into Group II. For those in Group II,
surgery was "easy and good," but the proof was not yet in that
they should have it, unless the nonprogressive symptoms were
unacceptable to the patient. There were only about a dozen such
cases in the first one thousand accepted for surgery. Group III patients were the best candidates. They were salvageable and it
seemed tragic to Harken and Ellis that they should wait, manag-
ing to survive on medical treatment, while the risks of their
having an operation multiplied as much as thirtyfold. Group III
patients did not have terminal changes, and their mortality rate
from surgery was down to 0.6 percent. Meantime their symptoms
were progressively limiting. "Often their life expectancy under
medical therapy is *hazardous*." Unless severe or irreversible secondary damage occurred, their clinical improvement after the
operation was "dramatic." For Group IV patients, Ellis, Dexter,
and Harken recommended further scrutiny to establish which of
them might be benefited by the operation, even though the risk
of immediate mortality was high.

Within ten years the control group in Denmark was cited as
proof of the accuracy of those judgments. All of Olleson's Group
IV patients were dead, most having died within two or three
years, compared with half of those operated on in Boston.
Seventy-eight percent of Harken's surgical Group III patients
were living a decade after surgery, as compared with only 48 percent of Dr. Olleson's medically treated patients. And the quality
of life for that 78 percent was incomparably better.

D.E.H. and his colleagues had been right to stress the
"awareness of our medical colleagues of a useful surgical technique in the Group III phase, before the terminal Group IV
period. The responsibility of the medical man has nowhere been

more clearly defined," they concluded, "nor the obligation of the surgeon more richly rewarding."

This one operation was indeed the important precursor of all that came later. "That was a brilliant generation," Francis Moore, chief of surgery at the Peter Bent Brigham Hospital, would say of those men and those who joined them. "Lots of people were part of it, like Jack Gibbon, Walt Lillehei, people abroad. There were other stars in the firmament, like Brock. But Dwight was the most inventive, imaginative, and creative. He was a great *practitioner* of surgery.

"At the Brigham, the house staff just loved him and his patients loved him. The medical service ran around trying to figure out what was wrong with his patients, and he would never take credit for diagnosis. He was very generous in consultations and I don't think I've ever seen a person who could grasp several points of view and immediately assemble them into a meaningful concept the way Dwight could. The other great figures in surgery, the great pioneers like Halsted, Cutler, and Cushing, never acquired big practices the way Dwight did. My God, he brought thousands of patients in here! I've often thought that was one of his problems, this huge number of patients. Cushing, for example, had a tremendous magnetism for patients, too, but they never bothered him as much as they did Dwight. Dwight had a big emotional stake in each one."

"It was my first day," Dr. George Cahill, who later became a renowned authority on diabetes research and director of the Hughes Medical Center in Boston, would remember. "I had just come up from Columbia Medical School and didn't know anyone. The ward I was assigned was for patients of Lew Dexter's and Sam Levine's, who were my heroes as cardiologists. I looked up at one moment and saw this entourage coming at about eighty-five miles an hour down the corridor with this big redhead in the lead. There were three or four house officers and four or five visiting foreigners in the group and they plowed into my ward and the redhead said, 'Which one is Mrs. Whosis?' I told him, 'Third bed on the right,' and with that, the whole crowd went there and the big guy said, 'Hey, young man, lend me your stethoscope.' So I gave him the only badge of office a medical intern has and he listened to about two and a half heartbeats and said, 'Yes, we'll operate tomorrow.' " (Harken would indignantly deny that he had ever said he would operate after listening to "two and a half heartbeats," but forgave Cahill his humorous exaggeration.) "Then he stuck my stethoscope in his pocket and off they went. There I was, sort of castrated without a stethoscope, so I chased them along the corridors and stopped a nurse to ask her who the redhead was. *The* Dr. Harken no less! I didn't dare interrupt him so I lurked about while he got dressed and they all went into the OR. One of the surgical staff told me which one was Dr. Harken's locker and I went in to look for my stethoscope when Dr. Harken reappeared. Apparently he had forgotten something. 'Hey, there,' he said, 'what are you doing in my locker?' I said, 'Trying to get my stethoscope, sir.' With that he opened it up and about a dozen of them fell out and he said, 'Here! Take 'em all!' "

Cahill grew to love both the chief cardiologist, Sam Levine, and the chief surgeon, Dwight Harken. The relationship between the two men, he said, was wonderful. Levine, so much honored as a pioneer in cardiology, was "a lovely, lovely man, very conservative," who had grown up as a Boston newsboy and worked his way through Boston Latin School and Harvard. "He gave the impression of being a kind of Talmudic scholar, exquisitely sensitive, and there, on the other hand, was Dwight Harken, a dynamo from the Midwest, like he was walking down Main Street, playing a trombone and a drum at the same time!"

One day Cahill saw the widow of a patient who had died a few days after his operation sitting with Levine and Harken after the man's death. They were all three crying, he said.

"I never knew whether or not Dwight actually had coronaries then," Lewis Dexter, his associate at the Peter Bent Brigham, said. "Just thinking about him makes me tired. He never seemed to get that substernum distress he complained about except on special occasions. When he was losing an argument, for instance, he would clutch his chest, but not when he was running up stairs, expending enough energy to climb Mount Everest. Doctors are horrible hypochondriacs. Dwight's heart was probably superb."

It had to be rugged to sustain his typical schedule in the 1950s and 1960s and into the 1970s. He never relinquished thoracic surgery to concentrate on cardiac, and one typical week, selected at random from his records in the 1950s, included: eleven mitral valve operations at the Peter Bent Brigham; twenty-six patient office appointments; bronchoscopies at the Waltham, Melrose, and Mount Auburn hospitals; an exploratory thoracotomy and a lobectomy at the Brigham; a thoracotomy at Milton; a de-epicardialization at the Mount Auburn. These, plus a midweek trip to New York City as a consultant and for the New York Heart Association dinner; a lecture in New York on the surgery for acquired valvular heart disease; a lecture in Boston to third-year medical students on pulmonary tuberculosis; a talk at the Quincy Medical Club; consultations at the Rhode Island Hospital in Providence; five admissions at Mount Auburn, Waltham, Melrose, and Boston City; grand rounds and a presentation at the Peter Bent Brigham.

The mitral valve operations were the most important. Medical treatment would in the future improve and would reduce the late manifestations of this disease due to childhood rheumatic fever, but among the generation on whom the pioneers and their colleagues all over the world were operating, many lives were saved or prolonged. Harken certainly had the most to do with spreading the blind surgical techniques that helped stenosis.

"If our conservative approach today had existed at that time," Dr. George Cahill remarked in 1975, "we clearly would now be a decade behind at least. Dwight Harken alone moved heart surgery up a decade, and a person with less flamboyance, less ego, less drive, less confidence—and less freedom—couldn't have done it."

Communication by medical literature was even slower than it is now, but a grapevine existed. Visitors to Boston, Philadelphia, and London went on to or went back to other countries. Soon the leaders in all the best centers knew in precise detail what the others were doing from the accounts of these visitors. If the visitors were suspected of being incorrect in their reports, the long-distance telephone was much used. A great deal of experimentation was going on in those days of freedom from government regulations. There is little evidence that men with the courage it took to perform pioneer surgery were irresponsible. Only a very few were ever accused of taking unjustifiable risks.

Many surgeons had been working on the problem of aortic stenosis. Laurence Ellis, in his meticulous way, traced one hundred patients backward from the autopsies at the Mallory Institute, through hospital, clinic, and to their homes. He gained a clear idea of just how significant the classical triad of symptoms— angina, syncope, congestive heart failure—was. He evaluated the relative importance of the irregular heartbeats. All symptoms could be ominous, but failure, when irreversible with medical treatment, was critical. Sam Levine with Charles Sackett further studied the natural history of aortic valve disease. The important warning signs differed because the pain from aortic valve disease could be tolerated for months and so could syncope (fainting). But once a sufferer had started going into failure, life expectancy was less than a year. Given the statistics, Harken realized that an operation did not have to be very safe to be considered a lot safer than the disease.

To enter the mitral valve, surgeons could take advantage of the little ear of the atrium. The aortic valve had no such available portal, and hemorrhage would be much harder to avoid under the powerful pressures of the left ventricle. Solely with digital guidance, the hazards were enormous. Harken worked out plans for an aortic operation, which he hoped would succeed. Dr. Sidney Burwell, a courageous physician, explained to a lady patient of his with aortic stenosis that Dr. Harken had an operation for her condition that he considered logical, but that had never had human trial. The risk could not be assessed. The lady knew that otherwise she was certain to die and chose to take the risk. After he talked to her, Harken said to Burwell, "She is a dear, brave lady."

Sue Williams, a superb nurse-anesthetist who was to assist at the operation, visited the patient. The lady confided that she was leaving some insurance money for Dr. Harken's use so that others might benefit in the future should he fail this time. She also gave Nurse Williams a note for her surgeon "in case."

When Harken put his finger through the "dear, brave lady's"

headwell (left ventricle) to reach the stenotic valve that day, a flood of blood from the left ventricle burst through the restraining purse string sutures, pumping out and around his finger. Harken put two, then three, then four fingers into the expanding breach as the heart muscle tore more and more widely. Vast quantities of blood were transfused under pressure, but no amount of fresh blood could keep up with the loss. The lady's blood volume diminished, bled out, and she died with Harken's hand in her heart.

"She trusted me. I loved her," said Harken and went home. Without even speaking to his stalwart wife, Anne, since he could imagine no comfort and wanted to die himself, he went upstairs in their new house on Lowell Street, into the bedroom, and to bed.

Sue Williams arrived at the house soon afterward and gave Mrs. Harken the patient's note. Anne Harken invaded his despair and read the message to him as he lay in the dark, his face to the wall. It said: "Thanks for the chance!"

Back at work again, D.E.H. was unusually tender, even with his colleagues. One thin, tall, blond Scandinavian doctor was working with him. The Dane had explained to nurses that there was no use trying to fatten him up. "My father, mother, all terribly skinny, too." That Friday Harken said to him, "Paul, you look tired. Awfully tired. I have been overworking you. I think you need a vacation. Let's see. It's now three o'clock. You knock off at five and don't come back here until Monday morning at seven! That'll give you a good, long rest." On Monday he said with satisfaction at his generosity, "Paul, you surely look well. Just great!"

At the Boston City Hospital William Swan, a surgical resident from Tennessee, developed a technique affording access to the aortic valve. By isolating a little knuckle of the aortic wall with a side-gripping clamp, just above the aortic valve, he could make a little slit in the wall of the aorta without losing blood. To the open edges of the aortic wall he could sew on an "operating tunnel"—a cloth tube two centimeters long and just large enough to admit the surgeon's finger. A tourniquet placed around the tunnel prevented blood loss as the finger was inserted into the aorta and the side-gripping clamp released.

As soon as he learned of this technique, for his first use Harken got Anne to make him a homemade tunnel, out of an old nylon shirt. For the tourniquet he boiled one of his daughter's tennis shoe laces. The makeshift device worked fine, and later he had operating tunnels made at the hospital.

"Perhaps the zenith of blind tactile intracardiac surgery was achieved in 1952," wrote Robert S. Litwak in his review of heart surgery, "by Charles Bailey and his colleagues." To close atrial septal defects, Bailey sewed peripheral portions of the right atrial wall to the defect's edges. In Boston Robert Gross and his colleagues sutured an open-ended funnel-shaped atrial well to a part of the right atrial wall, which they had excluded for the suturing process by a side-gripping clamp, much as the operating tunnel had been sewn to the aortic wall. Because the blood pressure in the right side of the heart was much lower than in the left (aortic systemic) side, Gross could let blood well up into his operating shaft. It rose to a level equaling the relatively low atrial pressure. Then it was possible to locate the defect by direct palpation, circumscribe it with sutures, and effect closure with a plastic patch or direct suture. John W. Kirklin, then at the Mayo Clinic, seemed consistently able to perform this operation better than the others.

Many such ingenious operations were devised by such master surgeons as Bailey, Gerbode, Glenn, Glover, Gross, Harken, Kirklin, Lam, and Potts, but not many of the procedures would remain "the best there is" for long. And often they were too complicated to permit simplification and widespread use.

The innovations of that tremendous decade would be discarded in the 1960s with open-heart surgery. Yet the "blind" surgeons could do certain things hitherto considered impossible, particularly opening up stenosed orifices in the mitral valve and, less satisfactorily, in the aortic. Harken's "bottle baffle" technique even converted an incompetent mitral valve into a more competent one. He planted a smooth Lucite bottle-shaped object beneath the valve to limit the area of valve leaflet insufficiency, thereby reducing the leak or regurgitation.

The most important addition to medical and surgical knowledge was the clear evidence that the heart was as tough as it was sensitive. In the early days the surgeons could work intermittently interrupting circulation in the working heart for what Harken called "indefinitely"—actually, only ten to twenty minutes. Between valve maneuvers the finger was retracted to the neutral atrial position. Shutting off the blood flow from the heart to the brain continuously for more than a minute or so at normal temperatures was very dangerous, though, and sewing up anything without direct vision was crude and imprecise.

There was an urgent need to *see*, and before the heart-lung bypass machines were made really useful, two interim techniques were used that provided singularly exciting dramas and one raging controversy.

8.

Ten Minutes to Look

Lewis Dexter, chief of cardiology at the Peter Bent Brigham Hospital, would say, "Cardiac surgery is the greatest thing that has happened to heart disease in all history!" Leroy Vandam, world leader in anesthesiology, would boast, "Improvements in anesthetic techniques have contributed in large part to the advance of cardiac surgery." These claims were acknowledged by the surgeons. In no field was the prime importance of anesthesiology better recognized, but the public rarely gave this aspect of surgery the credit it deserved. Perhaps the explanation lies in Vandam's own words: "You *know* what you are doing is not therapeutic! You are giving people drugs, poisons, necessary evils, so something else can be done. It's always a big challenge for us in major operations, keeping patients alive."

The history of anesthesia is a vital part of the history of all surgery. Sometimes a discovery made in that field preceded and made possible an extension of surgery, while sometimes the two sciences worked in tandem, with developments in one paralleling those in the other. When heart-lung bypass machines were improved and their use became widespread in the 1960s, anesthesiologists followed the cardiac surgeons, hard pressed to keep up with the need for drugs that not only maintained the proper level of unconsciousness but maintained the other body functions as well. Their drugs had to go into the blood, which was passing through the machine instead of the patient's heart and lungs. Drugs would be fed into the machine while the surgeons were given constantly extended periods of time during which they had direct vision into the opened heart. But before the cardiopulmonary bypass machines were in common use, there was one dramatic anesthetic technique employed in a few operating theatres that gave the surgeons six to ten minutes to look.

This method was hypothermia. By cooling the patient's body to very low levels, the demand on his heart to provide oxygenated blood was greatly reduced. As in animal hibernation, the human body could be, in effect, suspended, its metabolic requirements lowered while unconscious. Cold as an anesthetic was thus supremely utilized for the first time in the histories of both anesthesia and surgery in the 1950s.

It is surprising that in the distant past the anesthetic properties of cold were so seldom if ever mentioned by medical men and historians. It must have been pragmatically observed that chilling reduced at least surface pain, and the object of anesthesia was always to alleviate pain. Drugs were used for this purpose as far back as there is written history. Homer mentions a substance, probably some form of opium, called "nepenthe," a word meaning to "remove sorrow" and "forgetfulness." Analgesic drugs were known to be "poisons," as Vandam said. The Greek words *pharmakeutikos* and *pharmakon*, from which "pharmacology" and "pharmacist" derive, included the meanings "to practice witchcraft" and "to use poison."

The human desire for the alleviation of pain was catered to long before the danger to the body of extreme pain was medically recognized. The anesthetic as well as, quite likely, the pleasure-giving properties of such common plants as hemp, opium poppies, and mandragora root were historically recognized. In the third century B.C. Hoa-tho, a Chinese physician, kept his surgical patients insensible with a preparation of hemp. The first century A.D. Roman naturalist Pliny the Elder referred to mandragora as being employed for relief of pain in surgery. In fact, that strange weed, mandragora, was used as late as the 1900s as an emetic, antispasmodic, purgative, and narcotic, but now is best remembered for the superstitions that grew up around it. Its bifurcated root resembled human legs and in the Middle Ages the mandragora or mandrake was said to "shriek" when pulled up from the ground. Dogs were recommended for uprooting it rather than human hands. In Europe and England it was ground into love philters, and in the Middle East it was said to enhance a woman's chances of pregnancy.

The poet John Donne wrote in 1620 that "Annibal, to entrappe and surprise his enemies mingled their wine with Mandrake, whose operation is betwixt sleepe and poison." Another reference to its narcotic and dangerous properties is in a line of John Webster's play *The Duchess of Malfi*, written in 1623: "Come violent death, Serue from Mandragor to make me sleepe." William Shakespeare made such grand and poetic references to mandragora that the name was misused for a long time as a general term for all soporific drugs. "Give me to drink mandragora / That I might sleep out this great gap of time / My Antony is away," says his Cleopatra.

In 1782 a German medical paper recorded that Augustus, king of Poland, was given a narcotic and was unconscious during an amputation, but most surgical patients until the late 1800s seem not to have been so fortunate. Barber-surgeons in those days apparently just strapped their patients down and went to work.

The first of the modern anesthetics, nitrous oxide, still in popular use as a light anesthesia for short-term relief, was discovered in 1800. Sir Humphry Davy, a British chemist and physicist, experimented with it on himself to relieve local pain. He suggested that it be inhaled by patients during surgical operations "in which no great effusion of blood takes place," but a cautious medical climate prevailed. It may have been just as well. Enough nitrous oxide to render a man unconscious also renders him dangerously short of oxygen.

In 1844 Horace Wells, a dentist in Hartford, Connecticut, made himself famous by using nitrous oxide on himself, for lack of any other volunteer, and while unconscious underwent tooth extraction. He proposed making his fortune with "painless dentistry" but one fatality caused him to abandon the idea.

During the late 1800s Paul Bert in Paris conceived the idea of a primitive room-sized pressurized operating chamber. Two men pumped lustily to keep the atmospheric pressure in the chamber high, increasing the nitrous oxide effect and allowing adequate oxygen while patients were unconscious inside it. Bert was certified insane by the French authorities, labeled a criminal maniac, and forbidden his experiments. He put his chamber on wheels and moved it ahead of the police around the environs of Paris. Plenty of patients were glad to evade the law and have fractures set, amputations performed, or teeth pulled without pain, and they followed him on his peripatetic rounds.

Vapor of ether was discovered in the early 1800s by Michael Faraday in England while he was experimenting with chemical gases. In spite of his demonstration that it was marvelously anesthetic, ether was for a long time considered no more than a scientific curiosity. A dentist and physician, W. T. G. Morton, would give his classic ether dome demonstration of the uses of ether vapor at Boston's Massachusetts General Hospital in 1846. Morton used ether himself for dental surgery, but its acceptance in the United States was slow. Ether was employed regularly on the Continent and in England long before it was here.

Scottish physician Sir James Simpson used ether in childbirth after he assured himself that it did not interfere with uterine contractions. A Liverpool chemist, one Waldie by name, suggested to Simpson in 1847 that he try instead a newly discovered substance called chloroform. For many years after that chloroform was thought to be absolutely safe in proper quantity, which ether was not, and it became the anesthesia of choice for surgery and childbirth until 1876. In that year London's Dr. J. T. Clover introduced an ether inhaler that regulated the strength of the vapor, reducing its hazards.

Surgeons were now enabled to operate more slowly and deliberately. They were no longer judged largely by their speed. Their surgical patients may have lost as much as they gained since prolonged surgery opened the body to more infections.

Hospitals were beginning to burgeon in urban areas, and within them gangrene, pyemia, erysipelas, tetanus, and puerperal fever were rampant. These nineteenth-century hospitals were infamous as charnel houses. Patients sent to them were more likely to die than to survive. The well-to-do avoided them like the plague (and for the same reason).

One of the great heroes of surgical history is Britain's Joseph Lister. An effective fanatic, he introduced carbolic acid for antiseptic cleansing, the heat sterilization of surgical instruments, and the basic principle that surgeons should wash their hands between patients. When Lister's principles were accepted, "Listerism" would make surgery less routinely lethal, as well as painless when combined with anesthesia.

Only rarely has piety or superstition prevented the use of analgesics for painful medical procedures, even though stoicism was always a much admired virtue. But briefly in the nineteenth century certain religious sects in the United States held that human suffering was the will of God and that to alleviate that of women in childbirth was sinful. That same period, however, has been labeled a dope fiend's paradise. Opiates were frequently prescribed for minor ailments, and patent medicines containing opiates, such as "Ayer's Cherry Pectoral," "Mrs. Winslow's Soothing Syrup," and even "McNunn's Elixir of Opium," were available in general stores without prescription. These were also widely advertised as painkillers, cough mixtures, "women's friends," and all-purpose cures. In England dosing children with laudanum was an even commoner practice, and "Godfrey's Cordial," a mixture of molasses, sassafras, and opium, made a fortune. "Some persons take opium as a luxury," noted a British physician in 1873, "though by far the greatest number do so for some old neuralgia or rheumatic malady, and began under medical advice."

For surgery and childbirth, chloroform and ether were to be utilized almost interchangeably before it was finally learned that chloroform was toxic to the liver. In the 1911 *Encyclopaedia Britannica* the British authority on anesthetics, Herbert Challis Crouch, wrote: "The question as to which is the better anesthetic, ether or chloroform, for long operations is a moot point. In the hands of an experienced anesthetist there is probably little to choose as regards safety and the anesthetic advantages of the latter are incontestable. In the hands of the less experienced, ether is the more suitable drug."

His long article also included mention of a newly discovered injectable substance, urethane, a carbon compound tried so far only on lower animals because it depressed the respiratory center. Spinal anesthesia, he prophesized, might in time find its proper use, and he discussed hypnotism as a method of anesthesia, but only for selected cases. Nowhere did he mention cold or alcohol, the latter long pragmatically recognized as having anesthetic properties.

It was well known that exposure to cold could carry the body through all four stages of anesthesia, which had been roughly defined since 1900: first stage, disordered consciousness and purposeless movements; second stage, complete loss of consciousness but reflexes and muscle movement still strong; third stage, surgical anesthesia with muscular relaxation, loss of many reflexes, but with the vital centers of the medulla remaining active; fourth stage, paralysis of the medulla, respiratory and circulatory paralysis, poisoning of the heart muscle, resulting in death.

Freezing to death was not an uncommon occurrence in the Scandinavian countries during the long and lightless months of midwinter. Cold and alcohol could prove a lethal combination because the dilation of the surface blood vessels plus the anesthetic action of alcohol made cold more rapidly fatal, but in some cases, alcohol could delay death by freezing. Acting as a light anesthetic, drunkenness prevented panic and averted shivering, and by causing dilation of the surface blood vessels, it allowed more uniform cooling of the deep structures in the body.

In March 1776 there was an instance, authenticated by the Swedish Academy of Sciences, in which a man lived although he had been frozen to the point where he had "no heartbeat, no breath, fixed open eyes, and joints locked in what appeared to be rigor mortis." He was a peasant who had left for home on foot after drinking heavily. Knocked from his unsteady feet by a high wind, he fell beside the road in the snow. Many hours later he was found and taken home for dead. When the local doctor arrived, the peasant had already been laid out in his coffin. This village doctor detected a small region of warmth in the "corpse's" frozen abdomen and called for hot towels. Those, with massage, miraculously revived the man.

The next year John Hunter, Scottish pioneer in comparative anatomy, lectured in London on a visionary theory of "frozen sleep" to anyone who would listen. "All action and waste would cease until the body was thawed," he said, "and I think if a man would give up his last ten years to alternate oblivion and action by being frozen and then getting himself thawed every hundred years he might learn what had happened during his frozen condition." To win converts, he offered to demonstrate on animals, and, according to a contemporary report, froze in succession two carp, two dormice, some snails, and other animals, but when he tried to bring them back to life, he failed. Hunter found no takers for his offer of frozen immortality.

During the Napoleonic wars military surgeon Baron Larrey was so appreciated for his skill and compassion that his regiment refused to attack unless he was with them. Once they passed him bodily over their heads across a bridge to ensure that he could tend the wounded when they met the enemy on the other side. When Napoleon's armies were defeated by their greatest enemy, the Russian winter, Larrey used its snow and ice to lessen pain and staunch hemorrhages when he amputated.

Not until the twentieth century were cold's sleep-inducing, analgesic, and healing properties studied scientifically. But this same scientific century also created a high degree of public gullibility toward pseudo-sciences. When microorganisms that were still vital after being packed in glacier ice for millennia were discovered, the sensational press printed tales of "mammoths" and "dinosaurs" similarly resuscitated. "Frozen sleep" made mythical news.

One American, Edward Hope, claimed that he had mastered a process that would suspend human beings in frozen sleep for a hundred years and more. Anyone thus suspended could escape the normal process of dying permanently. Battening particularly on the hopelessly ill, he promised that they could remain alive in this suspended state until cures for their diseases were discovered. He built refrigerated vaults and sold stainless steel coffins in which frozen bodies could be stored. The freezers would be kept at a temperature of −320°F., the bodies in a perpetual bath of liquid oxygen. He claimed that if the freshly dead were frozen and stored, they could be resuscitated even after a thousand years—or as soon as whatever they were dying of was curable. The people thus suspended in time he called cryonics, the process itself "cryonic suspension." Hope charged $5,000 each for his freezers and sold insurance policies to cover maintenance at a cost of $700 for each future year.

Cryonic societies sprang up. The *Journal of Cryonics* was published, featuring warnings such as: *Remember! If you do not make arrangements for your cryonic suspension you will be buried or cremated when you are dead.* In 1972 there were at least thirteen cryonics already frozen in their tombs and an uncounted number of paid-up Cryonic Society members hoping for this earthly immortality.

Cold as both painkilling and potentially life-prolonging was subject also to serious study and purpose. There were many efforts to achieve the equivalent of hibernation in humans. Animals with this capacity reduced their body temperatures close to that of their environment and slept through winters. It was discovered that a physiologic mechanism, absent in other species, was necessary to hibernation, but that artificial chilling could induce prolonged sleep in warm-blooded nonhibernating creatures without the side effects of drug-induced sleep.

In 1938 Drs. Fay and Smith in Philadelphia asked themselves why body cancers rarely spread to the limbs, which were cooler than the trunk. Cancers themselves had higher temperatures than the healthy surrounding tissues. Was it possible that cooling the whole body would inhibit cancerous growth? Experimenting with hopeless human cases, they cooled patients to 80°F. and kept them in cold sleep for as long as eight days. The patients were brought out of this condition with no signs of damage, but their tumors remained unaffected, although, inexplicably, the pain from these tumors was eased for periods of days after they were awakened.

In Holland Professor Ite Boerema had noted that electric

shocks, which brought down blood pressure, did not damage the blood, while deep anesthesia, where there was anoxia (lack of oxygen), did. He thought anesthesia by cold might be another approach. Taking laboratory animals down to 65°F. by siphoning blood from the large terminal (thigh) arteries and passing it into an especially prepared glass container immersed in ice and then returning the cooled blood to the adjacent femoral vein of the bodies, he found that if the animals were cooled too slowly, it was difficult to revive them. If the cooling was done too quickly, their hearts fluttered, faltered, and failed. If he had the timing right, he could actually isolate animal hearts from the circulation up to twenty minutes without any evidence of brain damage.

Another experimenter, Dr. Andjus in Belgrade, cooled rats to below 55°F.; when revived, only one out of five showed ill effects. Yet by all the then accepted definitions of death (to be revised repeatedly in the future), the rats had been dead; they were without brain signals and as stiff as boards. Hamsters, natural hibernators, did even better. Taken as low as 41°F., they were as normal and alert as ever when brought back to normal temperatures, and suffered frostbite only if they were roughly handled while frozen.

The distressing question arose: How many men who had been pronounced dead by freezing had not been dead? How many airmen, fished from the bitter winter waters of the English Channel, who could have been resuscitated, were prematurely given up for dead?

In *The Risk Takers* Hugh McLeave recounts a singular case from 1951 that led in time to redefinitions of death. In Chicago a plump black woman, aged twenty-three, drank continually from midday to 9 P.M. in a bar and then staggered out into a cold winter night with a biting wind off the lake. She fell on the pavement, where she lay untouched until eleven hours later when a morning police patrol spotted her and sent for an ambulance. She was taken to the Michael Reese Hospital, presumed dead. Two doctors there checked her carefully. She was not dead. Her heart still beat, almost indetectably, varying between twelve and twenty beats a minute. For long intervals it appeared to stop. The doctors also detected the faintest signs of breathing.

Stimulants were administered by injection, oxygen supplied through a mask, and blood transfusions begun. When the senior surgeon arrived an hour later, she still appeared completely frozen, with an immovable head, unblinking eyes that felt like glass, no detectable pulse in her arms and legs, and a mouth that could not be forced open. Her temperature was 64.4°F. (34°F. below normal) and the only warmth was in her lower abdomen. There was no previous record of any person surviving with a temperature below 75°F.

Alcohol had probably saved the woman's life up to that point. Even in the hospital her death was narrowly averted. Her trachea (windpipe) was opened so as to pass an intratracheal tube to control respiration and oxygenation. The room temperature was lowered to 68°F., and her arms and legs lightly swathed in bandages. Late that afternoon her heart picked up its normal rhythm, except for frequent dropped beats. Her body temperature climbed to 80°F. Her eyes began to follow light and movement. By nighttime she had asked for her father and recognized him when he came in.

Within two days it looked as if her recovery would be complete. Even her memory returned, except for a twelve-hour alcoholic blackout preceding her collapse. She did survive, but a month later injury from frostbite necessitated amputation of her lower legs and fingers.

It was in 1950 that Dr. Wilfred G. Bigelow, scholarly investigator and master cardiothoracic surgeon, with his associates in Toronto, reported on experiments with hypothermia—chilling to produce total anesthesia. They had been given a grant to study the effects of cold. In the laboratory Bigelow's animals were taken down to 64°F. Heartbeats slowed from 180 to 25 a minute, body metabolic requirements fell, anesthesia was total; when revived, the animals showed no ill effects. Such a technique, Bigelow thought prophetically, might allow surgeons to operate on a bloodless heart. The basic rationale was to reduce the body's metabolism, particularly the brain, so much that the brain could withstand more than four minutes of circulatory arrest.

Medical advances, as Harken would often say, generally come about through evolution, not revolution. After innovative thinking comes careful laboratory trial. After laboratory trial confirms that the procedure is feasible and clinical studies indicate when the procedure is needed comes the quantum leap: human clinical trial. Orderly progress, not chance mutation, narrows the terrifyingly thin line between medical bravery and foolhardiness.

The laboratory and clinical studies were essential steps in developing hypothermia. It was in Minnesota's Minneapolis University Hospital that surgeons took the final step, using hypothermia on a human patient. Drs. Lewis, Taufic, and Varco, under the aegis of their remarkable chief of surgery, Dr. Owen Wangensteen, had followed up the Bigelow laboratory work on hypothermia and Wangensteen backed them in their decision to try it in the operating room.

The patient was a five-year-old girl who weighed less than thirty pounds. She had a defect in the interatrial septum. To mend it and salvage her life, the surgeons had to have a few minutes to see what they were doing. She was put to sleep with sodium pentobarbital, one of a group of drugs called barbiturates that had been found effective in calming nerves and inducing sleep. Curare, a drug used by South American Indians to poison their arrowheads, in the proper amount relaxed her muscles and prevented shivering, which could exhaust and warm the body. Her lungs would be ventilated with oxygen squeezed from a rubber bag and delivered through an endotracheal tube.

The careful cooling process took ninety minutes. They used rubber blankets, such as those Bigelow had developed for cooling his animals. A warm bath was ready in which to revive her—they hoped. When they opened her chest and occluded the vessels carrying blood to her heart, the little girl showed no signs of shock. The occluded right auricle was opened, the blood aspirated. In a race with the clock, under direct vision, the surgeon could then suture the inch-wide opening. Afterward the heart was quickly closed, the returning veins unclamped to refill the heart. The operation was a startling success. The child was up in a day. On the eleventh day she went home.

In Denver Henry Swan also tried hypothermia. He discarded the blanket and used ice water for a cooling bath for his patients. To achieve deep through-and-through warming, he successfully experimented with short-wave current applied through blankets. By the time Swan, from Denver, and Lewis, from Minneapolis, reported on hypothermia to the 1955 American Surgical Association congress they were ready to insist that the method was "highly effective and quite safe." Swan was eloquent in his description of the full range of possibilities made available by hypothermia. "Finger vision," he said, "is capable of limited success, and bears the same relation to real vision in surgery that it does in life—one can read Braille with moderate facility, but the chromatic values of the Mona Lisa escape one, and to shoot a winged mallard or to fly an airplane is impossible."

The cooling of the body would prove to have infinite uses in medicine. French Dr. Henry Laborit concocted a "lytic cocktail" using chlorpromazine, which tugged down temperature while reducing shivering (with other nerve-blocking agents), and would save lives, especially in brain surgery and on the battlefield. Later hypothermia would be combined with the use of the heart-lung bypass machines for open-heart surgery, greatly reducing the risks of cardiopulmonary bypass and prolonged anesthesia. Hypothermia as the means of anesthesia that made it possible to look into the heart had a day almost as brief as the time limit it imposed on the surgeon: "Safe for six minutes, possible for ten."

No anesthetist involved would forget the dramas of those operations. Leroy Vandam had many lively memories of his first year at the Peter Bent Brigham Hospital. As soon as he came there, he and Dwight Harken, the latter as "the individual most concerned with the application of hypothermia to cardiac surgery," were involved in a program to study and use hypothermia clinically.

Vandam had been a surgeon before trouble with his eyes had forced him to choose another branch of medicine for specialization. Anesthesia was his choice. The Peter Bent Brigham Hospital had been the first institution to hire a physician-anesthetist in 1914, at the insistence of Harvey Cushing, the great neurosurgeon. When Leroy Vandam was asked to replace William Derrick, who was moving to Texas, as a chief of anesthesia, he accepted.

"Anesthesia, where it is established, always comes up against

strong surgical figures," Vandam would say. "Dwight was one. All
the great early American anesthetists had been Midwesterners. I
think they had an inventiveness, an originality, an aggressiveness
and independence, plus a certain antipathy toward Eastern medicine, so they went their own way and did big things, and Dwight
came from that pioneering background, too.

"The pattern in the operating room is always set by the
surgeon. Some characters play music, and that bothers me. With
Dr. Gross there was almost deadly silence, while with Dwight—
with his personality and my personality and all the other people
there—it was not chaos but constant exchange, heated words on
occasion, moments of tension and anger and so on, but *never* to
the detriment of the patient. In fact, Dwight never allowed any
conversation that did not concern the patient."

One of their early disagreements was about Vandam's ac-
companying D.E.H. to outside hospitals. William Derrick, Vandam's predecessor, had done so.

"I did for a while," said Vandam. "Those were the craziest
and almost the happiest moments in my life. But they always left
me rather uneasy. We'd set out for Rutland in one of Dwight's big
Lincoln Continentals, with a secretary beside him and lunch
along. There were usually two or three prominent visitors with
us. He'd drive at a hell of a clip and when we got there everybody
was waiting, rather servile and frightened, with things more or
less ready, and if things weren't just right, they got hell. Dwight
was tense and we'd go ahead and do the chest operation and the
nurses were frightened and the nurse-anesthetist they had was in
awe of me. We'd do a procedure very well, and as soon as it was
over, take off again. It was helter-skelter, emotional, and fun, for
maybe $50 or $100 fee. I didn't get anything out of it intellec-
tually, I felt wrong about not knowing the patient, and it was a
disadvantage to my work at the Brigham. Anyway, gradually, as
other people got into cardiac surgery, you didn't go around like
that any more and do itinerant heart surgery."

Harken did not feel the same way. Vandam's memories of
the Rutland Veterans Hospital, the farthest away, he thought,
misjudged the situation. The exciting staff welcomed him, he said,
and maintained rigid vigil and meticulous patient care for him.

If there was perhaps some conflict between the two men, there was always apt to be between surgeon and physician-anesthetist. And D.E.H. was not only authoritative about anesthesia in his own right, but some irreverent residents had dubbed him in the operating room "Dwightie the Almighty." In the area of patient care at the Brigham, however, Harken and Vandam were completely in accord. Vandam not only visited and talked to each of their surgical patients before operations, but carried out a long-term study to establish the value of these visits and explanations by any surgical patient's anesthesiologist.

In *Introduction to Anesthesia,* on which Vandam collaborated with two other authorities, it is stated: "We prefer that patients come to the operating room awake though drowsy, free of apprehension and fully cooperative." Undue anxiety was a clinical enemy but, on the other hand, premature unconsciousness created additional hazards from the toxic drugs and could cause such complications as respiratory obstruction. "A degree of physical depression difficult to define is already present in these individuals," Vandam noted. Increased drowsiness from drugs alone in some cases made them even more anxious.

The results of Vandam's study proved the importance of visits. When patients with neither visit nor drugs arrived at the operating room, only 35 percent were no more than "understandably nervous." Sixty-four percent were agitated. Drugs alone rendered 48 percent "adequately sedated." A visit alone improved that to 65 percent, proof positive of its worth. The two together, visit and intramuscular pentobarbital, were the most successful. Seventy-one percent of patients receiving both were in the right condition.

"Just taking care of a patient during the operation is not enough," Vandam would say. "I admit anesthesia attracts a great many people because it can be practiced pretty casually, but I wouldn't be happy without patient contact myself. And in the last analysis, it is a knowledge of the patient and his disease that leads to correct choices. One cannot speak of an anesthetic agent that is useful and safe in all situations, but rather in terms of a method for the particular patient."

Blind surgery mortality had been reduced to a remarkably

low rate by both Harken and Bailey before either essayed hypothermia, which would give them precious minutes to look. Bailey
tried the cold-anesthesia method on complex cases impossible to
operate on blind, and lost thirteen out of his first twenty patients.
Harken was determined to do a lot better, and held many preliminary meetings of everyone concerned to plan for each procedure.

Each occasion in which hypothermia was used at the Peter
Bent Brigham Hospital aroused unusual interest. The amphithe-
ater was crowded and there were often ten times as many people
in the operating area as were needed. All the people who could
trip in had things to say. Added to the normal furnishings and
properties were iced water, a giant bathtub, and a windlass. Vandam described the scene with gusto:

"I anesthetized the patient, giving him the drugs for what
the French call artificial hibernation so he wouldn't shiver and
counteract the cooling process. When we get cold, you know, we
constrict, curl up, and shiver, which decreases heat loss, and we
also manufacture heat by a number of means, so we had to block
out all those defense mechanisms. Then we lowered the patient
on the windlass into the ice-water tub to cool him down, monitoring the esophageal and rectal thermometer probes so we could
take him out of the cold water just before he reached the desired
temperature. After you cool the surface of the body there is a drift
downward and it takes a while for the interior of the body to
equilibriate. One of the problems as they drifted was ventricular
fibrillation—probably why some of the pilots down in the English
Channel died very quickly, from unequal cooling. This was never
quite solved until Berkovits [the medical engineering genius with
whom Harken would work on many devices] gave us direct-
current defibrillation. Before that we had alternating-current defi-
brillators that were dangerous and damaging. It was always more
of a problem with cardiac patients anyway, with their diseased
hearts and poor circulation.

"Furthermore we had no way of warming up patients quickly
afterward. We had a hypothermia blanket with circulating warm
water and you had to watch out even if the water was only warm
because a burn will occur with too great a difference between the
temperature of the patient's skin and the blanket.

"I was in charge during the lowering of the temperature and the warming up. The patient was taken out of the tub and dried and put on the operating table. Meanwhile we were giving him drugs to keep him asleep, ventilating the lungs. Then the chest was opened. There wasn't much time after circulation stopped and the heart was open. Somebody counted off the half minutes out loud. Six minutes was 'safe' and we had to free the surgeon to concentrate entirely on his intricate and nerve-racking work. Surgical speed had to make up for lack of time. All the time we were monitoring, watching for side effects from the drugs that lowered blood pressure, et cetera. The anesthetist became the internist, you might say, keeping the body functions going, intra-arterial blood pressure, blood gases, how're we doing? How's the potassium changing? All that in conjunction with the surgeon, and if anything happens—if we can't get a heart started or it fibrillates—there's a group of drugs we give in rapid succession, but sometimes you can't get a heart started because the heart has nothing left when you come to repair it.

"It all takes many hours of preparation and lots of manpower, but by and large if a good heart operation is done, the patient is better off, has better circulation, almost from the beginning."

Operating with hypothermia never attracted many practitioners. Few surgeons had the requisite speed, skill—and daring. It was too cumbersome, and circulatory arrest with the heart isolated for only six to ten minutes was too little time to repair very complicated defects. When the body temperature dropped below 86°F., all too often the heart wriggled and the electrocardiogram recorded sinister "scribbles" indicating irritability or even ventricular fibrillation. Reversed by application of electric shock, the fibrillation might cease, but in some instances the rhythm never stabilized and the heart squirmed to a halt. Rewarming patients could bring metabolic changes with blood acid and base imbalance, bleeding, and sometimes death. Most surgeons and many procedures waited until the heart-lung machine was in routine use, a story of its own.

Boerema in Holland did continue to experiment with cold anesthesia. His objective was to cool patients down to 80°F. To warm them afterward he designed an operating cabinet in which controlled streams of hot air were blown over a box with a slatted open top over which the patient lay in a net. He did not close the wound after operating, but placed a transparent hood over the box while the patient was being rewarmed.

Next he invented a sort of diving bell in which his operations could be performed at three times normal atmospheric pressure and the tissues of the patient be charged with six times their normal level of oxygen. Within the bell, he thought, circulation could be stopped long enough for more intricate and time-consuming procedures. Boerema's team did not like experimenting with him on animals in the diving bell. There was a slight impairment of intellectual functions as they became lightheaded; the bell was cramped; and when they emerged, they had to undergo decompression drill to prevent the bends.

Nevertheless Boerema did operate successfully on a few human patients by combining hypothermia with high pressure, which made it possible to shut down circulation through the heart for longer periods without damage to other organs, particularly the brain. As with many innovations in one field, this one turned out to have better applications in others. High-pressure chambers would prove to be the most useful treatment for two other dangerous conditions. Saturating the tissues with oxygen killed non-oxygen-using (anaerobic) bacilli like tetanus, the gangrene bacillus. Also, lives were saved in cases of poison by coal gas, with its fatal affinity for hemoglobin.

Hypothermia as the means of anesthetizing a patient would be discarded when cardiopulmonary bypass machines were improved and rendered safer. After that the potential of cardiac surgery would explode. In time came recognition that hypothermia could be combined with the use of bypass machines. Lowering the body temperature decreased demand for oxygenated blood.

With prolonged open-heart surgery, the highly sophisticated anesthetist would become literally the guardian of life. The patient whom he had put to sleep and cooled was connected by his endotracheal tube to the machine that breathed for him and substituted for the heart pump. The anesthetist fed into the machine the anesthetic agents and elements that might be required. He was responsible not only for the level of the anesthetic state and lowered body temperatures, but also for the oxygen level of the blood, for the hemoglobin level, for the levels of carbon dioxide and acidity, and for blood volume. The parameters must be maintained to keep the patient's homeostatic stability. If the kidneys were not functioning properly, the anesthetist added diuretics; if the patient's blood had been too diluted by the circulating fluids that had been added to the pump, he added more red blood cells. Sometimes the heart required extra support by means of chemicals that enhanced the beat. Supervised by the surgeon and the pump team, the anesthetist monitored a multichannel device that showed the patient's electrocardiogram and registered all the other blood and body function levels. He had to be in continuous contact with the laboratory where oxygen levels and chemical balances were constantly checked. And when the patient was being rewarmed, the anesthetist had to check the heart as it returned to action and prevent it from becoming too irritable and ineffective.

The surgical heroes of each advance in cardiac surgery— from Alley of Albany through Zerbini of Brazil (see Founders Group list)—would owe a great deal to the spectrum of sciences, especially anesthesiology. On the other hand, anesthesiologist Leroy Vandam would add to his statement that "Improvements in anesthetic techniques have contributed in large part to the advance of cardiac surgery," the codicil: "Cardiac surgery had progressed so rapidly that anesthesia had been hard pressed to keep abreast."

9.

The Open Heart

The engineering of the human body is so complex and compact that to replace any of its organs by man-made devices taxes to the utmost man's resourceful brain. The spongelike surfaces of the lungs if spread flat would cover an area roughly equivalent to that of a doubles tennis court. Since their most important functions are to remove carbon dioxide and reoxygenate the blood that will recirculate through the body, driven by the heart pump, a heart-lung bypass machine must do the same. Lacking oxygen at normal temperatures, the brain dies in about four minutes. Time enough to operate on the heart for complex defects, with direct vision, required that an artificial pump-oxygenator replace both heart and lungs.

Dr. John H. Gibbon from Philadelphia dreamed of one, experimented in laboratories for years, and was the first investigator whose machine was used successfully on a human being. His success was followed by two failures. Stunned by the imperfections of his invention, Gibbon pursued his dream no further. Other daring pioneers went ahead.

In the 1060s Leo Eloesser was one of the greatest thoracic surgeons and an extensive contributor to the field. Litwak quotes from his "lyric" account: "Gibbon's idea and its elaboration take their place among the boldest and most successful feats of man's mind—with the invention of the phonetic alphabet, the telephone, or a Mozart symphony. Not a *Deux ex machina* but a *machine a Deo*."

John Gibbon's first, and only, personal success, was on May 6, 1953, 337 years after William Harvey published his conclusions about the circulation of the blood and the nature of the heart as a pump. It was twenty-two years after Gibbon had conceived the idea of such an extracorporeal mechanism to function for the heart and lungs. It was two years after Clarence Dennis had tried a locally developed pump-oxygenator in Minneapolis. Unfortunately Dennis's two patients did not survive. ("And when," says Harken, "in an often desperate attempt to save life, an innovative or experimental procedure is tried and the patient dies, from whatever causes, that procedure gains little support.")

The idea had occurred to young Dr. Gibbon one night in 1931 as he monitored a patient for Dr. Edward Delos Churchill in Boston. The woman was suffering from a massive pulmonary embolism. To operate on her was so dangerous that it would only be permissible if she were moribund. Churchill and his surgical team stood by in the hospital while Gibbon recorded her blood pressure, respiration, and faltering pulse minute by minute. When the time came and her condition was clearly irreversible, Churchill was alerted. He removed the embolus in six and a half minutes, but the patient died.

"I wish," Mary Gibbon, John Gibbon's wife and research partner, would write decades later in her "Recollections," included in Robert S. Litwak's history, "that her family might know of the thousands of lives that have been saved throughout the world because that woman died when and where she did!" It was while he watched her that John Gibbon grew obsessed with the belief that it should be possible to draw blue blood from the patient's distended veins into an apparatus where the blood could discharge its carbon dioxide and pick up oxygen the way it did in the lungs, then be pumped back into her arterial system. This would bypass heart and lungs in functions and in fact.

While he was still on Dr. Churchill's service in Boston, John Gibbon married Mary Hopkinson, a laboratory technician working for Churchill. Then Jack and Maly Gibbon went back to his

home city of Philadelphia, where he talked about his idea to anyone who would listen. Mary Gibbon was his only real convert,
but in 1934 Dr. Churchill, who she would say was "less than
enthusiastic," did offer the Gibbons laboratory space with a fellowship at Harvard for John Gibbon and a technician's salary for
his wife.

Cats were used for their experiments. Three a week were
maximum. One would be fetched from upstairs cages and anesthetized, usually with sodium barbital. A primitive method of recording cardiac reaction, by kymograph, a rotating drum that
registered wavelike tracings, was employed. Gibbon performed a
tracheotomy, opening the windpipe, and connected the cat to a
machine for artificial respiration while he and Maly exposed the
pulmonary artery. These preliminaries took four or five hours.

Mary Gibbon's account contains a description of those days:

> It was mid-afternoon before we were ready to start the really
> critical part of the experiment, gradually closing the clamp around
> the pulmonary artery and at the same time gradually withdrawing
> blood from the jugular vein [into the apparatus]. We would keep
> the clamp completely occluding the pulmonary artery for as long as
> we thought the cat could stand it, or nothing went wrong with the
> apparatus, but the things that were apt to go wrong were infinite.

When they removed the clamp, they put the cat back on its
own circulation to see if it could maintain its blood pressure at a
near normal level and its respirations at a near normal rate. If the
cat did so successfully, "The animal was nursed tenderly over a
period of an hour or so. Then the experiment was terminated, the
cat was sacrificed and an autopsy performed, the kymograph
record was shellacked so that no diener's [cleaner's] hand or
broom should smooch our record, the instruments and general
mess cleaned up, and we could go home . . . a long day."

They were to return to Philadelphia, where Gibbon had a
hospital appointment, at the end of the year. Gibbon reported
that "no evidence indicated eventual failure." Prolonged healthy
survival, he was certain, could be attained following extracorporeal circulation that replaced the functions of the heart and
lungs. But, he admitted, there were several features of the appa-

ratus and method that could be improved on. Commented his wife, "That was the understatement of the year!"

In Philadelphia the Gibbons converted the famous Dr. Isador S. Ravdin to their cause. Through the University of Pennsylvania, he arranged for space for them at the Harrison Research Laboratories and for the assistance of a full-time technician, Charles Kraul, to help Gibbon. The war interrupted the project, as it interrupted most pure research. After the war Harken's unique wartime record of intracardiac invasion and the subsequent success of blind surgery for mitral stenosis, beginning in 1948, proved that the heart was tough and resilient. If heart-lung bypass could be made possible, the potential for cardiac repair would be enormously increased. In Sweden, England, and elsewhere other men were pursuing the same dream. In Pennsylvania John Gibbon went back to work on his apparatus, this time at the Jefferson Medical School.

Two pumps working in phase were required to stand in for the heart alone. One drew off venous blood charged with carbon dioxide and pushed it through the mechanical lung, reversing the venous to arterial blood by removing carbon dioxide and adding oxygen. The second pump pressed the arterial blood back through the animal's arteries to perfuse the whole body.

> As I look back on the earliest experiments [wrote Mary Gibbon] the problem of getting enough oxygen into venous blood was the ever-present backdrop to all twenty-two years that elapsed between the concept . . . and the first successful operation. . . . Sometime shortly after Hillary and Tensing climbed Mt. Everest [also in 1953] we had the pleasure of entertaining Dr. Charles Evans in our house, one of the pair on Hillary's team to make the first attempt on the summit. They did not make the summit, but left oxygen and other supplies above the highest camp for Hillary and Tensing to use in making their attack on the peak. I remember asking Dr. Evans what seemed to be the greatest problem in all that complicated and courageous effort and he answered me laconically in one word: Oxygen!"

Finally Gibbon designed a metal box, five and a half feet long and four feet high, with two roller pumps to squeeze venous blood through plastic tubes, and a plastic box with six wafers of stainless steel mesh that spread the blood over their surfaces while oxygen was blown over it. IBM built the apparatus to his specifications. Stainless steel cannulae, hollow tubes that would fit the blood vessels leaving and entering the heart, completed the basic mechanical setup.

The animal laboratory where Gibbon and his associates now worked out surgical techniques for using cardiopulmonary bypass became a very exciting place. They opened the hearts of dogs, stitched and patched inside while their dogs were on bypass, and then restored the canines to normal function with increasing success.

In March 1953 Gibbon and the surgical team declared themselves ready for human clinical trial. A fifteen-month-old boy was in the hospital with severe congestive heart failure. Diagnosis, without benefit of catheterization, indicated a hole in the child's heart between the two upper chambers (an interatrial septal defect). In the operating room the cumbersome apparatus was set up and the child connected to it. The surgeons successfully invaded the little boy's nearly bloodless heart, but the hole they expected to suture was not there. His condition was obviously due to other congenital factors. The frustrated team could only close up the heart, successfully, but after the operation the child died.

On May 6, 1953, the second use of the apparatus was proposed. An eighteen-month-old baby girl had been seemingly healthy until six months before, when signs of a heart defect appeared. Exploration was made by catheter this time, and it confirmed that she had a large hole between the upper chambers. Through this interatrial defect blood was recirculating round and round at a rate that would eventually cause heart failure and death.

For twenty-six minutes the child was kept alive, her blood circulated through the Gibbon machine, while the right upper chamber was incised, to expose a gaping hole between the two auricles. This hole was closed with silk sutures. Then she was successfully restored to her own circulation. Two months later the proof was in. The girl's complexion was a healthy pink, her symptoms were gone, and catheterization of her heart indicated that the defect had remained closed.

When the next two patients on whom the apparatus was tried died, Gibbon called it quits. Reviewing the era of open-heart surgery that began with Gibbon's Turning Point, surgeon Robert Litwak expressed amazement that so few other surgeons had recognized the clinical importance of that one success. It seemed even more incredible to Dwight Harken that Gibbon did not go on.

"Maly, you are going to have to explain to me why Jack quit," Harken said to Mary Gibbon after John Gibbon died in 1973.

"Well," said Mrs. Gibbon, "it was such an emotional experience. It was just overwhelming! You can't have any idea, Dwight, what an emotional experience it was."

"Don't use that expression, 'such an emotional experience,'" Harken protested. "You've missed my point. All of us who have done firsts and gone on and lost lives and spent a good deal of our own lives to create new things realize what it is like to go through all that. And we also know the feeling of triumph as well as the feeling of defeat and we resent it when a man does just one successful case and quits! One patient lives and you *can't* just sit down and say, 'Now I've done it, that's it, that's my contribution.' You are *obliged* to standardize the technique so as to serve others."

As long as he lived, John Gibbon received homage for his monumental first. Harken always insisted that his wife, Maly, had less ego, more courage, and got too little credit, and he was never satisfied with her "explanation." "Jack should have had people with him who could and would carry on his work if he didn't continue himself," Harken would contend. "Some of the machines that other people used were basically his, though, of course, many others involved different principles."

The machine's most difficult function was to replace the lungs in oxygenating the venous blood by exposing the blood to enough air. Dennis Melrose in England replaced the screen oxygenator with a rotating tunnel of discs. Later C. Walton Lillehei in Minneapolis would succeed in converting the blood into bubbles, and then breaking up the bubbles. The surface area of the bubbling froth was more like blood would be in the lungs. A modified form of the Gibbon machine would actually be used with the greatest success by John Kirklin at the Mayo Clinic. In fact, there are so many men on the honor roll of contributors to cardiopulmonary bypass that the list is very long as well as international: Brukhonenko, Jongbloed, Dennis, Crafoord, Björk, Kirklin, Glenn, Senning, Dogliotti, Dodrill, DeBakey, Lillehei, Melrose, Gerbode, Kay, Cross, Effler, and so on. To concentrate on a few is to neglect the many, but otherwise interest would be diffused in a welter of names and places, a confusion of credits, even a rivalry of claims. It is only possible to highlight a few steps in the progression of events.

Take the adventurousness and scientific thoroughness of the young British Oxford graduate, Dennis Melrose, the genius of a peripatetic Dutchman, Willem Kolff, and the skill and imagination of surgeon Donald Effler at the Cleveland Clinic in the early days.

In England, shortly after Gibbon's success, Melrose immediately recognized its importance. He went to Sweden, where Crafoord and his associates had designed a revolving-drum oxygenator for a heart-lung machine. Stainless steel discs inside a transparent plastic container collected the blood and squeezed it through a circuit while oxygen was blown against the flow. Also in Sweden, Viking Olaf Björk was keeping animal brains functioning up to thirty-three minutes using a disc oxygenator while cutting off circulation through the heart by clamping off the venous flow of blood into the right side of the heart.

After returning to Hammersmith in England, Melrose designed an extracorporeal pump-oxygenator that was an improvement on Gibbon's. At the same time he began experiments to stop or slow hearts in animals by injecting potassium citrate. The Melrose machine was acknowledged to be a beautiful piece of precision engineering. It utilized a rotating plastic cylinder packed with seventy-six discs, which reduced the amount of blood needed to prime it. The question of whether it would work was solved by clinical trial at the Hammersmith Hospital. After a few successes with it the hospital established a surgical team led by William Cleland to operate on open hearts, but the time limit was still severe and only defects requiring very little time to repair could be tackled.

Melrose's laboratory staff was beginning to succeed in keeping animal hearts in a limp, flaccid state, almost at a standstill, for fifteen minutes by the injection of potassium citrate. This made the hearts less difficult to work on than while they were contracting at seventy or more times a minute. It also expedited the evacuation of air before closing the incision, obviating the persistent danger of air locks and brain damage.

Dr. Willem Kolff was at the Hammersmith Hospital during the Melrose laboratory experiments. He was the extraordinary man who had built the first crude kidney dialysis machine during World War II while the Germans were occupying his native Holland. A tall man with a huge head, he had a combination of a medical mind and that of a bioengineer. He believed that most parts of the body could eventually be fabricated in the laboratory. After constructing an artificial kidney out of a few bits of metal, sausage skins, and a beer barrel, he was certain that the principle on which it operated was correct. Rather than let the Nazis even know about it, he persuaded some escapees to smuggle it out of Holland to the Hammersmith Hospital in London. After the war he emigrated to London. When he accepted an appointment in Cleveland, Ohio, and left England in the 1950s, he bequeathed his historic jerry-constructed kidney machine prototype, beer barrel and all, to the Hammersmith as a museum piece.

He had also sent one of his machines to the Peter Bent Brigham in Boston where the medical and engineering genius of Dr. Carl Walter recast it into a therapeutic triumph. This would lead from dialysis to the first kidney transplant by Charles Hufnagel and his colleagues, and on to the first successful kidney transplant at the Brigham.

In Cleveland Kolff and surgeon Donald Effler began laboratory experiments with a Melrose-type heart-lung machine. Kolff, with his habitual frugality and extraordinary talent for using materials at hand, constructed his machine at the Cleveland Clinic with its core of tin can wrapped in twenty-two feet of plastic tubing, a plastic refrigerator in its jacket, and a small pump. It cost pennies in contrast to the few expensive machines used else-where. He and Effler also experimented with potassium citrate injections to achieve quiet hearts in open-heart surgery. In February 1956 Effler was ready for clinical trial using Kolff's machine and the potassium citrate solution, which by this time was also in experimental use at Hammersmith.

Before the first operation in Cleveland Kolff telephoned Melrose in England and the two men talked for half an hour about their methods. On Melrose's advice, relayed by Kolff, Effler gave himself a limit of fifteen minutes' working time in the heart. The first patient was a seventeen-month-old boy with a septal defect. The child was connected to the machine, and as soon as the heart was exposed, Kolff switched it on. A syringe was ready with potassium citrate, diluted with blood treated with an anticlogging agent. The needle was skirted to prevent its penetrating too deeply. The solution had to be perfectly placed. The child's aorta was drawn forward and clamped. Effler pierced it with the needle and emptied the contents of the syringe. The small heart began to pulse more slowly. Then the two pumping chambers, the ventricles, stopped, the auricles arrested until only the tip of the right auricle was still quivering. The heart seemed to lie dead in its niche. Effler placed retaining sutures to hold it open and made his incision. Normally the hole in the septum between the ventricles would have gaped; now it lay flaccid, like a frayed buttonhole in the stilled heart. In addition to making the vital repair, the surgeons had time to inspect the pulmonary valve and upper heart chambers before closing. Thirteen minutes. Now, would the heart start up and take over again?

The clamp was released. Blood washed the potassium mixture out of the coronary arteries and heart muscle. The heart began to move. In a few seconds it was beating steadily. Fourteen days later the patient was playing vigorously on the ward.

After a run of seventy-three such "stopped-heart" operations in the next fifteen months, with only reasonable mortality, Effler reported that the series had established "the safety and benefits provided by the Melrose technique of elective cardiac arrest, justifying its use in surgery on the open heart."

Writing his own epitaph recently for the Founders Group

list, Donald Effler said of himself, "The S.O.B. had enough talent to do a given operation well and was smart enough to reduce it to its simplest form." That was by no means a modest boast, though it sounds so to the layman. It is a basic standard for great surgeons and was very much deserved by Master Surgeon Effler.

Most of Effler's seventy-three patients were children. Children were not only the most heart-rending victims of cardiac defects, but the most amenable to the developing open-heart procedures. Congenital anomalies, with which a baby was born and which so often forecast poor and short life, could often be corrected, though the risk of *doing* was always to be balanced against the risk of *not doing.* Furthermore children recovered more readily from trauma than adults. Following open-heart operations, they also suffered far less from the emotional sequelae that might plague adults who had open-heart surgery. Many surgeons would find their small patients not only the most touching and appealing but also the most rewarding. In cardiac surgery Robert Gross at Children's Hospital in Boston, Conrad Lam in Detroit, and Walton Lillehei in Minneapolis were among the American surgeons who would contribute brilliantly to surgery on children with congenital defects.

At Hammersmith by 1959 the Cleland surgical team had had a series of successes with children and their fame spread to the U.S.S.R., where nothing had yet been done outside the laboratory on cardiac bypass. The Russians sent to London for a Melrose machine. It arrived, but the Soviet doctors reported that the machine did not work. Technicians from Hammersmith flew to Moscow to check, but found nothing wrong with it and left. The Russians still could not seem to make it work properly. A request followed—unequaled from that country's defensive, closed medical society since Peter the Great brought in an anatomical museum from Holland. The British surgical team was asked to come to Moscow and bring with them a complete surgical setup to demonstrate bypass surgery.

Surgeon William Cleland took with him Dennis Melrose, surgeon Hugh Bentall, anesthetist John Beard, cardiologist Arthur Holland, technician John Robson, plus Cleland's favorite scrub nurse. The team was uneasy. A death would be mortifying.

How poor would the selection of patients offered to them be?
How many would be hopeless risks? Suppose they lost a Soviet
child?

Dozens of young patients waited at the Moscow Institute of
Thoracic Surgery. With infinite care, the team from Hammersmith chose four.

The first one on whom they operated was a quiet little six-
year-old girl, born a blue baby. The Blalock-Taussig operation for
her condition, tetralogy of Fallot, was only palliative. With direct-
vision intracardiac surgery, she could be cured. The risk of doing
was directly related to the risk of not doing. The observation
gallery was crammed with surgeons from all the Soviet centers. A
few specialists from the Moscow Institute were on the operating
floor with the British team. With them, by extraordinary permission from the Kremlin, was a photographer from Tass to record
the proceedings.

Those in the gallery of onlookers gasped and murmured as
Cleland picked up his syringe of blood and potassium solution.
Inserting the short needle into the base of the aorta, he forcibly
injected the potassium citrate solution. As he did so, the heart
action flagged, then ceased. Cleland incised the right ventricle and assistants retracted the open heart walls. The septal
defect came into view. Through this had shunted the blood stolen
from the body that had damaged the lungs by its extreme pressure and volume. An obstructing muscular ring or band had to be
resected, the hole between the two chambers of the heart sewn
up, and then the right ventricular wall sutured. Nothing could be
hurried for fear sutures might damage the aortic valve or the con-
ducting system of the heart during the maximum half hour allowed for the critical work.

After the reconstruction was completed, the clamp on the artery was released; the patient's heart hesitated briefly, as did the
hearts of the Hammersmith team. Then, as blood washed out the
arresting chemicals, the heart began to beat slowly, taking over
from the Melrose pump-oxygenator. Within two or three minutes
it was beating strongly. The child's chest was closed and she was
wheeled out of the theatre receiving oxygen. Surgeons throughout the world sighed with relief when the news came. The

Melrose machine was tricky, but that team could make it work as no other could.

For two days the little girl's body showed the stress and strain before she began to get better. A week later she said joyfully to her doctors, "I shall dance! I say it to myself every minute. I shall be able to dance!"

Four successes brought the Hammersmith team well-deserved official acclaim and a surfeit of Russian hospitality. Moscow was now added to the list of cities where open-heart surgical centers were being established.

The heart-lung bypass machine posed considerable danger to patients. Safe oxygenation of the blood remained a problem, and so did damage to the blood from its contact with artificial surfaces. No other surface was as kind to blood as the body's natural vessel linings. Contact with other surfaces broke down red blood cells, precipitating microemboli that could damage the brain. The next important development was called the low-flow theory—that the body could be supported on much less blood than was considered necessary as measured by normal flow.

Anthony Andreasen, a British surgeon, believed that open-heart surgery could be performed using one heart to do the work of two. He had thought a great deal about the possibility of open-heart surgery since, as a medical student, he had been impressed by Alexis Carrel's work and theories. As a doctor with the Indian Medical Service between 1933 and 1947, he set up laboratories to experiment with blood circulation. Then as a surgeon with the Indian army during World War II and as professor of surgery at the medical college in Calcutta during the sanguinary civil war after India's partition, he observed many severe heart injuries. He noted that men survived hemorrhages that left them with very little blood, which supported his theory that one heart might support two human bodies.

After India gained its independence, Andreasen went to the United States, but got little attention. He then went to England where the Royal College of Surgeons gave him a £400 grant in 1950 to work in a small laboratory for animal experimentation at Downe, Kent, near the laboratory where the team from the Hammersmith Hospital was devising its heart-lung machine. Andreasen had an assistant, technician Frank Watson, who was remarkably ingenious at contriving apparatus out of bits and pieces—what medical reporter Hugh McLeave described as "string-and-sealing-wax" work. Envious of the Hammersmith team's liberal resources, Andreasen applied to the Medical Research Council for more money. The Council sent a representative down to talk to the two men, but according to Andreasen, he spent seven minutes in the laboratory and not much more time listening. His answer to their application was "No," and when he was asked why, he said, "The day of the individual experimenter is over. It is teams of experts now."

Andreasen went ahead, somehow, experimenting to see whether low blood flow would maintain life without injury to organs, and discovered he could keep animals alive on a flow between a tenth and a seventh of normal. He published his results, but almost the only man who paid the paper serious attention was a surgeon from Minneapolis, C. Walton Lillehei, who flew over to see for himself. Shortly thereafter a discouraged Andreasen gave up for lack of funds and, at the age of forty-eight, went out to Africa to organize medical services for a mining company in Sierra Leone. Later, when he was with the medical service in Ghana, he saw in a magazine pictures of an operation using his cross-circulation technique. It was Lillehei who became embroiled in the controversy that surrounded that method of saving lives.

C. Walton Lillehei is credited in the Founders Group list as "creator and innovator of perhaps more techniques and concepts than any other living heart surgeon." He was one of a number of creative surgeons to emerge from the Department of Surgery in Minneapolis while it was under the aegis of Dr. Owen Wangensteen. Wangensteen would call himself the "water boy" to his "geniuses," who also included Norman Shumway and Christiaan Barnard, who became famous for heart transplantation.

Wangensteen was made professor and chief of surgery at the Minnesota University Hospital in Minneapolis in 1930, when Walt Lillehei was a twelve-year-old boy displaying his technical dexterity by disassembling and reassembling his father's Model

T Ford. The position had been turned down by two chosen candidates, one recommended by Harvey Cushing at the Brigham in Boston and one sent from Johns Hopkins. Both men thought Minneapolis was "nowhere" and that nothing much was likely to go on there. Owen Wangensteen, who showed the men around, was unable to infect them with his own love for the desolate beauty of the surrounding countryside or impress them with the vitality of the northern city or persuade them that the research department there was capable of fine work, since it had been revitalized by George Vincent, president of the university between 1911 and 1917. In the end, "for want of a better," the Board of Regents at the university appointed Owen Wangensteen to the position.

Wangensteen insisted from the first that all his surgeons participate in laboratory research. He believed in interdisciplinary education for students, staff members, and interns and instituted a series of conferences with physiologist Maurice Visscher, who had worked in London with the famous Ernest Starling in 1904 and 1905. (Starling was the man who had pronounced the "law of the heart," which essentially states that the more the heart fills, the more it distends, and, until it goes into failure, the more energy it takes to contract. That landmark in comprehending heart function seemed remarkably simple and obvious once it was propounded, as would many stunning original theories.) When he was over eighty, and still active, in 1977, Owen Wangensteen would say, "Those conferences with Maurice Visscher were really the basis of what would go on."

Not long after his appointment in the mid-1930s, the Board of Regents regretted having chosen so feisty and independent a chief. Wangensteen had hired another man for his staff and garnisheed the salaries of the attending physicians who practiced in the city to pay him. In the brouhaha that followed, Wangensteen was nearly fired. He was sufficiently intimidated to refuse another young man who applied for an appointment, although he recognized the applicant's unusual potential. The rejected applicant, who had been born in Duluth, Minnesota, returned to Boston, where he had graduated from Harvard Medical School and interned at the Massachusetts General Hospital. His name was Robert Gross.

The year 1945, just after the war, was another bad time for taking a new man on. Nevertheless when C. Walton Lillehei applied to Wangensteen for an appointment, the chief of surgery just said to him, "Well, we'll find some money for you—don't know where," and to his secretary, "Get Walt a white coat."

Lillehei, like Harken, was a man distinguished by two outstanding personal characteristics aside from his genius. His energy was abnormal, almost superhuman, and his concern for patients was profound. Unlike Harken, Lillehei, even during the later years when he practiced in New York and was a world-renowned figure, continued to consider the Midwest his home. Born in Minneapolis of Norwegian stock, he was christened Clarence for his father, a dentist who practiced in the city for fifty years, and Walton, which was his mother's maiden name. The Clarence was reduced to a first initial and he was called Walt. His Minneapolis high school teacher predicted that if Walt Lillehei went to medical school, he would not last six weeks, but C. Walton and his brothers, James P. and Richard C. Lillehei, all became famous doctors. After graduating from the University of Minnesota's medical school in three years instead of four, Walt Lillehei interned at the Minneapolis General Hospital, and obtained an appointment to the London School of Hygiene and Tropical Medicine.

Pearl Harbor precipitated him into the U.S. Army Medical Corps as a first lieutenant, and he made the initial landing in North Africa attached to an armored infantry unit. Of his experience in the war he would write:

> The mobile desert warfare that followed demonstrated the complete inadequacy of the medical setup in those prehelicopter days, with critically wounded soldiers often spending twelve to twenty-four hours without medical treatment in an ambulance bounding across a roadless desert to reach the nearest surgical hospital. Consequently the ambulance en route frequently became a hearse.
>
> This situation was too disastrous to be tolerable. As a Clearing Company Commander by then in Tunisia, I helped improvise the first mobile surgical units on the spot with borrowed and scrounged equipment, and with surgical teams on temporary assignment from the rear area hospitals. The subsequent moun-

tainous terrain of Sicily and Italy reinforced the necessity of this concept. By Anzio this temporary setup was finally formalized, and by the time the war ended in Italy, I had received the Bronze Star and had attained the rank of Lt. Colonel as Commanding Officer of the 33rd Field Hospital.

When he returned to Minneapolis and Wangensteen took him on as a resident, Lillehei plunged into laboratory as well as clinical work at his chief's instigation. Even if they did not achieve any specific goal, Wangensteen felt his men would be better judges of all research for this exposure. Wangensteen was also unimpressed by arbitrary limitations imposed by conventional thinking. He believed that if you brought enough attention to a problem, and were not concerned about whether it was supposed to be possible or impossible, you might solve it. According to Richard Varco, another impressive cardiac surgeon at the Minneapolis Hospital, Wangensteen improved on the oft-quoted dictum pronounced by John Hunter in the eighteenth century. Edward Jenner had come to Hunter and told him he *thought* cowpox inoculations could eliminate the scourge of smallpox. Hunter said, "Don't think! Do the experiment." Wangensteen's revision was "Do the experiment. And do think!"

In 1950 the Variety Clubs of Minnesota, that state's branch of the worldwide organization of entertainers and media people, noting the prevalence of heart attacks among their members, offered the University of Minnesota $1.5 million to build a heart hospital. It would be the first medical institution in the world devoted exclusively to the heart. The Board of Regents turned the offer down. Medical fragmentation was already alarming the establishment. What if future bequests were offered for other single organs? A rumor began to spread, most probably instigated by the Machiavellian Wangensteen, that the Variety Clubs would give the hospital to the Mayo Clinic instead, and long-time rivalry reversed the Regents' decision. In July 1951 the Variety Club Heart Hospital opened, connected to the University Hospital buildings by ramps and tunnels. Part of the deal was to provide extensive laboratory research on heart disease. There were eighty beds in the Heart Hospital, forty for adults and forty for children.

Only four to six were designated surgical beds since there was very little cardiac surgery of any kind at the time.

Wangensteen's own absorbing interest was cancer research and surgery for cancer. He had done some pericardial surgery such as Churchill's, and had performed the first patent ductus arteriosus closure, Gross's operation, in Minnesota, but "that's as near to being a cardiac surgeon as I ever came," he would say.

His protégé, Walt Lillehei, had meantime obtained his master's in physiology under Visscher and become Visscher's assistant in the physiology research laboratory. Visscher set Lillehei to work on the problem of producing heart failure in dogs so that what happened to the important kidney function could be studied. These animal experiments would later win for Lillehei the Theobald Smith Award given by the American Association for the Advancement of Science, but before he could complete them he was diagnosed by the pathologists at the Minneapolis Hospital as suffering from lymphosarcoma. Dr. Wangensteen sent biopsy slides to pathologists at the Mayo Clinic and at the Sloan-Kettering Institute in New York. They confirmed the first reports and Lillehei was given only a 5 to 10 percent chance to live for a maximum of five more years. He opted for drastic surgery to be performed the day after he completed his senior residency.

Dr. Wangensteen, ever an apostle of the impossible, headed one of the three surgical teams who removed a record amount of malignant tissue, one team for the head, one for the neck, and one for the chest. Although in the nature of the miraculous, Lillehei's recovery was slow. He himself insisted on radiation follow-up treatment, although there was no evidence of spread. The experience taught him to delegate duties to others when possible and, he said, "I probably remember a little bit better than others to cut the penicillin injections from four to two a day as soon as possible." It may have added to the dimension of his concern for patients, at whose postoperative bedsides he would spend so many all-night vigils.

After completing his senior residency and his doctorate in the clinical science of surgery, Lillehei was offered and accepted an assistant professorship under Wangensteen. "We're making out our schedule of special interests, Walt," said Wangensteen.

"What shall I put down for you?" "Open-heart surgery," said Lillehei. "Good old Wangensteen," Lillehei would comment in 1977. "He didn't bat an eye. I think any other professor or chairman of a department would have said, 'Are you crazy? Never been one done.' He just put it down."

The only residue from his operation was that, for the rest of his life, Lillehei would look as if an exact copy of his former self had slipped slightly in reproduction. The lines of his upper body and neck were what artists call "out of drawing"—not deformed but somewhat awry. The piquant oval face and bright green eyes, which narrowed when he was concerned, did not change.

After Lillehei returned from his trip to England to see Andreasen he was very excited by the low-flow theory. By accident he discovered the very important fact that laboratory animals survived when the inferior vena cava was clamped off if just the tiny azygos vein was left open. "We weren't paying much attention, really," said Lillehei, but when they found out that anesthetized animals stayed alive on the flow from the azygos vein alone and awakened with no pathology, no brain or other organ damage, research was galvanized. To measure that flow in the first days, Lillehei used that every-handy rubber sack, the condom, to collect the blood. An amount of only 15 percent of normal was proving sufficient to sustain life. "Everything" hitherto had pointed to one hundred cubic centimeters a minute per kilogram of body weight as minimal to sustain bodies engaged in no activity at normal temperatures.

When Lillehei proposed that it might be possible to use one heart to temporarily sustain two bodies, even Clarence Dennis, the first man to use a pump-oxygenator on human beings, thought, said Lillehei, "I was some kind of nut."

Claude Beck, in Ohio, had suggested the idea of cross circulation earlier, and proposed that another pair of lungs would provide a good oxygenator, but nobody, including Lillehei, yet envisioned cross circulation between humans. Human donor hearts were not expendable. Laboratory dogs' were. In the Minneapolis laboratory dogs were paired: donor-dog and patient-dog. At first, efforts to connect them to each other were often fatal. The connecting tubes frequently got displaced, destroying the patient-dog's lungs in about thirty seconds. Lillehei and his cohorts learned to use the groin for donor-dog linkage, instead of the crowded area around the heart. In the groin the dogs' blood vessels, as in humans, were very close to the skin surface so that a small incision would do. Cannulations could be kept away from the immediate area on which the surgeon wanted to operate.

As it was improved, the method proved to be extraordinarily simple. The venae cavae of the patient-dog were occluded so that no blood went to the heart. A pump with one motor and rotating parts pumped first to one side, then to the other, regulating the blood that passed between the dogs so that the same amount went each way. Otherwise one animal got all the blood and the other went into shock. With the small amount needed—measured by the azygos flow, fifteen to twenty cubic centimeters per kilogram—going through the donor-dog's lungs for oxygenation and returning to the patient-dog, the patient-dog's body was perfused while its heart was empty and dry. The surgeon could work in the empty heart.

Not only did donor heart and lungs constitute the perfect machine for oxygenation, but all the homeostatic (body-stabilizing) mechanisms were preserved. The body needs, for the liver, pancreas, the endocrine organs, acid base and electrolyte balance—about which too little was then known—were automatically guarded. Healthy dogs with a basic metabolism similar to that of human beings, but even more delicate, began to show survival rates dramatically higher than those reported at medical meetings for humans who had been on the heart-lung machines.

In fact, except for hypothermia, open-heart surgery had come almost to a standstill because the mortality rate was too high. There was general pessimism and most medical practitioners had succumbed to the "sick heart syndrome," believing that open-heart surgery would always be limited to simple defects requiring only brief surgical procedures. Patients in whom radical surgery was justified were already ravaged with congestive heart failure and they were unlikely to survive major procedures. Pioneers who refused to accept such limitations, men like Jongbloed in Utrecht, Björk in Stockholm, Kay, Dodrill, Dennis, were castigated.

"Of course," Lillehei would say reminiscently, "we didn't

know but what the others were right! But we began to think that with cross circulation we could possibly close a ventricular septal defect, a hopeless lesion to repair at that time by any available means. Still we made a conscious attempt not to broadcast what we were doing very widely, but eventually you have to get the interest and cooperation of pediatric cardiologists to try."

The laboratory workers in Minneapolis asked the residents and pathologists to call Lillehei or an associate every time a child or infant died of congenital heart disease. They cooperated to provide fresh young hearts from the cadavers immediately after death. These were very different from ones that had already been fixed in formalin; the latter were discolored and like shoe leather that had been out in the rain and dried. The surgeons performed surgical cardiotomies instead of autopsies on these hearts, which gave them limited but extremely important experience. "Does give you a false idea how easy it is sometimes," Lillehei would say, "but anyway, it gave us confidence." He felt the time had come for clinical trial on congenital defects in young hopeless patients.

Two pediatric cardiologists, Ray Anderson and Paul Adams, were invited to investigate what was going on in the laboratory. They were so impressed that they agreed to watch for suitable patients who would otherwise die of conditions that could not be corrected by available procedures. Children in heart crisis at this time were treated medically and sent home. They almost invariably returned in short order. Those in heart failure were given digitalis, but rarely lived long if the failure persisted because, despite antibiotics, they often developed pneumonia and died of it. In March 1954 a two-year-old patient of Dr. Anderson's came in for the fifth time. He was clearly going to die. Lillehei went with Dr. Anderson to see his family. For the child, the risk was more than justified. The worrisome moral issue was that of jeopardizing a perfectly healthy donor, whose heart would operate as the bypass mechanism while the child's heart was open. There were risks to such a donor including a chance of air embolism. A possible exchange of imperfectly matched blood in some of the less understood subtypes and antibodies was a concern. The first-class blood bank man at the hospital would minimize the chance of such blood incompatibility, though to some it seemed serious. There was even a slight risk involved in administering light general anesthesia, thought best for the donor, although the groin cannulation could be done under local anesthesia.

One parent of a child usually proved to have matching blood. Both parents of the two-year-old boy brushed aside the risks to themselves and had their blood analyzed. The father proved to be the match. His heart was in perfect condition, which qualified him. He was happy to give his son, who had been so ill during his short life, any chance he could.

Wangensteen gave his enthusiastic consent to the experiment. The research was sound. The time had come. In fact, he spunkily suggested that Lillehei and surgeon Richard Varco, second senior man on the team, work up several cases before trying the first in case the first one failed and such efforts might be forbidden. Word did leak out and opposition mounted. Take a healthy human being and subject him to trauma for such a venture into the unknown? A harebrained scheme, declared the superintendent of the hospital, who was a potent figure. Lillehei was afraid that the operation would be canceled. The night before it was scheduled he left a note on Wangensteen's desk asking for final confirmation and consent. In the morning the answer was delivered to Lillehei. "By all means! Go ahead! O.W."

The surgical team, Lillehei, Varco, Warden, and Cohen, connected father and son. The pump was started. Through arteries and veins, the father's blood circulated through his son's body for twelve and a half minutes, the donor's heart, lungs, and homeostatic mechanisms taking over. The surgeons opened the right side of the child's heart, exposed the hole, and closed it with sutures. The heart improved immediately and took over. The method worked. Unhappily, the child's body, so long sapped of strength, could not resist pneumonia, which struck on the eleventh day after the operation. The father of the first child never regretted his effort to save him, even after the child died.

Wangensteen had been wise. Two other cases had been worked up and both of these were triumphs. In one an atrioventricular canal was repaired, an area that had previously been inoperable. Lillehei and his team were justified, and on August 31,

1954, they decided to tackle a blue baby. They knew this would cause additional controversy. The Blalock-Taussig operation was widely used and mortality following the procedure had become very low indeed. That operation, which added another defect to the congenital four, was marvelously palliative, but not curative. The Minnesotans thought they could surgically correct, and thus cure, the four classic defects of tetralogy of Fallot, and that the resultant return of the circulation to the normal physiologic state was a much better concept.

At the moment when the donor was hooked in, the heart chambers of the eleven-year-old victim of tetralogy on whom they hoped to operate faltered and stopped. Without waiting to try manual systole, Lillehei ordered, "Start the pump!" The donor heart took over for the patient's. The surgeons closed the hole and stretched the fused pulmonary valve. The patient's heart took over again. Fourteen days later the boy left the hospital. On his follow-up visits he told his doctors how much he enjoyed playing baseball for the first time in his life.

"It's true," Lillehei would admit, "that of our first ten operations for tetralogy of Fallot, four died. That was three times worse than the Blalock procedure at the time, but we were sure—and said so at several national meetings—that it was nevertheless a much better concept, which it would turn out eventually to be."

The Minnesota team took movies and prepared a report on forty-five operations using cross circulation for presentation to the First International Symposium on Cardiac Surgery in Detroit in 1953. Just before their turn came, Willis Potts, a pediatric surgeon, delivered a scholarly dissertation on an excellent modification of the palliative Blalock-Taussig operation for blue babies. Next came the color motion pictures of operations on ventricular septal defects and tetralogy of Fallot in open hearts while the patient circulation was maintained by the donor, an adult who was usually a parent. They were awesome, and clearly demonstrated the successful use of cross circulation. Excitement and some dismay rippled through the hall of assembled surgeons, so many of whom would again be present in 1975 at the Second International Symposium in Detroit. Willis Potts ran down the aisle, showing, said Harken, "a laudable spirit of fair play, intellectual honesty and sportsmanship combined with his wonderful sense of humor. Potts called out, 'Does anyone here remember an old operation called the Potts procedure for blue babies?' "

Cross circulation as a means of bypass for open-heart surgery had a very brief day. Evidence in favor of it was conclusive. Survival rates were high and blood damage minimal, but not only was the method difficult to organize, it was subjected to constant ethical criticism. John Gibbon protested at the American Association for Thoracic Surgery in Montreal, "We are still convinced that it is preferable to perform operations without involving another healthy person. There must always be some risk to the donor!" And if the donor was a parent, the moralists asked, what choice did he or she have in the face of parental obligation? It was really a no-choice situation.

Lillehei was sued for half a million dollars by the mother of a child who lived as the result of the operation; the donor-mother, however, suffered temporary paralysis. She outgrew it and the case was dismissed, but a lawsuit for such a sum, "a whole lot of money then," commented Wangensteen, created a very wary atmosphere. The team in Minneapolis, along with many others, turned their attention to improving the heart-lung machine.

The next major evolutionary step in heart surgery was the bubble oxygenator and a cheap, efficient, cleanable machine. This was developed in Minneapolis by Walton Lillehei and an unlikely young general practitioner named Richard Dewall.

Dewall had been in private practice in Minneapolis but had ambitions to go into surgery and into laboratory work. He kept turning up at the Variety Club Heart Hospital and in the face of his persistence Wangensteen had trouble saying no to him. Also, Lillehei needed another man in the operating room during cross-circulation procedures. Two members of his team had to concentrate on the donor, and if anything went wrong, the donor had to be saved even at the expense of the patient. The anesthetist could not "float" because he manned both the anesthesia and the pump. Dewall began arriving for procedures to take over the pump, and Wangensteen hired him.

Lillehei was already working on an improved heart-lung machine to replace the controversial cross-circulation technique.

Low-flow had gained some support but would later seem more an ingenious and interesting effort than a historical step in the cardiac surgery story. Lillehei did not agree with established authority that oxygenation by bubbling and debubbling was impractical. He was not convinced that the bubbles could not be removed to the point where nothing would be left that would prove injurious to the brain and other vital organs.

In the nineteenth century physiologists had succeeded in perfusing isolated organs with oxygenated blood. They had oxygenated blood by bubbling air through it and had studied its oxygen uptake. In the 1950s Juro Wada, a Japanese visitor at Boston City Hospital as a research worker, had experimented on rats. He bubbled their blood with oxygen, thus saturating it, and then debubbled it, but at the time no one appreciated the great significance this experiment would one day have for cardiopulmonary bypass. Isolated organs were one thing. The heart, which sent blood everywhere in the body, was another. Getting *all* the bubbles out was the major problem.

Lillehei remembered saying to Richard Dewall, who was proving to be a very innovative fellow, "Well, listen, Dick, we've got this idea about a bubble oxygenator. Easy to get 'em in, but we've got to get 'em all out. I've just heard of a new substance called silicone or antifoam. Corning Antifoam. They're using it for pumping milk and making cream in some dairies. Seems you just add a minute amount and it dissipates all the foam."

Dewall took over research on Corning Antifoam in connection with bubbling and debubbling blood. The substance seemed to be totally inert, and when ingested in the minute quantities used to make cream, had no discernible effect on human bodies.

"Turned out the stuff reduced surface tension of any fluid, and sure enough, it worked out very well in blood, but it didn't entirely solve our problems," said Lillehei.

Together Lillehei and Dewall designed and constructed a reservoir made out of a coil, a disposable piece of plastic tubing that eliminated complex difficulties in cleaning heart-lung machines between uses. The blood with antifoam was run through a helix type of spiral. "A simple thing, a bunch of tubing, a few needles and clamps, and a bottle of oxygen," said Lillehei. "We started using it in March 1955."

At first the patients the team chose were the ones smallest in size. "We were feeling our way along as far as flow was concerned. For patients whom we thought were too big for those first of our bubble oxygenator heart-lung machines, we used dogs' lungs. About fifteen times in all.

"That worked very well, actually, but it was very tricky. After about thirty minutes the dog's lung would start to fill up with fluid and then you'd be in trouble—the patient wouldn't be oxygenated. We never used chimps. Dogs were fine. But you had to get all the dog blood out first because mixing dog and human blood would be a disaster. We just washed the dog blood out with saline—it would go right through the blood vessel wall into the air spaces. Then we used dextran in great quantity to wash the dog's lungs. You'd be amazed what a country dog's lung looked like when washed. Absolutely chalk white! It's not the same with city dogs. We'd get our dog's lungs so absolutely white we knew they were free of blood and we could use the dog for thirty or maybe forty-five minutes. Then the lung would begin to fill with fluid, so we were working against the clock and we didn't like that.

"Then we got more experience with our heart-lung machine and it worked for all sizes of people. It was so simple and extremely effective. We got the thing fabricated in a unified way so it could be made by a company, sterilized, and shipped out. The surgeon didn't even have to set up the tubing.

"In 1957 we began working on the mitral valve. That was again rather controversial because Bailey and Harken had made so much progress with mitral stenosis, but they couldn't do anything about insufficiency, so we started working on that. Then came the sheet oxygenator, prefabricated. Hang it on a scale so you could tell the amount of blood out of the body and then throw it away after the operation. That was a tremendous step forward because one of the problems responsible for early mortality was that you simply couldn't clean all that stuff adequately in the machine, get the blood protein off, and sterilize by cold solution as opposed to heat. Some of the material in those other pumps had direct contact with the blood and were damaging it a lot."

Efficient, cheap, and disposable equipment for cardiopulmonary bypass would make possible the great evolutionary years of open-heart surgery. The idea that the "sick human heart" was inoperable would be essentially dispelled. More and more would be learned about the body and the blood, about heart block, heart assist, monitoring for the hitherto uncontrolled electrolyte and acid base balance. The anatomic and pathologic variations in congenital and acquired heart defects would be diagnosed and classified. Risks taken by the pioneers would be found justified by those who followed more safely behind them.

C. Walton Lillehei remained front and center among the pioneers, and hence a target for critics of each development. His list of credits extended to the development of the simple disposable membrane oxygenator with Lande in 1967 and the development of numerous artificial valves for total replacement in mitral and aortic positions. He also developed, with Bakken, a miniaturized transistorized electrical pacemaker in 1957. The final tribute to him in the Founders Group list is that he "made possible the extension of the opportunities afforded him by Wangensteen to his own illustrious disciples, including Shumway, Gott, Barnard, and others."

It seemed extraordinarily tragic to Harken and others among his friends and admirers when a conviction for income tax evasion tumbled him from the reluctant regard of envious men. The state of Minnesota revoked Lillehei's license to practice for a year. New York State, where he had gone as Lewis Atterbury Stimson Professor of Surgery at the Cornell Medical School, refused to condemn him, but his career was interrupted. Many colleagues considered him to have been a "crook" and he was replaced on the faculty at the University of Minnesota.

"I don't know," said Wangensteen, a loyal and mighty defender of his own, who testified for him at the trial. "The amount the university accrued in time may have been a lot. Walt went to lawyers and was advised to sue. After all, it was in their interest! He suffered greatly and people should forget about it. New York didn't discipline him, but the self-righteous Scandinavians here did. Walt was probably the most productive intracardiac surgeon of our generation."

Lillehei continued to live in St. Paul, and to travel from there to lecture all over the world. His brother James remained in practice and his brother Richard became internationally known as a shock expert. As his high forehead gathered additional wrinkles, Walt Lillehei kept his zest and his green eyes grew greener when he said, in 1978, "Ninety-eight percent of open-heart surgery is still done with bubble oxygenators, although we and others have done a lot by now on membrane oxygenators."

Bubble oxygenators were in dominant use as late as 1979, but further experiments with membrane oxygenators were indicating that they were safer. The advantages were not altogether clear, but presumably there was less drying of the blood, less precipitation of infinitesimal particles, and less trauma. The membrane obviated direct interface with the wet blood and the atmosphere, just as the membranes of the lungs provide a wall through which carbon dioxide can escape and oxygen enter without direct contact.

The membrane oxygenator was still in a stage of complexity, which would in time be reduced, just as the bubble oxygenator had been steadily improved. The debt heart surgery owed to C. Walton Lillehei for his years of work on bypass machines, on devices, on procedures, and as a surgical theorist and thinker, was overwhelming. He, in turn, credits his boss, Owen Wangensteen, and his close associates in Minneapolis for the atmosphere, time, and encouragement that permitted him to make his contributions.

10.

Replaceable Parts for the Pump

In the early days machines to bypass the heart and lungs took such a morass of tubes, wires, and apparatus that an operating theatre resembled a combination of a disorderly laboratory and an automobile repair shop. There was so much noise that in Harken's OR a supernumerary sat on a high stool signaling the execution of procedures by numbers. A British open-heart team used earphones. Even after many years of steady improvement, heart-lung machines would remain no smaller than a coffin, although the racket they made was reduced to little more than a pot makes on the boil. Since these substitutes for human function remained outside the body and could be easily repaired, size and durability were not vital.

Replacing parts inside the body was another matter. The heart's small valves, for instance, were inimitably efficient when they functioned normally. They opened and closed as the heart - beat the eighty times a minute, forty million times a year, or roughly three billion times, give or take a few million, during the Biblical three score years and ten.

When in September 1952, following years of research, Charles Hufnagel in Washington, D.C., implanted in a patient a self-contained prosthetic artificial ball valve outside the heart, below the subclavian artery in the descending aorta, it was a

Turning Point. This was the first successful artificial valve implantation in a human being. The patient had severe aortic incompetence, and this valve assisted circulation by significantly lessening the flow work load for the heart with its leaking valve.

For a while it was the best solution available, but Hufnagel had few emulators. The operation was too complicated, too limited therapeutically, and another glaring defect was the noise the implanted valve made. Placed as they were, the early Hufnagel valves made patients who lived with them in their chests sound like Captain Hook's nemesis, the crocodile who had swallowed an alarm clock. They could be heard across rooms and through doors and could hear themselves eighty times a minute, tick-tocking away. It was the aural equivalent of Chinese water torture. There were suicides.

Furthermore it was found that these valves were somewhat thrombogenic, but this took time to discover, as the valve was placed beyond the arch of the aorta from which arise those arteries supplying the brain. Hufnagel implanted many of these between 1950 and 1960 and many of his patients seemed much improved. In six of his early patients Hufnagel valves would continue to function for from fifteen to twenty-three years with "continuing benefit," a tribute to the valves' durability.

They were not installed, of course, inside the heart, so this was extracardiac, not intracardiac, surgery. In terms of the heart area, measured in millimeters, valves in the aorta, rather than in the natural location, were very far away. The valve reduced the reflux (regurgitation) and thus lowered flow work to the left ventricle. It did not reduce pressure work, sending blood to the body, and it is pressure work that requires more energy, more oxygen, for the myocardium. Heart muscle failure is heart failure.

There were other efforts to use homografts (tissue valves taken from another body) in the descending aorta to correct regurgitation from aortic insufficiency. Gordon Murray, a surgical genius in Toronto, worked in the laboratory on these before Hufnagel's success with a prosthetic valve. Canada's giant in the field of heart surgery, Wilfred Bigelow, thought there was a link between Gordon Murray's work and the first human homograft aortic replacement by Donald Ross of London. Harken tried to check this link, and confirmed it with Bigelow, but Ross could not recall it. Both were men of sterling integrity, said Harken, but as in the case of much human recollection, their individual memories differed.

As open-heart surgery became more and more practical, many men were working in the laboratories on artificial heart valves to go within the heart. In Albany, New York, Dr. George Bauer, a direct descendant of Martin Luther and a medical research engineer, would claim he had constructed the first one, but it was never tried.

Scientific advance is many layered and splendored. This was an era in cardiac surgery when surgeons, biomedical engineers, and medical scientists, learning from the mechanical sciences, evolved the wonders of replacement. Inert, "tissue-neutral" plastics were developed that did less damage to the blood interfaces when inserted in the body. Anticoagulant drugs reduced clotting. Titanium, silicone, Dacron, stroboscopic photography, all contributed.

In his Boston laboratory in the mid-1950s Harken worked with engineer W. Clifford Birtwell on an improved valve utilizing Hufnagel's principles. Harken designed it and Birtwell built an ingenious machine to test wear and stress. He accelerated the opening and closings of the valve to seventeen hundred cycles a minute, which was so rapid that stroboscopic photographs had to be taken to find out whether the molded silicone ball, inside a highly polished titanium (with three times the strength of steel and one third the weight) cage wearing a Dacron fixation shirt, was moving. The ball might seem to be moving but would actually be cycling incompletely. Also the "shaker" that banged the valve open and closed as a living valve would function, only a hundred times as fast, needed monitoring to see that the testing was continuous and that the current did not go off or the valve break. Birtwell and Harken put the testing machine in the boiler room at the Davol Rubber Company plant where Birtwell worked at the time. The boiler room was tended round the clock, seven days a week, and each boiler room attendant was taught to monitor the test.

In the ten years between 1950 and 1960 Harken had seen

eighty-seven patients with calcific aortic insufficiency and a constellation of symptoms. He thought they should have a prosthetic valve—if there were one. Of these patients, seventy-seven died within seven months. *"Perfection* may be the enemy of *good"* was one of his repeated maxims. "I realized I did not have to have a perfect valve. When what you do is safer than the disease it corrects—and is the best thing available to do—do it!" He began trying his valve in dogs, with some success, but animal results were never definitive.

On May 5, 1957, Dwight Harken flew from a medical meeting in Chicago to Osceola, Iowa, to join the town in its celebration of Dr. C. R. Harken's fiftieth anniversary in the practice of medicine. The light private plane was piloted by Dr. Donald B. Miller, a thoracic surgeon from Burlington, Vermont. At 5:30 in the afternoon Dr. C. R. Harken waited at the field under serene skies to meet his distinguished son.

As the Piper Tripacer came in, it tore into a high wire just beyond the field and plowed to the ground, flipped over, and came to rest a few feet inside the airport fence. It did not explode, and the two men, hanging unconscious head down from their seat belts, were cut free and laid on the ground. Dwight Harken slowly regained consciousness. He was blind because of blood in his eye chambers and unable to speak. He heard his father say, "Well, you made a most unsatisfactory landing!" and then his father's voice commanding that Miller be taken to the hospital because his pulse was failing and saying that he would go with him. Shortly after, Dr. C. R. Harken's son was lifted into a station wagon and also driven to Osceola. Dwight Harken's face was cut wide open, his teeth were smashed, and his right eye was badly damaged.

By the time he got to the hospital, Dr. Harken, Sr., was already making arrangements, alerting the best neurosurgeon in Iowa for Miller, who had cracked his head, and the best plastic surgeon for Dwight. He arranged for the highway between Osceola and Des Moines to be cleared of all other traffic by the police and sent the two visiting surgeons off in two ambulances, which sped silently along the trafficless highway at top speed. Dwight Harken got the headlines and concern for him was worldwide: "Noted Surgeon in Air Crash" and "Air Crash Injures Hub Heart Expert" were the banners on the front pages of the Boston *Globe* and the Boston *Herald* on May 6. The Des Moines *Register* in Iowa led with the story opposite "Soviets Hurl New A-Threat."

C. R. Harken's son was moved, impressed, and appreciative of his father's medical and human ethics in leaving his son on the field while he cared for the more severely injured man with him. D.E.H. himself was accused, sometimes bitterly, by his wife of neglecting his family for any patient who needed him. His argument was that saving lives was a concern that took precedence over everything else.

Domestically he felt himself to be a very different sort of father, if anything fatuously proud and affectionate, and Lord knows he was devoted to Anne. No one ever questioned that, and when Anne was able to get away she always accompanied him on speaking tours and international visits, to his delight, but when the children were young his inhumanly rugged schedule did take him away from them.

"We knew he loved us," his daughter Anne Louise, nicknamed Jill, would say, "but we didn't know him terribly well. When fathers were supposed to play baseball at my school, I volunteered Mother instead because she did everything for us. At Christmastime he would take me with him to bring flowers to all his patients and he obviously loved them a lot and they loved him."

Alden Harken, who would become a top-flight heart surgeon and investigator himself, said, "We were connoisseurs of hospital parking lots at an early age. When he took us with him on weekends that's where we ended up. There was a playground and a forest outside one of them, and a small store where we were allowed to buy Crackerjack. I learned to ride a bike in the Boston City parking lot. Jill and I used to sing endlessly while we waited for him, 'Where oh where can our father be?'"

When their father did concentrate on them, once in a while, both remembered him as "terrific fun." If friends were there and they asked him to "Crack some jokes, Daddy," or to walk on his hands, he always obliged. Other times he would concoct innovative and active amusements to "give Moms a rest." (As time went on, the Dwight Harken family, instead of drifting apart, would grow closer and closer together.)

At the time of his air accident Dwight Harken was forty-seven. Many people considered that his injuries would put an end to a career that had reached such a peak. "We see so far because we stand on the shoulders of giants" was a favorite quotation of his, and now his would be the shoulders on which other men stood. He had made his contribution.

"Obviously this will be a year on the sidelines for me," he wrote to his father in June 1957 from Chesham, New Hampshire, where the Harkens had a nineteenth-century summer house. Actually he did not remain on the sidelines very long. A special lightweight frame had been built to his measurements and flown to Des Moines for him from Florida to support his back, which had been broken. Temporary plastic teeth would be replaced by good permanent dentures. The atropine effect in his right eye persisted, but he could see to operate. In very little time he, and he was glad to report, Miller, were both back at work.

A British thoracic surgeon, Oswald Tubbs, had been planning a professional and social visit for months. When he heard of the accident, he assumed that seeing the Harkens would be purely social. "Not at all," he would delight in relating later. "Dwight knew I wanted to see his closed operation for aortic stenosis. He had his remarkable team at the Brigham—who could, if need be, conduct the operation themselves—open the chest and sew in the operating tunnel to the base of the aorta. Then Dwight explained that his broken back did not mean he could not stand, and that he did not need to see in a blind closed operation! So he went on and did a brilliant operation, with his right index finger held high, his back straight, and his eyes closed."

Now Harken felt that it was his ethical obligation to try his new valve as soon as the right patient with the terminal symptoms appeared. Clinical trial for the first time meant that patient, surgeon, and valve had to arrive at the crossroad together.

Mary Allen had been born with "heart murmurs." Ninety percent of such murmurs were estimated to be innocent and successive doctors assured Mary's parents that she would grow out of it.

At the age of eighteen Mary was working as a salesgirl in a Jacksonville, Florida, department store. At the end of each day when she walked to her bus stop, she was overtaken by severe breathlessness. After she got on the bus, she sat down quickly in the nearest seat and seemed to recover at once. A new driver on her route, Bill Richardson, noticed the pretty raven-haired girl who usually sat just behind him. He spoke to her and within a few weeks had changed his schedule so that he could pick her up in his car when she left work. Mary was always exhausted when she left the store, but once beside him in the car she was her animated self. In due course the personable young man and the pretty girl were married. They had a daughter and bought their own home in Jacksonville.

Bill was devoted, Mary beautiful, and their child grew happily. The only bad thing seemed to be Mary's repeated spells of weakness, with dizziness and breathlessness. Doctors continued to find nothing wrong and to discount her heart murmurs. Mary began to believe that her symptoms were imaginary, but Bill Richardson was quite sure they were not.

He stretched his moderate income to take her to New Orleans to the Oschner Clinic for tests. Harken would later believe that they found out what was wrong there, but did not tell the young couple because the condition was considered hopeless at that time. In any case, Mary felt wholly discredited; "psychosomatic" was a word that meant "crazy" to her.

In the summer of 1957 Mary Richardson suffered a minor injury and went to a general practitioner in Jacksonville. She did not mention her shameful bouts of weakness and breathlessness, but when the doctor listened to her chest with his stethoscope, he advised her to see a heart specialist. Mary returned home euphoric. The doctor thought she might be sick, not making it up. Bill telephoned the doctor, who recommended a cardiologist, Dr.

Hanson. They put the visit off until Bill came home one day to find Mary unconscious on the floor. Hanson diagnosed "aortic stenosis," and suggested an operation by the best, and, in fact, essentially the one man in the field, Dwight Harken in Boston. Bill sent Mary there with her mother.

The first time Harken saw Mary Richardson she was curled into the fetal position on the couch in his office waiting room. Pain had struck. He sat down beside her and coaxed her to talk. "All right, Mary," he said. "I believe every word of your story and we're not going to waste any time!" Within two hours Mary Richardson was in bed at the Mount Auburn Hospital. She knew now what aortic stenosis meant and felt comforted. "He treated me like a daughter," she would say.

Catheterization of the right side of the heart was by then relatively routine, but right-sided catheterization and right-sided angiography did not detect aortic insufficiency. It was obvious and easy to thread a catheter into any vein in the body and push it along until it went into the right atrium or right ventricle and out to the lungs. There was no such way to go on through the lungs and into the left side of the heart. Left-sided catheterization had been delayed until a way was found to perforate the atrial septum or thread a catheter through an artery, back through the aorta, down through the aortic valve, and into the left ventricle, testing the left-side pressures. This was a much more complex procedure and Mary hated the thought of it. However, Harken confirmed by catheterization the diagnosis of aortic stenosis and he suspected insufficiency. All they could do was to relieve the stenosis effectively by blind surgery, and hope that the valve, which was almost but not quite ready, would be available in time to save her next time around.

After the blind operation Mary's gratitude was touching. She did little complaining about the pain from the division of her sternum (breastbone), which still troubled her weeks later. She was too happy over her glorious emancipation from the terrifying fainting attacks, anginal pain, and breathlessness. Before she left the hospital for home, Harken put his arm around her and made her promise to let him know at once when and if she did not feel well. Any further dizziness, fainting, chest pressure or pain, breathlessness, would mean that she should return immediately.

"I was so full of nervous energy I soon forgot that Dr. Harken told me to stick to a salt-free diet and sleep a lot," she would tell medical reporter Jurgen Thorwald when he interviewed her for his book, *Patients*. "I now think Dr. Harken had me in mind for his artificial valve operation, but wasn't ready when I went in. He just wanted to keep me alive long enough to try it."

Mary grew desperately ill again, returned to Boston, and to save money went into a twelve-bed ward at Peter Bent Brigham Hospital. Tests began at once. Cardiologist Lewis Dexter assured Mary that catheterization was now much easier to endure and that she would not mind it. She did not and, with courage and complete faith in Harken, agreed to another operation.

This time he tried a procedure developed with his colleague, Warren Taylor. The aortic base that contains the leaflets of the aortic valve is so big, and the leaflets are so small, that when the leaflets do not come together and close as they should, the surgeons could put a band around the base and snug it up, making the base smaller, so that the leaflets approximated better, thereby improving their competence. When he attempted to place a "hangman's noose" at the base of her aorta and under the coronary artery origines, Mary's heart stopped twice and was resuscitated twice. The heroic effort failed. "Hang on," Harken told Mary.

Harken had tried his new valve just once on a nearly moribund patient, who had died. He did not want to try it again so soon, but he and Dexter agreed that Mary's only chance, now, was the valve. At least the courageous little dark-haired woman from Florida was in better condition than that tragic first patient had been. Her left ventricle was only moderately enlarged. It should withstand the major surgical change he would make, to a new aortic valve, and Harken had learned a lot from his failure. Also, the cardiopulmonary equipment had improved and experience with it had come a long way.

On March 10, 1960, Mary was brought to the operating room. She was anesthetized with the greatest of care. Patients

with heart failure from aortic insufficiency were notably poor anesthetic risks, and if the heart fibrillated, nearly impossible to
resuscitate. Adhesions from previous surgery compounded the
difficulty by preventing quick exposure of the heart. The process
was tedious, but exposure of Mary's heart was finally accomplished and she was ready to be placed on bypass.

Cooling was in use by this time and the machine's cooling
device lowered her body temperature to 82°F. Her heart went
into the fluttering, fibrillating, nonpumping state as the heart-
lung machine supported her life. Harken made his planned
inverted-Y incision at the base of the aorta. The flaccid, incompetent, stretched, perforated, and torn leaflets—which had degenerated since the first and second operations—lay limp. Excision
was rapid and simple. Suturing into place the new valve was
tedious, complex, and terrifying. (The process would be greatly
simplified later by Starr of Portland.) With all possible speed,
Harken completed the valve replacement and closed the aorta.

As the device on the heart-lung machine warmed Mary's
body and heart to near-normal temperatures, to the overwhelming joy of surgeon and team, Mary's heart recovered on its own.
Ordinarily the heart had to be shocked back into effective beating
rhythm. Mary's blood pressure returned to normal; her pulse-
tracing contours were like healthy ones.

There was jubilation among everyone in the OR, except for
the cameraman assigned to document this first. In his terror and
concentration the surgeon had forgotten the camera and neglected to afford the necessary exposure, most of the time block-
ing the lens with his body. Very little film documented that race
to success.

Bill Richardson would tell writer Thorwald that the swinging
door to the room where he waited was thrown open. He said he
saw the surgeon in a white coat thrown over his operating greens,
which were still stained with Mary's blood. "When I saw his smile
I knew it was all right. He had his chest thrown out *this* far, he
was so proud. 'She's fine, just fine,' he called out. 'We put in a
new valve and it's working beautifully!' " (Harken disputes Bill
Richardson's memory, since he does not believe he "overreacted"
at this early point.)

This Harken achievement, plus Albert Starr's successful implantation of an artificial mitral ball valve—also in the normal anatomical site—in Portland, Oregon, which soon followed, constituted another Turning Point. (In the 1970s a few people would even live with all three of their heart valves replaced, generally with better valves than the ball valves.)

Bill Richardson haunted the hospital during Mary Richardson's recovery. Word got around that he was the husband of the patient from Florida on whom Harken had performed the great first. He learned from doctors and nurses what a historic figure his Mary was before she was even conscious enough to know what had been done. "The first thing I remember," she would say, "was waking up and hearing this funny clock. I asked Dr. Harken what it was and he just laughed at me and said, 'There's no noise there at all,' but I still heard it." Bill could not hear the curious new sound unless he put his head on her chest. When he did, it was not much louder than when he had listened to their daughter's heartbeat in Mary's womb.

On April 2 Mary confronted a group of photographers. She stood beside a nurse who held a Harken valve on display. This was the first time Mary saw a replica of the caged ball that was keeping her alive. Mary, in common with many heart surgery patients, had a brief time of amnesia, retrograde before the operation and covering a period following it. Actually the operation had been fully explained to her and afterward she was quite conscious when Harken took Dr. Samuel Levine in to see her and had him listen to her heart. "Something mechanical there," commented Levine, and Harken explained the new valve. He had not yet showed it to her for the simple reason that the one in her chest was the only one in the world. By the time she faced the photographers, another had been made and this one was displayed. The next day Mary Richardson flew home to Florida, climbing the steps to board the plane without assistance.

Two failures followed Harken's success with Mary Richardson. The fourth operation was performed on Alfred Gallo, a forty-seven-year-old workman whom Harken had been treating for aortic valvular insufficiency with diminishing hope. Gallo wanted him to try replacement, and this time it worked. Gallo, with his new valve in place, went home a few weeks after the operation in remarkably good shape. If it had not been for the two of them, Mary Richardson and Alfred Gallo, Harken would certainly have suspended his efforts.

"A piece of Dwight Harken dies with every patient he loses," a colleague would say. In those early days there were deaths from fatal hemorrhages, from low cardiac output or circulatory weakness, from the succession of alternating-current defibrillating shocks sometimes needed to restore orderly heartbeat, each shock destroying more heart muscle. Mortality rates from valve replacement slowly went down, and in 1978 the rate was below 10 or even 5 percent in the great heart centers. Both Mary Richardson and Alfred Gallo lived to read in the newspapers about actor John Wayne's recovery from mitral valve replacement.

Samuel Levine, one of the best-loved, most competent cardiologists of all time, thereafter enjoyed telling the story of a presentation by D.E.H. at a meeting of the American Heart Association in 1960. Charles Bailey hooted at the idea that "the same man who recommends taking foreign bodies out of the heart now tells us that we should put them *into* the heart!" Harken replied, according to Dr. Levine, "It's all quite simple, Charlie—you just have to know when to put them in and when to take them out!"

Mary had had to have her valve taken out and a second one installed when the sutures in the first valve gave way. Then, in 1968, she suffered a stroke, the ever present danger for those harboring mechanical valves in spite of improved anticoagulation. She survived an unrelated abdominal operation in 1970, and the division of nerves to relieve pain in her shoulder following the stroke. The good and active years following valve replacement were over and her life was fairly restricted by the time the writer Jerry LeBlanc interviewed her in 1971, eleven years after she became the first person to live with a caged-ball aortic valve inside her heart. Thorwald quotes his report:

> Mary Richardson, blue-eyed and pale-faced, walks very slowly, delicately, yet with a kind of grandeur about her. Even though her left side has been paralyzed since 1968, she limps along with a look

of triumph about her, a small smile coming through despite what is an obvious struggle for her, just moving around. She emanates a sort of gratitude for the very act of human existence. Every beat of her heart is a victory for her.

Valve research and the clinical use of prosthetic valves to replace diseased ones accelerated. Research and clinical use of better and better prosthetic valves were gratifying, but criticism, consumerism, casual use of anticoagulants, and a litigation-minded public, plus painfully counterproductive FDA action, would by 1979 threaten the very availability of artificial valves.

In 1973 Harken, who as an avocation had become editor of the journal *Medical Instrumentation*, had already noted the proliferation of mechanical heart valves, the fruits of massive, continuous, and well-directed research. He had also noted the emergence of carping criticism. "How wrong of the government officials and extragovernmental critics of medicine to naïvely and maliciously assert that there has been more research on toilet valves than on heart valves," D.E.H. wrote in his opening comments for the fall issue, "when in fact there has been little solid investigation of 'water closets' since the original work of Sir Thomas Crapper in the 1870s."

The mechanical valves were given many names, and ferocious rivalry developed among the medical instrument manufacturers and among surgeons whose names were associated with the artificial valves they developed. Lengthy follow-up studies were made to support the characteristics of the Harken valve, the Starr-Edwards, Kay-Cross, Wada-Cutter, Smeloff-Cutter, Björk-Shiley, Lillehei-Kastor, and many other valves.

In 1975, at the International Symposium in Detroit, the outstanding ones were reviewed and defended. It made a sensation when Dwight Harken quietly announced that he had withdrawn the Harken aortic and mitral valves, which were still in use and ranked with the best, from the market. He had been frustrated in his efforts to introduce a much better artificial valve because the new government demands for testing were so extensive that he found the process exorbitant and unproductive. "It is my feeling that the flexible stent biologic porcine glutaraldehyde valve [a pig valve effectively cleansed of antigens] now represents the best currently available. Its lesser problems with anticoagulation, thrombogenic and embolic complications, in contrast to those of the current mechanical prostheses, prompts this conclusion and this action." The announcement was made in full knowledge that the tissue valves might in time wear out and require replacing.

The development of biologic valves had paralleled that of mechanical prostheses. They were an obvious alternative. Some forms were readily available, some types cheaper, and possibly with them the patient would not require anticoagulants for life. The biologic valves had proved, however, much less durable and there was still the question of rejection. D.E.H. thought wear was the major problem.

Autografts, constructed of the patient's fascia lata (tissue from his own thigh), were tried early on and found acceptable to the patient's immune system, which rejected many foreign biologic substances immediately. Unfortunately fascia lata valves shrank when implanted, so the valves became inefficient very rapidly.

Homografts or allografts, valves taken from human cadavers, were all too frequently rejected by the host body and were exceedingly tricky to harvest, sterilize, and keep sterile. To install them required a base on which the surgeon could sew. Nevertheless some surgeons used them with considerable success, Barratt-Boyes and Kirklin doing better than the others.

Xenografts, valves taken from other species, such as pigs, sheep, and calves, were at first rejected out of hand by human hosts. Methods were found to remove (digest) from them the allergens that caused rejections, especially those present in the fibrous collagen frameworks (connective tissue). A flexible base called a stent was added to the xenografts to facilitate suturing them securely in place.

At the Mayo Clinic and later in Alabama, John Kirklin, a pioneer in biologic valve replacement, particularly homografts, used them extensively. In other countries sometimes special factors influenced the surgeon's choice among artificial, mechanical, and biologic valves, either homografts or xenografts.

For instance, in New Zealand tissue valves taken from

human cadavers were easier to acquire. An arrangement with the coroner provided a surgeon with fresh hearts from victims of accidental death. Sir Brian Barratt-Boyes, a leading cardiac surgeon there, found that if the human valves were harvested promptly under surgically aseptic conditions so as not to require chemical or other sterilization, they lasted fairly well. They were cheaper, an important consideration, so he used mechanical valves only in occasional cases where biologic valves proved unsatisfactory or unavailable.

In Australia, on the other hand, coroners were neither sympathetic nor cooperative. Lawyers protected the bodies of the dead. When Australian surgeon Rowan Nicks returned from a training visit to America, he could not get research money. When he tried a mechanical valve, which Charles Hufnagel had given him, on a dog in his makeshift laboratory, the animal recovered, but its legs were paralyzed. He waited until better mechanical prosthetic valves were available. They proved to do much better in humans than in dogs. They were sterile and there was no problem with rejection.

"Pop them into position, once you had the technique," Nicks would say on a later visit to Boston, "and if you put them in safely, you knew the mechanics of them were tested and near perfect. I personally think that man's ingenuity is much greater than people credit."

Walton Lillehei put it another way: "The more artificial device work we do, the more we believe in God!"

The entire March–April 1977 issue of *Medical Instrumentation* was devoted to valves. Articles on every aspect of these replacement parts were contributed by the men most authoritative in their fields. One omission was noted by editor Harken with an apology: "To discuss heart valves without Albert Starr is like publishing a monograph on silver without mentioning Sterling!" but Starr's contribution had arrived too late for publication.

C. Walton Lillehei's article met the deadline, but was much longer than his three-page allotment. It ran to ten. Even that much space, Harken commented, was "only a pump primer for Walt. This will come as no surprise to those who have shared panels with him. The only difference between him and the many who run over their time is that he says worthwhile things in that time."

Lillehei pointed out that the technical problems with mechanical valves had been largely overcome. Operative risk had fallen to an acceptably low level. Clinical relief was consistent and often "dramatic." He concluded: "We anticipate that refinements will further improve the results of valve replacement surgery particularly in those two areas where most desired—namely flow through small sizes and thromboembolism. However, the final answer will come only in the crucible of clinical experience."

Contributor Alain Carpentier, professor of cardiac surgery in Paris and outstanding pioneer in tissue valves, credited with several firsts and many improvements, agreed with Harken that glutaraldehyde xenografts had become the most reasonable choice in valvular replacement. He estimated that the durability limit of ten to fifteen years was offset by the low rate of complications and freedom from anticoagulation hazards. "In our opinion," Dr. Carpentier concluded, "the patient should take part in choosing between a bioprosthesis and a mechanical one. This critical choice will depend upon the relative importance to each individual of an improved quality of life with a bioprosthesis versus the lower risk of reoperation with a mechanical valve."

Harken's editorial last word was, as usual, outspoken. Over 300,000 people were wearing valves that had either improved their lives or had saved them. Nevertheless drawbacks persisted: the need for anticoagulation; wear and tear, which necessitated replacement, especially for tissue valves. In order to dramatize the need for further efforts toward perfection of all the extant valves, Harken wrote: "They have one thing in common: *There is something wrong with all of them!*"

"Nothing is perfect," said the Philosopher in James Stephens' *The Crock of Gold* as he ate his breakfast porridge, "there are lumps in it."

The one point on which all the surgeons agreed in the 1970s was that regulation in the name of consumerism had gone so far that research was slowing down and little new could be tried in the crucible of clinical experience. To frustrate further good in the name of perfection seemed to them a poor exchange medically because it confined them to using the tried and proven—and faulty.

During the much freer 1950s and 1960s good had come in many areas of medical treatment. To keep up with what was better and best became a bigger problem than ever. Improved surgical procedures and streamlined diagnostic techniques had spurred advances in anesthesia, drugs, intensive care, coronary care, blood gas, and electrolyte analysis. Breakthroughs in one area always begot breakthroughs in other areas. Each departure from already established practice did demand evaluation. If the departure was an improvement, it obligated dissemination.

In order to disseminate the advances made in the United States, the State Department sent out medical teams as part of its cultural exchange program. The cardiac teams, representing extraordinary recent advances in the care of the heart, were widely welcomed. The teams were generally balanced, with two clinical cardiologists, one physiologist, and a surgeon. They went to both developed and developing countries, extending and exchanging knowledge.

Inside the United States a group of restless, aggressive young cardiologists formed the American College of Cardiology with their own continued professional education as its primary purpose. For a long time the academic community distrusted the organization as second best and even a threat to the American Heart Association. Dwight Harken felt that the two organizations should be complementary, not competitive. If the founders and leaders of the American Heart Association, whose purposes included fund raising and public education, were also to become members of the College of Cardiology, which concentrated on professional education, the destructive rivalry would cease. He accepted the presidency of the ACC in 1964.

With his usual organized energy he went straight to the top. Dr. Paul Dudley White, founder of the American Heart Association, and honored with the title "Father of American Cardiology," was the most influential cardiologist in the country and a friend with whom he had worked. (When President Eisenhower suffered a heart attack, it was, of course, the eminent Dr. White who was called to the White House.) Dr. White joined the American College of Cardiology, and so did cardiology's most revered lady, Dr. Helen Taussig, along with many others such as Drs. Sprague, Herman, Katz, Blumgart—all on Harken's "blue ribbon list." To augment this list, Harken searched the cities of the United States and the medical academic centers to find out who were considered both "the best" and the "most popular" cardiologists. He himself knew the surgeons. To those selected, he wrote: "We need you in the College now. Some day you may need the College." The American College of Cardiology soon gained a momentum and prestige it has never lost. On its own, the organization instituted an exchange program with other countries that was much more extensive than the government's. Government sponsored or privately supported, the American College of Cardiology circuit courses became and remain a remarkable success. For this Dr. Eliot Corday of Los Angeles deserves credit. This great cardiologist and ambassador made the contacts and gave briefings and instructions that were careful and clear. "Corday's way" was summed up in his statement: "We can serve others by taking them what they want, what they need!"

International friendship grew naturally among medical men. Paul Dudley White wrote more extensively of his visits to other countries in his autobiography than of his medical career. Dwight, with Anne Harken, traveled more than half a million miles on such trips and entertained, unforgettably, innumerable visiting physicians and their wives who came to Boston. Medals, plaques, scrolls, and such from foreign governments, academies, and societies accumulated and Harken was made an honorary member in medical associations everywhere.

In the 1970s the American College of Cardiology undertook to establish a unique center for harvesting, distilling, and transmitting information by intramural and extramural means: Heart House. A site in Bethesda, Maryland, was acquired, close to the National Institutes of Health and the National Library of Medicine. Heart-research would not be done there, but research on how to communicate all that was going on, on exploration of the most efficient modern modes of communication, would. The buildings would house the national offices of the College of Cardiology, and their national and international programs would be administered there.

Harken was made chairman of the campaign committee and was directly and indirectly responsible for raising the money. He retired from operating in 1975 and devoted the considerable spillover of energy this released to Heart House. Such a center had been one of his fondest dreams and final goals. He thought that Heart House, which opened its doors officially in October 1977, might constitute one of the truly major breakthroughs in the twentieth-century attack on cardiovascular disease—the greatest epidemic of all time.

11.

300,000 Pacemakers and 75,000 Bypasses

No other means of mechanically aiding the ailing heart is so nearly ubiquitous as the pacemaker for regulating its electrical system. No other surgical procedure for heart repair is currently performed nearly as often as the bypassing of blocked coronary arteries. The rapidity with which both went from concept to commonplace is startling no matter how accustomed one has become to the pace of twentieth-century scientific advances.

Paul Zoll is called "the Father of Pacemakers." While monitoring Harken's patients during cardiac surgery at the 160th General Hospital during the war, he became more and more aware of just how unexcitable and insensitive the heart could be. There must be some *reasonable* way, he thought, of reversing cardiac arrest.

Claude Beck, in Cleveland, Ohio, had already pioneered the resuscitation of hearts by opening the chest, grasping the heart in the hand, and pumping it to simulate its contractile propulsive forces and to cause the circulation of blood to resume. To open the chest for that purpose was a radical procedure, and it became a macabre jest at one time to warn people they should not have a heart attack, faint, or fall down in Beck's city. If you did, it was said, you might wake up with a bloody shirt and your chest split wide open.

Restoring circulation by squeezing rhythmically for the heart with the hands inside the open chest was sometimes useful. An arrested heart would under certain circumstances also respond to a fraction of a milliampere of electric current, applied directly in the open chest, but a much larger amount of current was essential to stop the fibrillating disorganized heart. Stopped it must be, all the muscle over the heart at the same time, if the heart was to start again with all fibers of muscle participating at the same time in orderly sequential beats.

"It did seem to me very much too bad," Zoll would say later in his quiet, pensive mutter, "that a patient should die of inadequate heart rate or ventricular standstill when the heart is basically so responsive to electrical stimulus." After the war he would go to work on an external shockmaker. He would try to build a machine that would supply the necessary electrical energy to start a balky, irresponsible heart.

The first recorded use of electricity in medicine goes back to 47 A.D. when a freed slave of the Emperor Nero's accidentally came into contact with a live "torpedo fish" or electric ray. According to the writer Scribonius Largues, it cured the man's pain from gout. Largues's contemporary, the physician Discordes, subsequently recommended using the electric eel for headaches. In the second century that extraordinary Greek, Galen, applied the live fish to the human body as an anodyne.

The Reverend John Wesley, founding father of the Protestant Methodist Church in the eighteenth century, was an advocate of "electrotherapy." He wrote of a case in which a man had heart attacks. "I advised him to take no more medicine but to be electrified through the breast. He was so. The violent symptoms immediately ceased and he fell into a sweet sleep."

In 1774 an essay was published entitled "On the Recovery of the Apparently Dead" by Charles Kite, a member of the Royal Humane Society in England.

"A Mr. Squires," wrote Kite, "very humanely" tried the effects of electricity on a child who had fallen from a window and been taken up for dead. "Twenty minutes at least had elapsed before he could apply the shock, which he gave to various parts of the body without apparent success; but, at length, on transmitting a few shocks through the thorax, he perceived a small pulsation; soon after that the child began to breathe, though with great difficulty. In about ten minutes she vomited. A kind of stupor remained for some days, but the child was restored to perfect health and spirits in about a week."

(Harken warned against anecdotal medical testimony, frequently inaccurate, poorly recalled, and colored by will, emotion, dramatic or selfish motivation. The child in Kite's anecdote could not have had complete circulatory arrest for twenty minutes. She may have had undetectable breathing and heartbeat, and afterward there may have been some brain damage. Nor can it be certain that the electric shock had anything but a coincidental relationship to her recovery.)

Kite concluded that this and other examples plainly pointed out that electricity was the most powerful stimulus that could be applied. "And are we not justified in assuming that, if it is able so powerfully to excite the action of the external muscles, that it will be capable of reproducing the motion of the heart, which is infinitely more irritable, and by that means accomplish our great desideratum, the renewal of circulation?"

In the nineteenth century the diagnosis and description of ventricular fibrillation were worked out and it was also discovered that there was a period when it could be reversed by the application of current, less than a killing dose. In due course a portable electrified "reanimation" or resuscitation chair was advertised for sale, and, in the late 1880s, a book by Richard Reece, *Medical Guide for the Use of Clergy, Heads of Families and Junior Practitioners in Medicine and Surgery*, included an explanation of its use.

Resuscitation by electricity often amounted only to the equivalent of the "thoracic thump"—banging a victim on the chest, as modern rescue teams are taught to do. Until recently, Harken would say, there was "precious little" distinction made among simple syncope (fainting), cardiac arrest, ventricular fibrillation, and even convulsive and epileptic states. To develop such distinctions took a tremendous amount of widespread experimentation, and there were hazards and deaths-by-intended-cure all along the way. Men perfected an electrical apparatus for killing criminals before they succeeded with an apparatus to save lives.

Twentieth-century research included that of William Kouwenhoven, pioneer in the field of biomedical engineering, who won high honors for his life study of defibrillation. In the 1930s Albert Hyman invented an "artificial pacemaker"—not for chronic pacing but for electroresuscitation. Wilfred Bigelow and his associates in Canada experimented not only with cold sleep but with pacemaking in laboratory animals as well. They passed a transvenous electrode beyond the sinoatrial node (the intracardiac rate control center) to administer current and, in a letter to Dr. David Schecter at Mount Sinai Hospital in New York years later, Bigelow indicated that if they had just gone *one* centimeter farther, they would have had a pacemaker.

Paul Zoll, working at the Beth Israel Hospital in Boston after the war, tried but quickly concluded in the laboratory that passing an electrode down the esophagus behind the heart was impractical. He invented an external shockmaker, a needle to be inserted under the skin at the apex of the heart, another electrode to be applied to the skin surface at the fourth rib interspace. The first clinical test was scheduled for a seventy-five-year-old man who had suffered heart block for two years. Heart block, of course, was caused by malfunction of the electrical conduction system of the heart. When the heart impulses in the system developed partial, intermittent, or complete breaks in the circuit, blocks occurred. In his case, the rate was slowed, and unfortunately repeated injections of heart stimulants given to keep him alive proved insufficient and his heart failed before they could try the shockmaker.

In September 1952 a male, ten years younger, arrived at the hospital with congestive heart failure from heart block. For six days repeated injections of drugs helped him, but the two main pumping chambers were beating at only half the normal rate and often his heart would stop for up to a minute. Zoll's shockmaker was attached to him. It was connected to the electrical supply, which could deliver steady shocks, lasting 2/1000ths of a second, fifty to a hundred times a minute. The shocks were administered only when the ventricles came to a halt, and showed up plainly on the electrocardiogram. On the 7th of October the patient's heart failed and the machine was switched on. For fifty-two hours only outside stimulation drove the ventricles. On the 9th of October the ventricles began to beat spontaneously, at forty-four beats to the minute. The machine was shut off. Two days later the electrodes were removed. Shortly thereafter the patient was able to leave the hospital.

"That is where it all began," Paul Zoll would say, sitting quietly behind his desk at the Beth Israel in 1975. He was more interested in talking about patient care and psychology than his role in the pacemaker story, which had made him famous and won for him the Mary Lasker Award. "The whole business of control of cardiac rhythm began, really, with the external pacemaker in 1952."

Zoll's contributions had not ended there. In 1955 it was at his and his colleagues' instigation that Dr. Frederick Vanderschmidt at the Massachusetts Institute of Technology designed an improved machine. Using the transistor battery, invented in 1948, Vanderschmidt's shockmaker would feed shocks of half a volt directly into the heart. Leads were introduced into animal hearts, and the upper chambers picked up the tiny natural shocks, amplified them, and passed them on.

The next step was taken in Minneapolis by C. Walton Lillehei and a television repair man, Earl Bakken. Lillehei was convinced that electrodes could be stitched directly onto the heart. Leads through the chest could then feed in a pulsed current. He needed a power source that could be regulated to control the frequency and intensity of the current. The amount of current required was very small and the power source thus should and could be very small. A physicist at the University of Minnesota promised him such an apparatus, but did not deliver.

Earl Bakken had a television repair shop in a garage at his house. Lillehei got in the habit of calling in Bakken when the electrical equipment in his operating room went awry. "The hospital technicians never seemed able to fix it when it went on the fritz," he said, "which it did, although it wasn't very complicated equipment in those days. Earl could always make it work. So I told Earl what I wanted for a power source and he said, sure, no problem. Three weeks later he came back with it. You could just set the rate wherever you wanted it and strap it on the patient. Worked fine. The next step was to make it a little smaller, coat it with plastic, and put it inside the body. So there you had it. The first implantable pacemaker! In 1957. Earl Bakken set up a little company to make the first ones. That little company he named Medtronics and by 1974 it had sales of about $100 million a year." (By 1978 the figure was $180 million.)

Meantime British doctors had developed pacemaking equipment that reduced the danger of applying shocks through the chest from outside. Shocks administered through layers of skin, fat, muscle, and pericardium had to be of such high voltage that chest and back muscles went into violent contractions and painful spasms. The shocks also caused burns. Batteries, which the patient could carry around with him, were made. These delivered lighter shocks to the chest heart wall. The batteries needed to be charged once a week. Next a battery was developed that lasted two years. Later there was even one that could be recharged by the patient. Implantable pacemakers were a further improvement, and it was quickly recognized that patients with hearts that stopped for long or short periods—heart block—needed them.

When implantation became common, statistics on longevity afterward were gradually assembled. The results were discomforting. A large number of those with heart block dropped dead within six months after pacemaker implantation. It was too easy to explain this incidence of mortality by another "sick heart syndrome," that these were very sick people with very bad hearts who could be expected to die. Something else might be wrong.

"You see what you look for and you look for what you know," Harken would say over and over. To find what you don't know you are looking for requires the serendipitous mind. Serendipity was one of Harken's favorite words—in fact, he was one of those who resurrected it from obsolescence. The word had been coined by Horace Walpole in 1754 from a fairy tale, "The Three Princes of Serendip." These princes had the gift of finding happy and agreeable things for which they were not seeking.

That there was a vulnerable point in the short period represented by each beat of the heart was known to modern physiologists. It showed up in the electrocardiographic tracings that documented the electrical action of the heart. The portion of the tracing known as the T wave represented a time of excessive excitability of the heart muscle. That was the vulnerable period when extra stimuli could cause ventricular fibrillation. Dr. Bernard Lown had already worked with biomedical engineer Barouh Berkovits to develop the cardioverter, an important apparatus for restoring effective rhythm to hearts with life-threatening arrhythmias.

It was serendipitous that the staff men at the Peter Bent Brigham Hospital noticed while running electrocardiograms on their patients with pacemakers that if the pacemaker fired simultaneously with the top of the upstroke of the heart's T wave, the result could be life-threatening. As is often the case, other men observed the phenomenon at the same time: Sowton in London, Fish in Indianapolis, Lemberg in Miami among them. The tentative conclusions drawn were that repetitive beats following a pacemaker stimulus falling in that vulnerable period could cause not only those beats but fatal ventricular fibrillation as well, which could account for the high mortality rate in patients with the early pacemakers. That it took months to happen could be because the stimulus of the pacemaker in the vulnerable period was not strong enough unless the threshold during that period was lowered by such things as electrolyte imbalance or digitalis.

The men in the Harvard group, headed by D.E.H., took the problem to Barouh Berkovits, then employed by the American Optical Company.

Barouh Berkovits is the only man without a medical degree included in the Founders Group list for his contributions to cardiac surgery. A quiet, heavyset man, he never blew his own horn, but Harken would never miss a chance to blow it for him. Rolling out his intriguing name whenever he reviewed the history of cardiac surgery, Harken would pay special tribute to the three major Berkovits inventions of which he himself had made the earliest possible use. In 1974 Dr. Harold Laufman, professor of surgery at

Albert Einstein Medical College and director of surgical education at Montefiore Hospital, in New York, gave money for an annual award that he hoped would become the Nobel Prize of Biomedical Engineering. In 1975 Barouh Berkovits was chosen by the Association for the Advancement of Medical Instrumentation as the first recipient. The citation opened:

> Barouh Berkovits has saved innumerable lives and an untold amount of human myocardium and returned useful heart function to numberless patients who would otherwise have suffered the consequences of cardiac insufficiency by making the direct-current defibrillator that replaced the alternating-current defibrillator with its danger of coagulation necrosis to the patient and the danger of shock to the operator.

It had been established by surgeon Armand Lefemine in Harken's laboratory that direct current could be used seventeen times with no more damage to the heart than resulted from one shock of alternating current. Three or four defibrillating shocks with alternating current could cook the heart; there was so much coagulation that it could not recover. When Berkovits created the direct-current defibrillator, Harken put it to immediate use at the Peter Bent Brigham Hospital. Soon it was the only kind used the world over.

The citation continued:

> The genius of Barouh Berkovits has made it possible to time the electrical force so that many patients suffering from limited cardiac output or life-threatening arrythmias can have effective rhythms restored by what has become a standard word: cardioversion.

Harken was the first surgeon to employ the Lown cardioverter and was extremely fond of his original model, a tall, top-heavy affair that had to be operated on its side. He moved it with him from the Peter Bent Brigham to the Mount Auburn Hospital, refusing to replace it with more elegant and newer models. Nurses and technicians complained about its ungainly appearance, although they admitted that it worked perfectly. Harken said they

complained just because they considered it beneath their dignity
to utilize his revered antique.

The award citation went on:

> Barouh Berkovits has been able to time the stimulating impulse of
> the cardiac pacemaker so that it occurs only when needed and dur-
> ing periods of the heart cycle when such needed impulse is safe,
> thus inventing the demand pacemaker.

The timing device employed in the demand pacemaker was
not dissimilar to the one Berkovits used in his cardioverter, but
by 1966 zealous advocates of patient protection were seriously
hampering the clinical application of new devices developed in
the laboratory. "Human experimentation" was the pejorative
phrase and malpractice suits, for enormous sums, were beginning
to skyrocket insurance rates for physicians, especially those who
worked in high-risk areas. Manufacturers of devices were also
threatened, and became wary of releasing innovative equipment.

Before he could obtain a demand pacemaker for implantation, Harken found it necessary to write a formal letter to Berkovits, its inventor, who was eager for clinical trial, to cover the
manufacturer:

> Dear Mr. Berkovits:
> A unique emergency situation has arisen with reference to de-
> mand pacemakers.
> You are well aware of the very extensive experimental work that
> has gone on and safety testing with your implantable demand pace-
> maker. You also know that we have used this as an external unit to
> make a patient ambulatory.
> The unique situation to which I refer, carrying with it a special
> obligation, has arisen in connection with [a patient]. One week ago
> today, I did a semi-emergency operation to bring her out of heart
> failure for a ruptured Sinus of Valsalva of her aorta that had rup-
> tured into the right atrium. This operation, under circumstances of
> heart failure, was rewarded by spectacular success in that she has
> rapidly come out of her heart failure and done very well. In con-
> nection with repairing the defect, it was necessary to use the zone
> of the bundle of His [a cardiac connective system] as the solidest

available tissue to close the aorticoatrial window. I did this with full knowledge that the sutures were producing heart block. We were monitoring the patient on the table at the time, but there was no other tissue to make our primary closure much less the essential secondary patch.

Since the operation [the patient] has done spectacularly well. On the other hand, she has had to be paced from time to time through the wire that I had implanted in the myocardium at the time of her surgery.

Now she competes with the pacemaker if we carry it at the rate of eighty or so and [it] gives her an uncomfortable or even hazardous tachycardia. Conversely, if we turn off the pacemaker, no matter how carefully we watch her, there is the opportunity for her to drop into an excessively slow rate with sudden death. This is the problem of uncertain but complete heart block.

This represents the ideal opportunity and indication for demand pacemaker. It is my firm conviction that the risks' residual with the use of the pacemaker that we have tried in the laboratory are far less than the conspicuous risks surrounding either carrying her on the existing types of pacemakers or having continuous monitoring in our coronary care unit as is required now. The impracticability of having somebody sit with this lady to monitor her with the existing equipment that ties her to the bed is obvious.

I therefore make this appeal to you and your distinguished company to make as a special project an implantable pacemaker that we can use in this specific patient. You are rendering a life-saving service to this patient and this unique opportunity renders a unique service to other patients who need pacemakers. The combination provides a maximum service to all. I hope that you will be able to cooperate with us in this very important project.

With kindest personal regards.

Sincerely yours,
Dwight E. Harken, M.D.

P.S. To be specific, we need an implantable pacemaker with an intravenous electrode.

I regard this as a personal obligation that you hopefully will share in offering this patient a demand implantable pacemaker.

Word got around in the medical fraternity that D.E.H. was going to implant the first demand pacemaker. Everyone who could got in on the case. Brigham cardiologist James Dalen described the scene. "Came the day when the catheterization laboratory, carefully prepared, was ready for me to help them fluoroscope her. The room filled up with eager visitors plus the scrub nurses and the technicians. When Dwight and his team arrived, he saw that one essential was missing: the patient! They had forgotten to bring her up. Dwight dashed away and returned wheeling her into the room himself."

The implantation was a success. The demand pacemaker was established as such an improvement that other kinds were discarded from use. The final accolade in Barouh Berkovits' citation from the Association for the Advancement of Medical Instrumentation read:

> With imagination and innovation he continues to extend these principles and to produce even better cardiac output by atrial and ventricular coordination.
>
> He has combined these and other forces in a continuing effort to improve his existing devices and to develop new instruments to relieve human suffering and save human life.
>
> He does all these things with such self-effacing modesty that his devices are better known than their developer.

I interrupt this narrative to include a personal anecdote, since it has a point and a moral. The point has to do with how commonplace a once creative step in healing can become, the moral, with the drawbacks of success. The profit motive in the proliferation and competitive manufacture of medical instruments or devices, once they had been popularized, delayed what both Harken and Berkovits fought for: the standardization of parts for all makes.

Before I watched a major procedure D.E.H. suggested that I look in on a change of pacemaker, a very simple affair now done under local anesthetic. I was given a sterilized gown, a covering for my hair, covers to go over my shoes, and provided with a mask. The atmosphere in the OR was thoroughly relaxed. The patient, an elderly and very deaf gentleman, lay comfortable and conscious, his head under a flap of cloth like a tent side. From a long incision, obviously only skin deep and bleeding very little, in his anesthetized right side protruded the end of a small oblong battery with wires leading back out of sight. A nurse leaned down and yelled, asking how he did. "Fine, just fine," he croaked in reply, loud and cheerful.

A young surgeon who was officiating asked the scrub nurse for an instrument while Harken and another older surgeon chatted with me beyond the sterile line. Then the young surgeon raised his voice indignantly and another nurse went scurrying out. The manufacturer or somebody had sent or laid out the wrong screwdriver. He could not unscrew the tiny bolts that held the wires.

Harken exclaimed, "God almighty"; he and the Association for the Advancement of Medical Instrumentation and Barouh Berkovits had been pleading for standardization. Orderlies and nurses presented the surgeon with alternate screwdrivers, none of which fitted. The nurse by the patient's head yelled at him again. He seemed oblivious of the commotion and repeated that he was "Fine! JUST FINE."

Exasperation, without alarm, mounted. I was irresistibly and frivolously reminded of young mechanics wrestling with screwdrivers that did not fit car battery wires, except that these were so very tiny. Finally the correct miniature instrument was found. The surgeon quickly removed the old pacemaker power unit and inserted the new one in its pocket of tissue, screwed everything back tight, and closed the incision.

For one split second the electrocardiographic beat had faltered in its steady rhythm. Before the young surgeon reacted or the monitoring technician spoke up, I had noticed the two older surgeons tilt their heads and, like rabbits, lay back their ears. "You learn to sense it," Harken said. There was a run of procedures—checking tests and measurements for tissue sensitivity, and such obscure—to me—details as intervals, thresholds, millivolts, et cetera, et cetera. Then the patient was wheeled out, replying to the solicitous nurse, "I'M FINE—JUST FINE!"

Technically the procedure was simple. Electronically and as a piece of engineering, what a masterpiece the pacemaker was.

The pacemaker was one advance that kept malfunction in their hearts from killing people. Cardioversion, intensive care, counterpulsation, as well as constantly improved procedures for correcting defects and replacing valves in the opened heart, steadily improved the longevity statistics for the heart troubled. Courses in cardiac resuscitation by nondangerous means were offered for volunteers everywhere. Nevertheless one form of heart disease, that of the coronary arteries, became the number one cause of death in this and many countries.

Coronary artery disease, the narrowing or occlusion of the arteries supplying the heart muscle, was first described in 1912, but was all too often wrongly diagnosed as indigestion, rheumatism, influenza, pleurisy, or fibrosis. As diagnosis improved, mortality statistics indicated that in 1961 two out of every five male deaths in the United States could be attributed to coronary and degenerative heart and artery disease. Various theories blamed the cholesterol that collected in the arteries from animal and other "hard" fats, others blamed stress, smoking, and lack of exercise. In-depth long-term studies supported some of the theories. Further statistics confirmed that coronary artery disease had become the greatest single cause of death.

In 1958 Claude Beck, the cantankerous man from Cleveland who had pioneered manual systole in the open chest for heart stoppage, railed at his fellows during a meeting of the American Association for Thoracic Surgery: "There exists a strange complacency toward this disease! There is no relationship between treatment and death. Therefore, there is no responsibility for death. This futility has paralyzed thinking and has created a belief that to do nothing more than the old routine is to make no mistake. Nowhere in medicine is there such intellectual emptiness as exists in the understanding and treatment of this disease!"

Michael DeBakey in Texas had demonstrated that the obstruction of arteries was a segmental rather than a diffuse rusting of the pipes. He had devised grafts and sent blood around obstructed abdominal arteries. Beck himself had observed in experimental work that the heart muscle would open new tendrils to nourish itself with blood, given a chance. He believed surgical techniques could be devised to foster this process. Canadian surgeon Arthur Vineberg had realized that the heart muscle would carry on if nourished with fresh blood in the places where its own arteries had failed. He performed a palliative operation that brought blood in by planting a chest artery (the mammary artery) in a tunnel he made in the heart muscle wall. Some surgeons were attracted by the efforts of Beck and particularly by Vineberg's procedure, but after large numbers of these operations there seemed to be no solid scientific support justifying continuation. Later, studies of a patient of Vineberg's demonstrated that blood could be brought to the heart by his technique.

Cleveland, Ohio, became the focus of intense medical interest with the development of angiography for locating heart defects at the Cleveland Clinic. This began with an accident. One day in 1958 F. Mason Sones, Jr., and his colleagues injected the usual X-ray opaque dye into the catheter, which Sones pushed back down the brachial artery into the subclavian artery and into the arch of the aorta. He meant as usual to go through the aortic valve into the left ventricle. To his horror the right coronary artery appeared clearly on the screen. His catheter had slipped into the right coronary artery rather than into the left ventricle. He was visualizing the coronary arteries and, therefore, performing angiography rather than ventriculography. It had been thought that an injection of this nonblood material into the coronary artery might cause instability, damage, coronary occlusion, all sorts of problems. Nevertheless the patient remained stable.

It was also thought impossible to locate the tiny orifice in the base of the aorta. After that accident, Sones developed a catheter with a configuration that made it easier to find the coronary orifice. From then on he learned to reduce the injectate and was able to study the entire coronary circulation, sequentially, reaching into vessels as small as 100 microns. Sones' catheter brought forth the present era of revascularization surgery. His technique also provided for accurate diagnosis in coronary artery disease, and, more important, it defined the needs of the individual patient.

Sones' fortuitous discovery was made in 1958. In the 1960s

two pioneers attempted coronary bypass—David C. Sabiston in North Carolina, whose patient died shortly after surgery, and Michael DeBakey in Texas, who did not follow up on his success. In 1967, without knowledge of the other efforts, René Favaloro, in Cleveland, used a vein graft to achieve coronary bypass. It is Favaloro whom the Founders Group list credits for this Turning Point. He was the undoubted leader in the development of aortocoronary artery bypass surgery.

Arthur Vineberg, in Canada, had been unable to persuade the reluctant medical world that his theory of mammary implant was correct until it was angiographically documented that communication between the implanted artery and the coronary circulation remained patent (open). By his procedures a mammary artery was taken off the chest wall and stuck, higgledy-piggledy, into an area of heart muscle. A certain amount of blood that escaped from the artery into the wall of heart muscle did give a small bypass. Favaloro used a length of vein to literally bypass the block in the artery, specifically located by the new sophisticated angiography. Coronary artery bypass surgery was called open-heart surgery since it required heart-lung bypass to accomplish it, but the heart itself rarely had to be opened. The incidence of hospital mortality was remarkably low and the immediate relief of angina often spectacular. The operation became generally popular, and the number performed would in time exceed by far the total for all other open-heart operations combined. It was effective in many, many patterns of coronary artery disease, and for a major block of the left main coronary artery, called the "widowmaker," became all but mandatory.

Dr. René Favaloro left Cleveland to return to his native Argentina. On the medal presented to him by the American College of Cardiology was the inscription: "This man's fierce patriotism to his native country cost the United States one of the finest surgeons in the world."

Widespread use of a surgical procedure often breeds suspicion of overuse, sometimes rightly. The Veterans Administration undertook a study in one of a group of its hospitals and published results that created a media scandal. There were headlines such as "Coronary Artery Bypass Surgery Found Unnecessary" and some of the medical leaders broadly opined that medical treatment yielded results that were similar to those of surgery. The surgeons felt that the report represented much of the worst that could be done in so-called scientific reporting.

The study was of selected patients; eliminated were most of those with clear indications for bypass surgery, such as uncontrollable pain, left common trunk coronary artery obstruction, and unstable angina. The survival rate of the residual group of patients was studied by comparing those who survived with medical treatment (i.e., nonsurgical) with those who had undergone surgery by some VA surgeons, whose results did not compare favorably with surgical results generally held to be satisfactory. When a patient in the VA study group became unstable under his medical regimen, he could simply refuse to continue it or he could be switched to surgery. Even so, at the end of three years the surgical series, with poor surgical mortality, was doing as well as or better than the medical patients—and the odds were gaining. The quality of life in the surgical series was far better, with less pain and greater activity.

It was, said Harken of this particular study, as if the medical critics simply refused to read the fine print and as if the media read only the flyspecks on the page instead of the music. Also, there was at least one other report from another VA hospital that showed that surgical results were better than the medical results. The paper was accepted by the American Heart Association for presentation at the annual meeting. The authors were commanded to suppress the report, nobody would say by whom. A mysterious blank space was left in the AHA publication of abstracts.

René Favaloro returned to the United States to defend coronary artery bypass at a meeting of the American College of Cardiology following publication of the VA report. His former chief, Donald Effler of Cleveland (later Syracuse), chaired a panel on the subject. On a subsequent panel of experts discussing the subject of coronary artery bypass, Dr. John Collins from Peter Bent Brigham Hospital presented cost figures based on a group of one hundred coronary bypass patients. The surgical patients had spent so much less time in hospitals after their surgery than before that the savings, over a postoperative period of four and a half years, paid for the cost of the surgery. Favaloro made such a brilliant and impassioned speech supported by solid evidence that Dwight Harken was quoted in the April 3, 1975, issue of *Time* magazine as saying, "Any doubt as to the efficacy and desirability of coronary bypass surgery must now have suffered Sudden Death!"

By 1978 the total of coronary bypass operations exceeded seventy-five thousand. By this time one surgeon alone, Dr. Denton A. Cooley, had performed over eleven thousand of them. To the public Cooley and his former chief, Michael DeBakey, pioneer in revascularization surgery, had become the two best known names in the whole history of cardiac surgery.

12.

The Texas Titans

A recent *Information Please Almanac* listed twenty-five hundred "Famous Names," selected on the basis of public familiarity. Just six twentieth-century medical practitioners were included: Albert Schweitzer, Jonas Salk, and four heart specialists—cardiologist Paul Dudley White, and cardiac surgeons Michael DeBakey, Denton Cooley, and Christiaan Barnard. It was not surprising that two out of the six were from Houston, Texas.

Houston is the largest city in Texas, where the state flag flies over the Stars and Stripes on public buildings. The city's oligarchy is said to have fired a conductor of its symphony orchestra for boasting on the air that he had conducted the London Philharmonic while failing to mention his Houston post. Houstonians built the Astrodome, the largest indoor sports arena in the world at the time, and spent, within twenty-five years, a quarter of a *billion* dollars on a medical center that included five large hospitals. In the 1960s two immodest surgeons, Michael Ellis DeBakey and Denton Arthur Cooley, made Houston the best known cardiac surgical center on earth.

Personal publicity has been traditionally frowned upon by the medical profession, equated as it was with quackery rather than with ethical medical practice. Paul Dudley White was forgiven his emergence into fame because he was a distinguished elder, did not seek the notoriety, and used it to good purpose to educate the public on how to take care of their hearts and to build friendship with other nations. DeBakey and Cooley were criticized as propagating theirs—but not by Houstonians—and Christiaan Barnard anathematized for turning his first briefly successful heart transplant into media field days, starring himself.

In his keynote opening address at the Detroit Ford Symposium in 1975 Dwight Harken paused to needle his arch rival, Charles Bailey, for the news coverage Bailey had encouraged twenty-five years earlier. "It used to be the Barnum and Bailey syndrome," he observed, "then Barnum died. Now it's *Barnard* and Bailey." The sally was greeted with a roar of laughter. "The Barnard and Bailey syndrome is suffered widely over the world," Harken went on. "Indeed it seems endemic in Texas."

The men from Texas were among the panelists. When other speakers threw slides of their statistical results on the screen to evaluate procedures, the numbers often ran to hundreds. The figures from Texas were sometimes in the thousands. A wave of sound from the auditorium filled with cardiologists and cardiac surgeons greeted these Texas totals. It was composed of rueful laughter, disapproval, and perhaps envy. Houston seemed to be the center of assembly line surgery. There was no operation DeBakey or Cooley performed that at least a few other surgeons could not do equally well, technically superb though both men were, but there was no question who had done the *most*.

After his eleven-thousandth coronary bypass in 1977 Denton Cooley celebrated. "Denton operates so fast," Harken would remark, "that he could get away with anything!" and in introducing him at a medical meeting he called him a surgeon who "operates with Woolworth volume and Tiffany quality." Michael DeBakey, for his part, had once performed eleven elaborate operations in an eighteen-and-a-half-hour stretch, and then stuck his head into the empty corridor of the hospital at 1:30 A.M. "Anybody else out there want an operation?" he inquired.

Medical visitors could see more heart surgery in Houston in a week than elsewhere in months. They flocked in from all over the world to watch Mike DeBakey glare ferociously through his trifocals or Denton Cooley peer through elegant gold-mounted half-spectacles into the opened human heart. Professional comments were uniform in terms of technique: DeBakey's surgery was beautiful, Cooley's, miracles of speed and precision. Both men's reputations would be tarnished, as many others were, in the overenthusiastic rush to perform heart transplants following Barnard's first two, but in the judgment of history, so often at variance with contemporary judgment, they will survive. For many years Houston was Lourdes to heart-diseased pilgrims from everywhere, and even Texas-sized pride was satisfied.

The city of Houston, with its infamous climate, its terrain sprawled over miles of marshy ground that never lifts higher than fifty-four feet above sea level, had been built by such outsized, driving, operatic men. Blood feuds were part of its story. The open enmity that grew up between the two great Houston surgeons reached the proportions of legend. "Theirs was a feud," commented Thomas Thompson in his book *Hearts*, "more angry, more poignant and more useless than Freud's sorrowful estrangement from his disciple Jung."

Dwight Harken matched the "Houston hassle" with other feuds in the jealous world of surgery: Tudor Edwards and Roberts, at the Brompton in London, who refused to speak when they passed in the halls of the same hospital; the unforgiving bitterness between David Sabiston and Will Sealy at Duke University, both on the Founders Group list and both ordinarily kind, gentle, well-mannered men. In Cleveland, Mason Sones, whose work in angiography made coronary bypass surgery effective, and pioneer surgeon Donald Effler were only prevented from tearing each other to pieces by the strong, benevolent intervention of René Favaloro; when Favaloro left for Argentina, Effler left Cleveland and went home to Syracuse. The Bailey and Harken feud, though each was based in a different city, could flare up at any meeting anywhere. Their matches in medical arenas would have drawn blood had words been swords. Of the others Harken mentioned, he said, "All these were horrible feuds between wonderful men."

Thompson, while researching his book, which centered on DeBakey and Cooley, asked a Houston surgeon who knew them both well what the long relationship between DeBakey and Cooley had been before their climactic break.

"Professional," replied the surgeon. "No warmth. Mike, after all, had come from a Lebanese immigrant family and his mother taught him how to sew his own underwear and he worked in his father's drugstore and when he finally got to Tulane he was not popular. In fact, he was very much an outsider, the owl, the foreigner, the guy who didn't get invited to join a top fraternity. It wasn't that he was not well liked, I just don't think people paid much attention to him at all. Cooley, on the other hand, was the son of a rich society dentist in Houston and they owned a lot of the north side of town. Denton was always the most popular kid in the crowd, the leader, the one with charisma, the star athlete, the one all the fraternities at the University of Texas fought to rush. And Cooley was the handsomest son of a bitch ever to pick up a scalpel."

Whatever the truth of this assessment—and others have said that Michael DeBakey felt about his protégé Cooley as a father toward a son before the break—the poor boy and the rich boy made their separate ways.

Michael DeBakey was twelve years the elder of the two. He struggled his way into the Tulane University Medical School and there came under the influence and guidance of Alton Oschner. Oschner was to surgery in New Orleans and the world what Wangensteen was to Minneapolis and the world. He was a teacher, practitioner, and a great-hearted man of the highest standards who fostered and inspired ability whenever he found it, in the laboratory and in the operating room.

One of Oschner's devoted admirers was Dwight Harken. He loved to tell about the time when he emerged from New York's Times Square subway station in his usual hurry. His briefcase came unclasped and his papers spilled to the sidewalk. As he crawled about picking them up, a passerby came to his aid. Lifting his head to thank the man, Harken found himself face to face with the distinguished professor of surgery from New Orleans. "Never expected to bump into you quite like this, Dwight," said Alton Oschner. Another time Harken telephoned Oschner when he was mustering support for ASH, Action on Smoking and Health, to ask for permission to put his name on the ASH letterhead. "No time for any explanations," said Oschner. "I've got to catch a plane. But anything on which you put your name, Dwight, you may put mine on." When Oschner gave his trust to another medical man, it was without reservation or jealousy.

Oschner took under his generous wing the medical student from Lake Charles, Louisiana, who had worked his way through Tulane. Mike DeBakey responded by doing brilliant work in Oschner's laboratory. "If he had not become a surgeon," one colleague would say of him, "Mike could have been a great medical engineer." He absorbed Oschner's ideal of careful, intensive research and exquisite surgery, but Mike DeBakey did not learn from his benevolent mentor how to control his violent temper.

DeBakey's unusual ability was reflected by his postgraduate career. After internship and residency at the New Orleans Charity Hospital under Oschner, he had two years of resident service in Germany, mecca then for the medically ambitious. He returned to serve in the office of the American surgeon general, and between 1942 and 1946 was successively assistant director, acting director, and director of the Surgical Consultants Division. In 1948 Houstonians, determined to put their city on the medical map, hired him as professor and chairman of the Department of Surgery at the Baylor College of Medicine. The college had recently been moved to Houston and badly needed upgrading.

DeBakey's ruthless upgrading began at once. An organized effort by the staff and nurses to get him fired only backfired. The Houston establishment understood power and discounted love. DeBakey could exercise formidable charm in bullying the people who counted, and his gift for getting and spending money would prove awesome, even in Houston. His two bright, literate sisters from Louisiana came to work with DeBakey in Houston. They assiduously promoted his reputation, protected him from importunate lesser folk as he grew increasingly famous, and, since they both wrote well, turned his publications into models.

DeBakey's major contribution to medicine as a whole was in the field of vascular occlusive diseases—those that shut off the blood flow in clogged blood vessels. For this, he can never be ignored by history. In the autopsy room early on, he observed that obstruction in many instances was localized and segmental, thus subject to rational surgical intervention. This concept and his pioneer work on it would affect worldwide medical thinking and action. In the Houston laboratories he and his research group devised and revised grafts to make it possible to send blood around obstructions in the arteries. They soon discarded tissue from cadavers and contrived grafts of plastic cloth.

DeBakey's clinical resection and restoration of an abdominal aortic aneurysm was a widely heralded "first." Actually it proved to be a second. Charles DuBost in Paris had done one just before DeBakey. But there was soon no question who had performed the most: DeBakey.

In 1952 a second name began to appear on DeBakey's papers on the subject of aneurysms, that of Denton A. Cooley. DeBakey cast into deep shadow the men around him and Cooley did not really emerge from the shadow until his open break with his chief.

In its way, to grow up rich, handsome, and popular can be as much of a handicap as poverty and an unappealing appearance, but Denton Cooley was as ambitious as he was self-assured. After sailing through the University of Texas, he went on to the prestigious Johns Hopkins School of Medicine in Baltimore, modifying his Texas accent with the flavor of Maryland. After the war he served in the army as chief of Surgical Service at the 124th Station Hospital in Linz, Austria, and followed this with a year as senior surgical registrar in thoracic surgery at London's Brompton Hospital.

In 1952 Denton Cooley was appointed to DeBakey's faculty at the Baylor College of Medicine. He remained unperturbed under the ferocious surgical tutelage DeBakey provided, and DeBakey found him a worthy heir, the most skillful junior he had ever had. Cardiac surgery was not a large field in the 1950s and Cooley performed such heart surgery as was done in Houston for a long time. DeBakey was concentrating on arterial aneurysms, particularly in the abdomen, and the peripheral vascular surgery that would eventually lead to coronary artery bypass.

As much as possible Denton Cooley avoided laboratory work, which did not fascinate him, and consistently refused to assume any administrative responsibility. He began to build a private practice. By the 1960s, as mechanical extracorporeal circulation improved and DeBakey began to do open-heart surgery, Cooley's private practice was almost as large as, possibly even larger than, DeBakey's.

DeBakey had developed a roller pump for intravenous infusion, enlarged for use on Gibbon-type and other machines. Competing now in the open-heart field of surgery, he grew jealous of Cooley, of whom he had once been so proud. Cooley began to find it increasingly difficult to get beds for his patients within DeBakey's bailiwick. He moved more and more of his patients into St. Luke's Hospital, down the street, or to the Children's Hospital, also within the gigantic Houston complex. As he himself wrote for the Founders Group list, he began "aggressively"—his word—"to develop improved techniques for operating on congenital and acquired heart disease" and became a vocal early exponent of anoxic (lack of oxygen) cardiac arrest in open-heart surgery.

DeBakey dominated the public press after he performed an operation in which he took blood away from the lungs and returned it to the body through the aorta, bypassing mechanically the left ventricle. The patient died quietly two days after a photographic essay appeared in *Life* magazine.

Domingo Liotta, an Argentinian working in DeBakey's laboratory, had been the man most responsible for developing that bypass machine. DeBakey, whose gift for cultivating sources of money for his pet projects extended to Washington, was given a major federal grant for the purpose of developing an implantable artificial heart. Liotta was put in charge of that research program. The surgical dream of an implantable artificial heart was equivalent in the early 1960s to that of placing men on the moon. Liotta constructed a heart of metal and plastic and performed many experiments with prototype models on dogs. Canine survival had been poor when the bubble oxygenator was tried on dogs, yet the oxygenator had proved successful with human beings. With parallel reasoning, Liotta tried to persuade DeBakey to try his artificial heart on humans although the laboratory dogs were not doing well. DeBakey was understandably unwilling.

Transplant! If one man was dying because his heart was giving out and another was dying of other causes with a healthy heart, could not the healthy heart be used to save the heart victim? Norman Shumway had been working on the idea for years, first in Minnesota and then in California. Adrian Kantrowitz in New York was carefully preparing to try. Then Christiaan Barnard in South Africa, using techniques directly derived from Shumway during his training with Shumway in Minneapolis, performed one in December of 1967. The patient lived eighteen days. The media went all out encouraging public euphoria based on premature hope for the fatally troubled heart. A new medical hero was hailed.

The history of transplant, with its excessive hot and cold fluctuations, primarily concerns Barnard, Shumway, and other men, although Cooley was one of the first to follow Barnard in bold but extremely disappointing adventures in transplant. DeBakey waited longer before essaying several transplants, but his own dream, financed by the $2.5 million government grant, was to perfect the mechanical heart.

Through 1968 Cooley remained an ardent believer in the surgical "Easters" promised by transplant in spite of his own failures. At the same time he made a secret pact with Domingo Liotta, who was working with DeBakey on the other side of a widening rift between Cooley and DeBakey. Cooley paid Liotta with his own money, of which he had plenty, to moonlight for him on an artificial heart.

A Cooley patient lay in St. Luke's Hospital. He was scheduled for a transplant, but no donor had been found. The man and his wife pleaded with Cooley to somehow save his life. In the dead of one night the patient's heart went into irreversible failure. Cooley asked Liotta to bring "an" artificial heart. Beside the patient's bed they set up a huge console to power it. Thus powered, the artificial heart might keep the patient alive until a donor could be located.

Cooley removed the patient's heart and implanted "an" artificial pump and the next day went on television to proclaim his "first." On the same program the patient's wife, likening Cooley to a saint, made a tearful appeal for a donor heart to replace the mechanical one that was miraculously keeping her husband alive.

DeBakey heard the news in Washington. Monumentally outraged he fired Liotta. Liotta's defense was that his laboratory work was valueless "unless you have a man who will go ahead and take the risk!"

Cooley's patient lived with the implanted artificial heart, powered by the console, for sixty hours. A dying donor was flown to Houston by chartered jet. Cooley replaced the artificial pump in his patient's chest with the donor heart. Twenty hours later the patient died.

That was by no means the end of it. A malpractice suit was brought by the patient's wife. Endless questions of permission, comprehension, and so on were raised. The case was re-created on television. DeBakey's testimony was wary. On the record he neither condemned, nor condoned, the experimentation and could not *swear* the pump used was the one from his laboratory, although it looked very similar. Cooley was exonerated for taking extreme measures when the testimony of the anesthetist positively indicated that otherwise his patient would have died. Many of the specific and general questions brought up during the trial, both legal and ethical, would compound the many problems resulting from cardiac transplantation. The immediate result in Houston was that DeBakey and Cooley never spoke to each other again.

The Texas Titans went their separate ways, although it required care for them to avoid passing each other on the streets within the Houston complex. When they met, as they inevitably did, elsewhere in this or other countries, Cooley might have been willing to make token peace, but DeBakey looked straight through his tall enemy. Both were in demand as speakers, but they refused to share the same platform. The rift was total and exceedingly public.

Cooley, with no further connection at Baylor College, frequently had as many as a hundred patients at a time in St. Luke's or Children's Hospital. In one six-month period he performed a thousand open-heart operations, with a year's total objective of two thousand. He continually broke his own records for speed. Once he commented on his own skill while sewing in an artery from a patient's thigh connecting it to the aorta and a coronary artery. "You practice for this procedure," he remarked in his soft, detached voice, "by circumcising gnats."

DeBakey continued as head of his school, chairman of his department, directing his laboratory, and operating. Perhaps DeBakey operated less than Cooley, who did little else. ("Denton would rather operate than ———," commented one colleague, and another friend remarked that he suspected Cooley's wife of getting sick and going to the hospital in order to see her husband.)

Neither surgeon was ever accused—as some were—of performing unnecessary operations for the sake of monetary gain. If they seemed to worship numbers, the numbers were never questioned. However, Thompson, in *Hearts*, does quote one Houston physician as saying, "They weren't liars. But what you call an improved patient is a value judgment. You may cure a patient's headache, but have to cut his leg off!" Such phenomenal numbers did raise questions in some minds about the emotional area of doctor-patient relationships. This was a factor never to be ignored in healing. Healing could be left to the physicians, but surgeons Harken and Lillehei were two who inspired love, loyalty, and motivation in their patients to the extent that this became a potent metabolic and healing plus. But belief in the surgeon of choice is an act of faith and the source of that faith may be awe and distance just as it may be warm love and gratitude for personal care.

For surgery, especially complex and high-risk surgery, egotism is required. Both DeBakey and Cooley had it in such measure that in-jokes were told and retold about them. There was the Cooley scrub nurse quoted and requoted as having announced in the St. Luke's coffee shop, "I've had it with Dr. Wonderful and his God Squad. I'll take orthopedics!" Told and retold until it became hackneyed was the Christmas Day story on DeBakey. He arrived to find most of his staff missing. The cheeky resident on duty interrupted DeBakey's tirade against the laziness and incompetence of the absent. "Sir," he said, "they are at home celebrating the birth of *another* great man." DeBakey laughed.

He is not supposed to have laughed when a Boston story, possibly apocryphal, was told. DeBakey arrived, it was said, at a hospital to find its parking lot full. "Find me a place," he demanded of the attendant. "My name is Michael DeBakey!" "I couldn't find you a place," the attendant replied, "even if your name was Denton Cooley."

For many years if you asked any laymen what they knew about heart surgeons, even if the reply did not include Cooley's and DeBakey's names, it identified Texas. "Those guys in Texas," as one (inevitable) taxi driver put it, had a long day as the personification of heart surgery. Houston was satisfied. "Houston speaking" would become the voice that reached the men on the moon not long after Houston was replaced as the cardiac center of attention by Cape Town, South Africa.

13.

Second-Hand Hearts

The truth of it is that a borrowed heart, replacing the recipient's, remains the donor's heart. Its new possessor may live and function for years while its original owner has been for that long dead, but the heart continues to "remember." It may adapt well, adjust to its responsibilities in the host's body, even adopt its host's personal deficiencies, but both host and heart have to be continually coaxed into getting along together.

Immunosuppression is the most important aspect of that process of coaxing. All mammals maintain militant defense systems to guard against invasion by foreigners, "alien" cells. The defenders make no distinction between invaders with inimical and invaders with beneficent intentions. Sometimes we die in the battle from the instinctive unreason of our defensive systems.

Ancient medical dreams of grafting spareable bits from one human onto another were defeated by the phenomenon of rejection. Dr. Alexis Carrel, who is to transplantation what Robert Goddard is to space, defined the rejection process before 1912. However, medical literature, long before proof, recognized the potential of trades between littermates, approximated in humans by identical twins.

Extensive skin grafting between identical twins was successfully accomplished in 1927. Their cells were so genetically similar that the defense aroused was, at worst, half-hearted. Animal experimentation in transplanting organs after World War II was extensive, particularly with kidneys (of which, of course, we have two). The results were inconclusive. Transplanting a kidney, even using littermates, was a delicate operation. In the laboratory, techniques were gradually worked out.

At the Peter Bent Brigham Hospital in 1954 transplant history was made when a healthy young man saved his identical twin's life by permitting surgeons to remove one of his kidneys and give it to his brother. The two of them regained near-perfect health. The essential prerequisites for that operation were exceedingly rare: identical twinship with the occurrence of the lethal disease in one twin in a paired or supernumerary organ. Much more had to be learned before less perfectly matched organs could be transplanted.

One little known incident in the early kidney transplant efforts involves three Peter Bent Brigham house officers. In 1952 in a side room of the hospital at midnight, by the light of a gooseneck lamp, they worked over a dying, unconscious woman with no renal function to install a kidney from a fresh cadaver in her body. The artery and vein to and from the cadaver kidney were attached to the thigh artery and vein of the moribund patient. Miraculously the ureter of the newly attached kidney began to pour out urine.

Harken expressed his sense of wonder at the selflessness of the three young men in the exhilaration of innovation. They were uninhibited at the time by "human experiment" committees that would demand to know whether they had had informed consent, by laborious deliberations and legal concerns. What further advances and breakthroughs, he often speculated, might still be occurring if restraints and regulations had not become experimental straitjackets. Those three house officers went on to positions of importance. David Hume was professor of surgery at the University of Virginia's great medical school before he was killed in the crash of his own plane. Charles Hufnagel, a famous pioneer, became chairman of the Department of Surgery at Georgetown Medical School. Ernest Bandsteiner was made chief of surgery at the Rhode Island Hospital.

Kidney transplant would progress to the point where it would enable many people who would otherwise have died to live. Patients could be kept alive by effective mechanical kidney function until a suitable transplant could be arranged. Live donors having two could spare one. Single vital organs were—and are—a very different matter. The donor of organs such as the heart or liver must be legally dead since the donor would die without their function. Animal experimentation between littermates went on, and so did studies in overcoming rejection.

At a meeting of the American College of Surgeons in 1967 a report was made of liver transplants in two children, performed by Dr. Thomas Starzl at the University of Colorado. They had survived more than eleven weeks. In 1977 an update on liver transplants noted that out of 302, 47 recipients were still alive; the longest-surviving patient had functioning graft for seven and a half years.

At the same meeting in 1967 Richard Lower showed motion pictures of a dog with a transplanted heart. Lower had worked in Wangensteen's laboratory with Norman Shumway in Minneapolis and with Shumway at Stanford University in California, and moved to the University of Virginia with David Hume. Although it was not conclusive in human terms, the sight of Lower's brown and white mutt scampering about with a littermate's heart in her chest provided a sensation. Furthermore, during the year of her survival, the mutt had given birth to a litter of puppies.

In December 1967 Christiaan Barnard, at the relatively ill-equipped Groote Schuur Hospital in Cape Town, South Africa, performed his sensational first human heart transplant. Louis Washkansky lived for eighteen days with a healthy heart in place of his own, taken from the body of a victim of an automobile accident. Three days after Barnard's operation Dr. Adrian Kantrowitz, then in New York, replaced the heart of a child, but his recipient lived only a few hours. On New Year's Day 1968 Barnard's second heart transplant made Philip Blaiberg the most famous patient in the world. He would live for 551 highly publicized days.

Enthusiasm among surgeons reached its peak in 1968 and plummeted in 1969. From Minnesota, C. Walton Lillehei called

Barnard's a "fantastic piece of surgery," and from Houston, Michael DeBakey, pursuing his artificial heart, said, "This breaks the ice—it is a real breakthrough!" Barnard, who had clinically applied the techniques so long and patiently worked out by Norman Shumway, was given standing ovations at medical meetings, including that of the American College of Cardiology in San Francisco. Among cardiac surgery's old lions, Dwight Harken, then fifty-eight, was the only loud nay-sayer, protesting that there was no reality to the international euphoria, to the hopes being raised everywhere, until control of rejection improved. His voice was the only one raised against such procedures at the John F. Kennedy Symposium on Heart Transplant held in Boston in May 1968.

The year 1968 would see 101 heart transplants performed worldwide: 54 in the United States, 14 in Canada, 10 in France, 23 in other countries. Of these Blaiberg lived into 1969, and two, one operated on in Milwaukee, Wisconsin, one in Marseilles, France, were still alive in 1977. Most results were so discouraging that the total number attempted in 1969 was only 47.

In fact, the score of successes went much as Harken had predicted. Three past presidents of the American College of Cardiology, Burch, Corday, and Dack, all cardiologists, demanded an immediate moratorium. They cited Harken as the one prominent cardiac surgeon who had not been carried away on the tide of early enthusiasm. Simplification or anything resembling routine success had not followed the pioneering efforts. Money spent on the transplants had diminished funds available for research and development in more promising fields of heart surgery, as Harken had predicted. Legal and ethical questions remained unanswered. Many institutions quickly dropped from the field altogether. A single heart transplant meant mobilizing the entire hospital, and some major hospitals, such as the Massachusetts General in Boston, forbade their surgeons to perform any at all.

It would be a long time before the cardiologists and surgeon Harken, who had reserved the right to change their minds, began to do so. This happened when Norman Shumway's cautious progress in Palo Alto, California, justified the procedure as worth clinical experimentation.

Meantime the question of legal death for donors remained ill-defined. If a donor's heart could be kept beating, was he actually dead? In 1969 Dr. Lower and his Virginia team were accused of "murder" by a donor's brother and sued for a million dollars. There was the suit brought against Denton Cooley by his patient's wife, who claimed her husband was the victim of "human experimentation" because he was kept alive on an artificial heart until a donor heart could be transplanted, after which he died. In 1971 Cooley, whose twenty-two transplant patients were all dead, quit. He offered the public explanation that no more requests were coming in, that the families of brain-dead victims no longer offered their kin as heart donors. After twelve transplants, Michael DeBakey did no more. In 1971 only seventeen transplants were performed worldwide, and when the total did climb back into thirty or more a year, most of them were Norman Shumway's, whose research and techniques the others had borrowed.

More disappointing even than the dismal survival statistics was the quality of the lives prolonged by transplant. That is an ultimate test of the value of any medical advance. Even the most successful of the patients who lived on with borrowed hearts were tethered to their doctors and hospitals. They lived the precarious existence of the invalid.

There was no reason to assume that the heart tissue was privileged tissue or an exception to the rejection phenomenon, D.E.H. believed in 1968. In the transplanting of teeth, skin, biologic valves, and kidneys, rejection remained the biggest problem. Physicians still had a great deal to learn about the art of peacemaking between host bodies and transplanted foreign parts. The danger of rejection with foreign hearts was acute. It lessened if the patients survived the first year, but they had to be continuously and meticulously monitored, extensively medicated. Some could maintain a reasonable semblance of normal life— one resumed professional bowling—and many recipients, in spite of everything, became zealous missionaries for heart transplant.

When a human being's life is prolonged, there is no simple answer to the question "Was it worth it?" Of the first two heart transplant survivors, Philip Blaiberg would have answered with a

resounding *yes*. By the time world attention had turned to Blaiberg, Louis Washkansky's wife had said *no* for him.

Louis Washkansky was eager to be Barnard's guinea pig. It
was his only chance for survival. He gave his informed consent to
the surgeon. That is, informed up to a point. Barnard, in his con-
fessional autobiography, *One Life*, admits that he offered Washkansky more hope for more time than he expected himself.

The procedure for the first transplant is minutely described
in Barnard's book. So are the following days. After his slow recovery from the major heart operation, for one week Louis Washkansky shared the world's excitement, a happy Lazarus.

On the fourteenth-postoperative day lung infection set in
and frantic conferences ensued at the Groote Schuur. To decrease
the anti-immune drugs would increase the danger of rejection for
Washkansky's borrowed heart. Antibiotics in the amount that
might check the infection could bring his digestive system to a
halt; it was already on the brink of collapse. Washkansky was reported as miserable over the medical and physical indignities to
which he was subjected in the desperate attempt to save his life,
especially when he lost control of his bladder. He seemed to give
up hope and Barnard could no longer convey to him the comfort
he himself took in the fact that Washkansky's own heart would
have failed long since. The new one was holding firm, beating
steadily.

The layman reading the rest of Barnard's story of Washkansky's last days, with which he ends *One Life*, may react as one
does to human torture. Many of the other doctors at the Groote
Schuur urged restraint, wanted Barnard to permit Washkansky to
die. At this point Harken's sympathy with and understanding for
Barnard in the crisis was total and uncompromising. He had only
contempt for those doctors who would give up at this point, and
was bitter at the doubters who urged giving up. Harken would
say that he would never have forgiven himself for getting a patient into such a situation, but once the patient was there, by accident, or design, he would support the most desperate efforts to
save his life. "This is the reason that once the patient has cast his

lot with the conscientious, competent pioneer, that patient or his family should not shift to less concerned care!"

Convinced that Washkansky must be kept alive, Barnard connected him to a respirator. He talked to his patient, who could no longer speak, his vocal chords rendered immobile by the endotracheal tube. Barnard insisted that Washkansky's silent, frustrated movements meant "Tell me, tell me more." He begged Washkansky's wife, Ann, to keep up her husband's fighting spirit. Late at night on December 20 Washkansky's body turned blue from lack of oxygen in his congested veins. Although he was receiving pure oxygen, the discoloration intensified. Barnard quotes Ann Washkansky as saying that Barnard was now behaving "like a madman." Barnard refused to concede to the inexorable biologic processes killing his patient. The operation had been superb, successful. He determined to connect Washkansky again to the heart-lung machine, to perform a thoracotomy, and clean his blood with the oxygenator. It might add time for the antibiotics to work. "We can't let this man die. We can't!" Barnard said.

In his autobiography Barnard quotes the intense conversation that followed with Dr. Velva (Val) Schrire, Washkansky's cardiologist:

Schrire: Chris, you have no more time. It was up yesterday or maybe even the day before. It's all over.

Barnard: My God, how can you say that?

Schrire: Listen, Chris, Washkansky is clinically lost. Everybody knows it except you.

Barnard: Everybody doesn't know it. We had a chance until tonight. We still have a chance . . .

Schrire: To put him back on the pump is madness.

"I did not know how to reply," Barnard wrote. "Was I subjecting him to further pain merely because I refused to give up? How much of this was now myself—and how much Washkansky?" Schrire succeeded in restraining him from using the pump, but Barnard still refused to admit defeat. At five o'clock in the morning he was still injecting potassium, and continued to do so until toward 6:30 A.M. on December 21, when Louis Washkansky died. The young girl's heart, which had kept on beating for his those eighteen days, stopped. The postmortem would prove that Washkansky's lungs, filled with blue-green pneumonia, had little air space left. The borrowed heart was blue and dead. But the suture lines were perfect, no error, no clot. (Of this part of the book, Harken would comment that it must have been intended for an uncritical audience. "This is clearly a case where a heart-lung machine was justified, it should have been tried!" Harken did not condone trying transplantation at the time in that place but would condone nothing less than Barnard's total, all-out efforts and denial of death. He considered the pain Barnard was suffering the "most heinous creation of Satan in his most diabolic mood. I would ask all to understand it and wish no one to suffer it.")

Barnard walked alone at dawn after arranging for a postmortem. He went by the laboratory with its barking dogs, squealing pigs, screaming baboons, on to his office at the medical school. The copy of *Time* magazine with his picture on the cover was there; a telegram from CBS lay open, advising him that Drs. Michael DeBakey and Adrian Kantrowitz had agreed to appear with him on *Face the Nation* on December 24. What could he reply if he canceled? "Professor Barnard cannot come because his patient has died and he has lost confidence in himself?" His close friend, Dr. Jacques Roux, came in. He had heard the news on the radio and urged Barnard to do another transplant immediately.

"I'm going to America . . . I'm going to face the world . . . and then come back and do a transplant on Philip Blaiberg," said Barnard.

On the last page of his book Barnard reported the conversation he had with the second man he had scheduled for transplant, Philip Blaiberg:

Blaiberg: How soon can you do it?
Barnard: I have to go overseas for about ten days, but we'll do it as soon as possible after I get back. In the meantime I'll have you transferred to my ward.
Blaiberg: More than ever I want this to be a success—not only for my sake, but also for you and the other doctors.

Barnard: You can help us by doing one thing.
Blaiberg: Yes—what is it?
Barnard: Stay alive until I get back.
Blaiberg: Don't worry. You'll find me here waiting.

The day after Louis Washkansky was buried, Christiaan Barnard departed from Malan Airport. The public tide of excitement was still at full flood, the "Miracle in Capetown," as *Newsweek* had called it, was still considered one. If criticism might have been expected from surgical colleagues because he had used Shumway's techniques, Barnard undercut it by stating at once that he had learned 90 percent of his technology in the United States. He was greeted by Mayor John Lindsay when he arrived in New York, made dozens of public appearances, and accepted an invitation from President Lyndon Johnson to visit his Texas ranch. Young and personable, giving the outward appearance of modesty, disposing of questions about rejection with the acknowledgment that it was a problem, he remained the man of the hour. Back in Cape Town Philip Blaiberg waited.

Some reporters still stood by at the Groote Schuur. They were kept more or less informed by Marius Barnard, Christiaan Barnard's brother and a member of his surgical team. In Barnard's ward Philip Blaiberg was deteriorating so rapidly that the staff was afraid he would die before Christiaan Barnard got back. Velva Schrire, his cardiologist as he had been Washkansky's, knew that transplantation was Blaiberg's only chance. In 1967 Schrire had sent his own diagnosis to Cleveland, Ohio, for confirmation. No other operation could help Blaiberg.

Barnard returned late on December 30. Reporters waited at the airport and on New Year's Eve the newspapers sported banner headlines concerning the hero's arrival. Crowds gathered from time to time at the hospital, awaiting news of a second transplant.

New Year's Day was a very special holiday for the so-called Cape Coloreds, South Africans of mixed black and white blood. One such couple who went on a picnic that day were Clive and Dorothy Haupt. Clive Haupt collapsed suddenly and was taken to the Victoria Hospital in Cape Town. There Dr. Basil Sacks concluded that he had suffered a massive cerebral hemorrhage and there was no hope of saving him. Sacks informed the Groote Schuur that he might have a heart donor for Barnard. Dorothy Haupt and Clive Haupt's mother, who earned her living as a cleaning woman, were asked for permission. His mother was reported to have said, "If you can save the life of another person, take my son's heart."

Blaiberg was reported to have agreed that he would accept a Colored's heart, any heart. Perhaps because he was, like Washkansky, the son of Jewish immigrants, he did not share the deeply inbred racial prejudice felt by the Dutch-descended white Afrikaners. Haupt's unconscious body was transferred to the Groote Schuur and kept functioning until brain death, the decerebrate state, was determined. On the afternoon of January 2, 1968, Haupt's heart was removed to replace Blaiberg's failing one.

The operation required exquisite timing between two operating rooms, one for the excision of the donor heart, one for the removal of the recipient's and its immediate replacement with the donor's. Actually the procedure itself was simpler to perform than some complex valve replacements or coronary artery bypass surgery, though more dangerous to the patient. Barnard's procedure was technically identical to the one he had used for Washkansky. This time the donor's heart was a better tissue match, and after a single shock it began to beat again, strongly and regularly.

An Italian reporter waiting outside the hospital caught Barnard as he emerged from a side door at six o'clock. Jurgen Thorwald in his book, *Patients,* quotes the Italian as saying that the weary but elated surgeon shook hands with him and several other watchers, kissed two little girls, and told those assembled that the operation was a great success. Philip Blaiberg was already feeling well in an isolation room. Christiaan Barnard's brother Marius seconded this first bulletin. The team, he said, had learned a lot from the Washkansky experience and would be better able to avoid rejection in Blaiberg's case.

Eileen Blaiberg, the patient's wife, celebrated the transplant at home with friends and relatives. Champagne corks popped. "I, too," the Italian reporter would add in sad retrospect, "believed that this time Barnard had succeeded and that before long thousands of hearts would be transplanted throughout the world."

Laudatory and continuous publicity about Barnard and Blaiberg followed the case for the more than a year that Blaiberg lived. It was enjoyed to the fullest by Blaiberg, Barnard, and the patriots of South Africa. All of them had suffered, so to speak, from underprivilege.

Barnard was a South African Horatio Alger hero. He was raised in a desert settlement, the son of an impecunious Afrikaans minister who preached to a Colored congregation. His mother was in the tradition of valiant frontier women and ambitious for her sons. Their brains and her determination enabled her boys to overcome wretched poverty and achieve university educations and medical degrees. As a promising surgeon, Christiaan Barnard was awarded a fellowship to train in the promised land under Professor Owen Wangensteen. C. Walton Lillehei and Norman Shumway were there. Barnard scrubbed floors for additional income, and sent for his partially estranged wife, a former nurse, and their daughter. When he returned to South Africa it was with the gift of a heart-lung machine for the Groote Schuur Hospital. He performed the first heart valve replacement there for a black South African woman, and by the age of forty had built his own surgical team.

To study kidney transplantation, Barnard obtained a second fellowship to work with Richard Lower, a former colleague of Shumway's. After his return to South Africa he did a few animal experiments of his own and one kidney transplant. Then he had the daring and vaulting ambition to attempt the first human heart transplant. His detractors would add that he also had enough ignorance—but genuine pioneers, who might disapprove of Barnard's excessive love of publicity, resented even more deeply the nonspecific doubters who, they thought, were reflecting only their own lack of daring or competence.

For his part, Philip Blaiberg had grown up in the provincial Oudtshoorn, a barren region between Cape Town and Port Elizabeth. He made no claim to being other than an ordinary man and his modest career as a dentist in Cape Town was enlivened by a passion for amateur sports and by some mild mountain climbing. His joy in life was limited when he became a cardiac cripple and he was further saddened by the death of his twenty-two-year-old son from a bullet wound. In 1967 when cardiologist Schrire's verdict, confirmed in Cleveland, doomed him, Blaiberg succumbed to despair—until he heard a radio report about Washkansky and Barnard.

Cape Town had already become the place where a medical miracle happened. It had in Barnard an international hero as much admired as Lindbergh. Until then most international publicity given South Africa had been unfavorable. Now the world was astonished, and subsequent failures in the United States, France, Spain, Brazil, and Japan only added spice to South African pride in Christiaan Barnard as his second transplant patient, Blaiberg, continued to live and seemed to flourish. Small wonder, perhaps, that nation, surgeon, and patient placed so high a premium on recognition. Everything Barnard did was news, and he did everything.

> The young revolutionary [wrote the Italian reporter who continued to follow the Barnard story through 1968] who changed the whole nature of cardiac medicine was also breaking personally with the traditional proprieties of his profession. In Paris, Barnard appeared at the Crazy Horse, a strip-tease joint. In Monaco, 900 millionaires paid sizeable entry fees just to see him. Princess Grace danced the first dance with him at a ball. In Rome, the Pope received him in private audience; so did Gina Lollobrigida and Sophia Loren. In London, the participants in a Miss Universe contest voted him the most important man in the world. On February 15, before flying off from Cape Town on another tour, he visited Blaiberg to say goodbye to the living symbol of his success.

Whatever the accuracy of that exuberant report, Barnard certainly cut many a caper. And on that February 1968 visit to Blaiberg he had a press photograph taken with his patient, who was smiling and holding the jar in which his old heart was preserved.

Blaiberg was not only delighted to smile at his old heart in a bottle, he went to painful extremes to prove to the press how well he was. When he left the hospital to go home in March, he insisted on leaving his wheelchair at the exit and walked to the car while flashbulbs popped. He also walked from the car to his front door, although once out of sight of the newsmen, he had to be supported. Bales of telegrams and letters arrived for him as the world press assiduously reported his progress: his first haircut, what he ate, his first bath, the many medicines he took. His opinions were sought on every conceivable subject, and he delivered them portentously, receiving reporters and selected visitors in his living room. They were only required to wear surgical masks and to sit at a distance from him. When anyone, anywhere, expressed any doubt about his recovery or vitality, Blaiberg made feisty offers to meet the doubter at the airport, drive him himself to his apartment, and join him in a drink.

On May 3, 1968, Denton Cooley transferred a heart from a young woman to Everett Thomas. The donor was a suicide who had put a bullet into her brain. Cooley had operated on her heart in 1962, when she was ten years old, and knew it was sound. The recipient was a middle-aged man with three bad valves and poorly functioning ventricles. Cooley had cut the time for his transplants to under an hour, and the timetable on this one was capsuled and later published in *Hearts*:

> May 2, 1968. 11 P.M. Transfer of donor to Room 2. Transfer of potential recipient to room 1.
> 11:50 P.M. Opening of Thomas's thorax reveals hopeless destruction of his heart.
> 11:55 P.M. Donor's heart stops beating. [Brain death had already been determined.]
> May 3, 1968. 12:45 A.M. Dr. Cooley and Dr. Hallman remove Thomas's heart. Dr. Bloodwell removed donor's heart.
> 12:55 A.M. Donor heart taken to room 1.
> 1:01 A.M. Donor heart fitted and sutures placed by Dr. Cooley.
> 1:35 A.M. Completion of last suture.
> 1:37 A.M. Opening of aortic clamp. Wild irregular heartbeats [ventricular fibrillation]
> 1:39 A.M. A single electric shock suffices to induce rhythmic heartbeat.

On May 21 Cooley transplanted a heart to replace that of Louis Fierro, and on May 24 announced that Fierro was already in "fine fettle" and that heart transplantation was no longer experimental. It was now a revolutionary therapeutic means of saving lives. St. Luke's Hospital was setting up a heart transplant unit. The new antilymphocytic serum, added to previously used drugs, was proving "miraculously" effective against rejection. Only a lack of donors was holding up a series of miracles as heart patients rushed to St. Luke's to wait for them.

On June 11, 1968, the American media had another field day at a press conference in Houston. At St. Luke's Hospital Denton Cooley and "the fastest heart surgery team in the world" presented transplant patients Everett Thomas and Louis Fierro. Both patients wore hard hats sent to them by local construction workers. They looked frail under the hats, but Fierro quipped that he "felt like a millionaire" and Thomas said, "I'm the other millionaire."

"A heart," pontificated Thomas, tall, earnest, and deeply religious, "is simply a muscle pump and mine has been replaced. Now that I have a new fuel pump, I'm a new car. For me, heart transplantation is the greatest contribution to the preservation of human life and the donation of a heart the gift of gifts. We are going to be the Blaibergs of America and represent for our country what he represents: the advance guard of a new medicine."

On the same day, June 11, it was kept from the press that Blaiberg had gone back to the Groote Schuur Hospital, dangerously ill. The next day, June 12, at St. Luke's Hospital Cooley's fifth transplant failed. A second donor could not be found, so Cooley attempted to keep his patient alive by implanting a sheep's heart, which failed absolutely and almost instantly. (Many thought by doing this Cooley had gone too far, but Harken was more charitable. "After all, when your patient lies before you on your operating table, you find a one in a million chance very attractive—if you don't give the patient that chance at that point you have some cruelly haunting thoughts that you didn't do the weird thing because you were unwilling to make the effort. That emotion is toughest when hours of effort have left you exhausted, emotionally and physically spent.")

When Fierro and Thomas left St. Luke's in "fine fettle" they were given undemanding jobs where the public could see and talk to them. Both loved being on display. Thomas would frequently mention God and Cooley in the same breath. By October they were both back in the hospital. Fierro died on October 14. Autopsy revealed that the coronary arteries of his healthy borrowed heart had degenerated in five months to those of an arteriosclerotic old man. Thomas seemed to have developed an allergy or sensitivity to the antilymphocytic serum. In November, when Thomas's transplanted heart began to fail, Cooley in desperation attempted a second transplant. Thomas's third heart beat feebly and then stopped. Some of those waiting at St. Luke's Hospital in Houston for heart donors and their own transplantations went home in alarmed retreat.

In Cape Town Blaiberg was quietly released from the hospital again. By this time he was visibly crippled, but he tried to keep up appearances and convinced himself that he was making steady progress. He even insisted that he would go with his wife on a triumphal tour of Europe. The Groote Schuur team, with Barnard often away and not available to process his patient's well-being, persuaded Blaiberg not to leave while his surgeon was abroad. It would worry him too much. Eileen Blaiberg went alone, to enjoy and perpetuate the Blaiberg "miracle."

The ominous signs of damage to Blaiberg's body from the drugs he had to take included marked decalcification of the skeletal structure and, as doctors would suspect and tests confirm, his new heart was being mercilessly attacked by the same disease that had brought Blaiberg to Barnard initially: coronary sclerosis.

Christiaan Barnard and Eileen Blaiberg both returned to take over his care from Barnard's colleagues and from the Colored maid, Katie, who had long and lovingly cared for Philip Blaiberg at home. Dr. Barnard pleaded with Blaiberg's wife to consent to a second transplant. Katie, who had been closest to her employer's current suffering, backed Eileen Blaiberg's decision that enough was enough. Philip Blaiberg spent his last five days dozing and receiving oxygen and on Sunday, August 17, 1969, he died. His borrowed heart had succumbed to the arteriosclerotic process that, in its lifetime, had destroyed his own.

A year later an article on cardiac transplantation by Norman Shumway, the most important investigator of the possibility, and his cohorts at Stanford University was published in the September issue of *California Medicine*. Its conclusion:

> The initial enthusiasm, approaching hysteria, which greeted the first clinical cardiac transplants now seems to have been replaced by a generally pessimistic outlook. Both reactions are probably inappropriate.
>
> The journalists' "medical breakthrough" rarely results in a radical change in patient care. It is, rather, the cautious clinical application of information gained in the laboratory that results in the gradual development of new therapeutic methods.
>
> At this point, we believe cardiac transplantation remains within the realm of clinical investigation.

Shumway in California and Richard Lower in Virginia would continue these clinical investigations under scientifically stringent conditions. Harken, a man whose own clinical investigations in other areas had led him to oppose the transplants, reserved the right to change his mind, but continued in opposition to clinical heart transplantation. In June 1971 the editor of *Chest* magazine, Dr. Alfred Soper, editorialized:

> It is traditionally the diagnostician who stays the surgeon's hand, but fortunately there are scientists such as Dr. Harken who bridge both disciplines at historic moments. [This] reflection is not meant to deny the invaluable data obtained from cardiac transplantations which have been performed in the past few years. The courage which prompted the implementation of this procedure has contributed much to our knowledge and refusal to perform a limited number of transplants, under ideal clinical and investigational environments, would have resulted in irreparable loss. One need not, however, be a therapeutic nihilist to applaud Dr. Harken's continuing contributions in the sphere of surgical responsibility.

Harken amplified that complex statement. "When one obstructs for obstruction's sake he is apt to be right because more ideas are bad than are good. On the other hand, when one obstructs with reason and explains those reasons he then deserves the privilege of saying 'I told you so and I told you why!' " In a letter to the young nonmedical son of a friend who asked about transplants he explained carefully:

A long time before the world recognized heart transplants as a brave but disappointing adventure, I explained my specific reasons for not undertaking some. In public debates I pointed out that the model of the kidney where one could have one transplant rejection, dialysis with mechanical kidneys, retransplant with another kidney, and so on to three or four transplants, was the way to render service to patients while studying tissue matching and the biologic as well as pharmacologic control of rejection. The "one strike and you're out" techniques of using nonpaired vital structures such as the brain, the liver, the heart, all impress me as folly and exhibitionism.

One off the record comment I might make is that obviously there were people who said "Harken can't do transplants or he would." In order to scotch that rumor I did take a patient who was brain dead and had her kidneys removed for transplantation, put her on the heart-lung machine, took the heart out, stopped it for half an hour, put it back in and started it up again. (Of course we had performed this type of autotransplantation several times at autopsy in the pathology department. Actually the technique of the surgery has never been the barrier. This is what underscores the folly of celebrating or prancing with pride immediately after "successful" heart transplant.)

This autotransplantation is much more difficult technically than taking a heart from one donor and giving it to a recipient. One takes the heart out when he is obtaining a donor heart with wide margins for anastomosis (the joining together of two or more hollow organs) and leaves wide margins when excising the heart of the recipient. Therefore, one has much more tissue to work with when he transplants from one person to another and is expending the donor, than he does when he takes out and returns in what we call an autograft. One such autotransplant on a living body that had no kidneys and no brain was documented on colored movie film.

This procedure likewise proved the ability of the heart severed from its nerves to perform, and in those two cases the clinical investigation was done on brain-dead and completely un-conscious bodies and there was no suffering whatsoever then or afterward—nor, of course, lives saved.

In *Medical World News*, March 8, 1976, a report before the Society of Thoracic Surgeons in Washington by Dr. Randall B. Griepp was summarized. He believed that physicians should now start thinking of heart transplantation as truly therapeutic rather than highly experimental. Dr. Griepp worked with Shumway at the medical center in Palo Alto, California. The group had had ex-perience with 102 transplants on 97 patients.

Conclusions: A patient who survived the first year had about a fifty-fifty chance of living for five. Rehabilitation techniques had improved. Surveillance to detect early signs of rejection had im-proved through endomyocardial biopsy, possible under local an-esthesia. Medication was better understood and there had been considerable reduction in the incidence of arteriosclerosis in the transplanted heart graft.

The cost of a heart transplant was now only $30,000—"only four times that of replacing an aortic valve"—and had come down proportionate to the inflated costs of other heart operations. The 1974 Anatomical Gift Act in California permitted removal of a donor's heart while it was still beating if there was no evidence of brain function. This made it easier to obtain suitable organs.

Guidelines for selecting transplant recipients among patients applying to the Stanford University Medical Center in Palo Alto grew stringent. The form sent to cardiologists with potential can-didates filled eight single-spaced pages. Particular emphasis was placed on emotional stability. The basic commandments were:

1. Class IV cardiac disease, refractory to medical or surgical treat-ment. Bed-chair existence, and/or poor prognosis for six months survival.

2. Under age 55.

3. Stable psychological history.

4. Adequate finances and medical insurance for pre-transplant evaluation. [After that, grant money was available to cover the cost of care at the Stanford hospital.]

5. Availability of vigorous follow-up medical care when the patient returns home.

6. Strong positive attitude on the part of the patient and his family after discussion of the transplant procedures and its failures.

Underlined after the survival statistics, "which should be explained to the patient," was the caution: *"That cardiac transplantation is not a 'cure-all' must be pointed out to the patient."* That line may have more significance for some patients than for others. For most end-stage cardiac cripples, the choice for transplant was primarily for the chance to live at all. Statistically hope might not be high, but it existed.

The totals published by the American College of Surgeons/ National Institutes of Health on July 1, 1977 (see below), were accompanied by a newsletter that stated:

Now that the Kidney Registry has been transferred to the Department of Health, Education, and Welfare, the NIH feels that the activity of the Registry, currently handling heart, lung, liver and pancreas, is not of sufficiently high priority to warrant renewal of the grant. The Board of Regents of the College feels that the Registry has served a valuable function over the past eight years, but cannot justify the expenditure of College Funds to continue the current, limited activities. Please do not send any more reports or requests to this Registry.

Some surgeons were reported as glad: one less form to fill out. Others regretted losing a central source of information.

HUMAN HEART TRANSPLANTATION
Dec. 3, 1967–July 1, 1977

World Totals

Transplant teams	65
Transplants	346
Recipients	338
Living Recipients	77

Chronology and World Distribution • July 1, '77 (numbers in parentheses indicate survivors)

Year	World Totals	U.S.A.	Canada	France	South Africa	Other Countries
1967	2	1	0	0	1	0
1968	101 (1)	54	14	10 (1)	2	21
1969	47 (1)	34	1	0	4 (1)	8
1970	17 (3)	16 (3)	1	0	0	0
1971	18 (3)	13 (2)	1	0	3 (1)	1
1972	18 (4)	15 (4)	0	0	2	1
1973	33 (4)	21 (3)	1	8 (1)	1	2
1974	29 (10)	17 (8)	0	9 (2)	1	2
1975	32 (16)	23 (12)	0	5 (2)	3 (2)	1
1976	31 (20)	21 (16)	1	5 (2)	4 (2)	0
1977	18 (15)	10 (8)	0	3 (3)	4 (4)	0
Total	346 (77)	225 (56)	19	40 (11)	25 (10)	36

American College of Surgeons/National Institutes of Health

Update on Organ Transplantation in the World	Heart	Liver	Lung	Pancreas
Transplant teams	65	43	22	15
Transplants	346	318	37	57
Recipients	338	302	37	55
Alive with functioning grafts	77	47	0	0
Longest survival with functioning graft	8.7 yr	7.5 yr	10 mo	4.2 yr
Longest current survival with functioning graft	8.7 yr	7.5 yr	—	—

Cases reported to the Registry, July 1, 1977

American College of Surgeons/National Institutes of Health

Of the recipients alive in June 1978, fifty-one were patients of Shumway's. He also had by far the best overall record for length of survival. The record of eight years and seven months belonged to surgeon Henry at the Centre Cantini in Marseilles,

France, and recipient Charles Boulogne, a French Dominican priest whose transplant Henry had performed on November 28, 1968. Shumway's record patient, seven years and six months, was preceded on the list also by a patient of Barnard's, who had survived eight years and two months. Until November 1974, when he died, Richard Lower's patient, Louis Russell, a teacher in Indianapolis, held the record in the world. His operation, performed at the Medical College in Virginia, was the thirty-fourth transplant done in August 1968. Seventeen months later Russell was quoted in the *Louisville Courier Journal*'s December 4, 1969, issue as saying, "Now I'm No. 1. The thirty-three others have died. Nobody has borrowed time. There's none for rent and none for sale. When my time comes . . . I'm ready to go. I'm a Christian."

Transplant news was no longer sensational. The press was warier and press releases from the Stanford and Virginia centers, where the most transplants went on, were low key. In time donor shortage was eased slightly by the transporting of donor hearts from long distances. The Medical College of Virginia announced a heart brought in from six hundred miles away in May 1977. It had been flushed with cold saline solution and placed in a kidney transport container—kidney transport had already become fairly routine. A television documentary on transplant patients and procedures was made in Palo Alto, and from time to time reporters wrote stories about the survivors for magazines or newspapers. Most of them were more than willing to talk.

To use a colorful example, Richard Cope, one of Shumway's most grateful transplant recipients, like Philip Blaiberg, enjoyed publicity. He even violated the donor anonymity imposed by Shumway. During an interview on the *David Frost Show* he thanked by name the parents of the seventeen-year-old boy who had been fatally injured in a motorcycle accident and whose heart he harbored.

Richard Cope really had no business still being alive, he said, when he arrived in Palo Alto from Patchogue, New York, in 1970. He had lived through cardiac revascularization by mammary artery implant (the Vineberg operation) at the Mayo Clinic and a later attempt at revascularization in a New York hospital.

He was only forty-five and he wanted very much to live. Heading for California, he joined the pathetic gathering of patients waiting for donors. Shumway talked to Cope and said he would have to live permanently in the area if he had transplantation because of postoperative therapy. Cope said he would not stay. "The quality of life had to be there, and it wouldn't be there for me in Palo Alto!" His doctors also told him that the government would cover the cost of the transplant operation because it was experimental research, and also the postoperative therapy, but that he would have to pay his own bills if he left California. That was all right with Cope. He was an aerospace engineer with the Grumman company and the company carried major catastrophic insurance on him. When, after Cope's evaluation, Shumway was reluctant to schedule a transplant, Cope went home. California, he said, was no place to die—or live.

He came back again when there was no further hope for him and, on October 25, 1970, became Shumway's twenty-sixth heart transplant patient.

"I saw a heck of a lot of Shumway before the surgery," Cope would tell a *Medical World News* reporter for an article published August 23, 1974. "He is very gentle, very quiet, one of the sweetest men I know. Almost everyone holds him in awe, but I don't think he likes it. You can sit and talk to him, just like anybody around. He wears an old pair of sneakers and an old green smock, and far be it for him to look like a famous heart surgeon. A really terrific human being! I know that when he's lost patients, he's been so despondent that it's almost ridiculous. He is also very shy."

Cope's recovery was remarkable. He was soon up, "bounding around," and within three weeks was hiking, as measured by a pedometer, fifteen miles a day within the hospital. Less than five weeks after his transplant he booked a plane ticket home. His doctors argued that he must not leave because he required drugs that protected him against a host of possible infections that could prove fatal. They threatened to withhold the medications that he must take with him. He agreed to stick around—until January 19. "Then I split. If I was going to get a transplant to lie around in a hospital, or stay in California, I didn't want it. I wanted to come back home, work where all my friends are, everybody I know. I had to come back here where I have a wife, a family, a boat, and where I like to go fluking. That's living!"

His remarkable primary care physician flew from New York State to California to learn about Cope's treatment and how to recognize subtle cardiographic evidence of impending rejection. Six little green tattoos were placed on Cope's chest to indicate where to place the ECG leads. Every week Cope and his doctor touched base with Stanford by telephone. Every ninety days engineer Cope sent out his own carefully prepared charts. Otherwise he continued to make his own rules.

He played golf. Once he flipped over in a snowmobile. ("I thought everyone was going to have a heart attack!") He traveled whenever he pleased by air and took only one special precaution. "I make sure I have my pills in my hand! They may lose your luggage. They lost mine once with my medication in it. The guy said to me, 'We'll have it for you in a couple of days.' I said, 'Don't bother. I'll be dead in a couple of days.' So they put on a special flight to run my luggage up."

Cope's favorite story about himself related to the pass he wangled to leave the hospital, soon after his transplantation. His wife was in town and the pass was from 3 to 7 P.M. so that he could have dinner with her. Two weeks later his doctors offered him a weekend pass and asked if he would mind having intercourse with his wife wearing an electrocardiographic monitoring device. " 'We'd like you to try,' they said. I said, 'I already did.' They said, 'What do you mean?' I said, 'The day you gave me that pass to go out for supper. Works fine, doc!' "

Cope lived through rejection episodes on Long Island and one on a return trip to California. He shrank from five foot eight to five five as vertebrae collapsed in his back from prednisone-induced calcium depletion. The essential prednisone, while suppressing the rejection function, softened his bones to allow "backbone compression" and he suffered from cracked and broken ribs. Nevertheless, four years after his transplantation, Cope said, "I wake up, and it's teeming rain and I hold my face up to it. Hey, what a lousy day? Lousy? Man, if I open my eyes to that day, it's a great day!"

The transplant story is one of concentrated and continuing drama. Its final importance in the history of heart surgery cannot be estimated as yet. It did bring into sharp focus all the legal, ethical, and moral questions involved in surgery whose value has not been proved and underlined the question as to whether certain major procedures should only be permitted in centers specializing in them.

Almost the only aspect of heart transplant on which all the surgeons everywhere agreed was that the early publicity was disastrous. Pronouncements that were printed had all the validity of palmistry or horoscopes. Christiaan Barnard was much censured for his superstar encouragement of publicity. Owen Wangensteen, ever the staunch defender of his former young men, defended Barnard. "After his heart transplant, South Africa used him as an ambassador of goodwill, being out of the mainstream and having such a poor image in world opinion. He was personable, you know. I think they encouraged his publicity, pressured him. He might have been better off if he'd done no transplants. Chris was a *good* research worker. He had solid achievements. And he did see Shumway's work in the laboratory."

Norman Shumway's dedication and integrity were never questioned and he continued to keep a low profile vis-à-vis the press. By 1978 Harken agreed when Walton Lillehei said that Shumway was beginning to show some very good results. Both stressed what Harken had articulated a decade before when cardiac transplantation broke on the scene, that it should be pursued as an experimental clinical therapy in only very specifically equipped centers: centers where extensive heart surgery competence paralleled renal transplant experience with immunosuppression. Centers, moreover, where those basic qualifications were supported by willingness on the part of administrative, medical, and surgical faculties to forego much else to dedicate space, funds, and facilities to heart transplants.

Of Shumway himself, Lillehei said, "Remember, he's made many innovations in surgery for almost every congenital and acquired lesion. His technique for preserving the myocardium—still one of the big problems, how to get a quiet heart on bypass, with no beat, flaccid and relaxed without damaging the heart muscle when you cut off the coronary flow—by cooling the heart selectively [i.e., putting ice around it or flushing it with cool solutions to quiet it without reducing the metabolic requirements of the rest of the body]. That doesn't eliminate all possible danger, but prolongs the time you can work before you start to get great damage. He was one of the first to get mortality of tetralogy of Fallot surgery down. One of the evolutionary stages is to get the risk of the completely corrective operation lower than that of the palliative procedure. And he had one of the finest training programs for young surgeons. He's a tremendously important contributor to many things."

Heart transplantation was by no means on the way out so long as men such as Shumway and Lower continued to practice and hand on what they were learning about it. Nor would media interest cease. In the November 15, 1977, issue of the Montreal *Gazette* a half-page interview was published with Jerry Young's wife. Her husband was the recipient of his third transplanted heart in Stanford. Mrs. Young said she had been told that

> Jerry was dying for three years. He's been fooling us for three years, and I believe he's going to continue to do so. But it's taking a toll on all of us. He's managing to survive, but we're all dropping dead slowly. There's an old saying: "The sick bury the well." There is the burden of responsibility that remains and life goes on. Once you pick up responsibility, you can't put it down. I'm fighting for Jerry and me, then I'm fighting for three beautiful children.

In the same issue was a UPI story about the first heart transplant performed in China in the spring of 1978. The patient died after 126 days, but before that resumed his regular activities, including basketball. Ju-Lung Sun of Fu Wai Hospital in Peking made the announcement on a visit to the United States. His colleague, Ju-Sheng Tai, professor of cardiothoracic medicine at the Fu Wai Hospital, said heart-related diseases had never been as great a problem in China as in the West, and that heart disease was decreasing in China, as it was in the United States.

As for heart transplantation, Norman Shumway said it was a shame coronary bypass surgery had not improved first. "I think some patients have undergone transplantation who might have been salvaged through coronary bypass surgery."

The future holds the hope that not only will heart disease continue to decrease through better care, but that one day there will be an artificial implantable heart to replace the human heart. It is interesting to contrast the current views of two great cardiac authorities—C. Walton Lillehei and Donald C. Harrison—on that possibility and on the future of transplanting. Harrison has from the beginning played an important role in Shumway's transplant program in California. The following quotations are from each of these men speaking separately.

Lillehei: The risk of heart transplant now is lower than for cancer of the lungs, many cancers, but the real problem is that the number of donors is extremely limited. Much has been learned—as a matter of fact, it has been shown unequivocally that a simple mechanical pump can replace the heart because, at least at first, the transplanted heart is completely de-enervated. It's just running like a pump oblivious of the environment around. The nerves have all been cut, which proves that this independent heart—or pump—can sustain life very effectively. I would have thought ten or fifteen years ago that by now we'd have an inter-corporeal pump that we could install like we put in heart valves today.

Harrison: Most of the physicians and surgeons who got into transplant programs early did not have adequate background or understand immunology or know how to select patients. Carefully performed surgery and medical management on patients selected by appropriate criteria have provided experience indicating that clearly transplants can help some patients individually who are in the end stages of heart disease.

Such experience, meticulously documented, has had tremendous scientific importance; for example, in understanding how the heart functions and is controlled by the nervous system in man. We learned that the heart can function very well without its nerves. It doesn't speed up quite as fast. Neurohormones come into play when there are no nerves, but that takes more time than nerve impulses. Second, we learned a lot about the electrical conduction system in the heart. Many things we've learned are applicable to patients with intact nervous systems. The critical nature of immune rejection, how it occurs in the heart, we can study. At this institution there is a lot of interplay. Transplant has stimulated a lot of work in immunology and immunogenetics.

We've a whole host of drug actions. This is a fine pharmacologic model for the study of drugs that act directly versus those that act through the nervous system. We discovered early on that patients who had a lot of rejection episodes had circulating cytochromes, and triglycerides [among the chemical elements that were known to be related to arteriosclerosis]. They had developed a greatly accelerated form of arteriosclerosis. I mean they could go through the whole aging process that may take fifty years in a normal human. A de-enervated or a transplanted heart or an immunologically troubled heart telescopes the process of developing arteriosclerotic heart disease. We are beginning to work on the problem. All this is still in the hypothetical or conceptual stage, but this is a new way of looking at the whole problem of arteriosclerosis. Where else can you better study it than in a model like this? Dogs just don't develop arteriosclerosis, though chimpanzees do.

Lillehei: Blood damage from various materials has been a more difficult problem than we had anticipated. It's held up the mechanical intracorporeal heart. Three groups in this country, in Salt Lake City, in Mississippi, and in Cleveland, are doing a lot of work on this and there are two or three groups in Germany, who now get calves to live regularly for three or more weeks, a fair length of time, with a complete intracorporeal mechanical heart. Some have gone on longer, but various problems occur, such as mechanical breakdowns, which I think can be solved.

A most vexing problem is the cumulative damage at very low rates to the blood: it's being damaged faster than the body can remake it. Kidneys get plugged up by the debris from damaged blood cells, and then, of course, infection is a problem. But Jack Norman, at Harvard and now down at Houston, with a plutonium power source (very expensive research, of course) has shown clearly that it's easy—not easy but very practical—for dogs to get enough power from plutonium so that you don't need to visualize anyone running around with a set of power line wires to run an artificial pump.

I think blood damage is a simpler problem than rejection. For all the work that's gone on in immunology in the last twenty years, a tremendous amount stimulated by transplant, we're still using the same drugs we did years ago when I did ten heart transplants. Shumway and others have learned to use these more cleverly. It was kind of shotgun therapy before. Now it's becoming more laser beam. But they are the same old drugs so we haven't come too far in solving the problem.

We'll solve the blood problem, which is cumulative. A couple of hours on the heart-lung machine is bad enough, but a body can tolerate that. But it can't when it goes on for weeks and months. When we do solve those problems, we'll get the intracorporeal mechanical heart.

Harrison: An effort such as was put into going to the moon would certainly develop an artificial heart in the near future, by solving the engineering and material problems—making small enough power supplies, parts durable enough—and chemistry, to keep blood from adhering, clotting, cracking. But probably from a societal point of view, we're not quite ready to have an artificial heart. There would be a lot of questions about who would get them!

In transplant the donor problem is the limiting factor. You don't have that many people with brain death prior to heart damage. I would say if you could keep end-stage heart patients alive for a week or a month before you could find a donor—which is often possible even now with a little modification of some of the assist devices—we could prevent the tragedy of those ready for heart transplantation for whom we don't have a donor.

Say you had an artificial heart that really functioned. Talking about numbers, huge numbers, the number of people who will die of heart disease—even if you put an age cutoff below sixty— economically and philosophically, how could you choose? The problems with communities and hospitals that have arisen over who should be on chronic kidney dialysis would only be intensified by a factor of ten if you had an artificial heart!

Nothing short of total human annihilation will deter medical explorers from trying to conquer disease in new ways. Perhaps it is not an altogether miserable sign that the first heart transplants drew almost as much worldwide attention as declarations of war, or the explosion of atom bombs. Although exaggerated, the news was a portent of hope and healing, not of destruction. In its own way, heart transplantation also emphasized the individuality of every human being, down to each of his separate cells. But if individuals with the commonest of potentially fatal diseases, malfunctioning hearts, can have replacements, provided they can get them, what then? Knowledge is not wisdom. There is always the age-old problem of choosing who shall live and who shall die.

14.

Mended Hearts

Preserved in Dwight Harken's files is a note on a rough piece of paper torn from a pad. The handwriting is neat and childlike.

> The Chilean doctor told me when Dr. Harken operates I will be all right, but if he does not operate I will live three or four months only, because I like some times dancing, I like play, I like all young woman like and I can not
>
> I cannot carry medium packages because I get out of breath
>
> I can not life 6 month on the bed with my husband because I have dysponea
>
> I can not play with my girl because I have dysponea
>
> Dr. Harken I am very happy because you came to see me, my life are in your hand
>
> Remember you promise help me because I am helpless, remember my life in this condition is not life—I am a temperament woman and I can not, do you understand me? Will you help me?
>
> Please help me, all my life I am remember

That is no more a "typical" plea than there is any such thing as a "typical" patient, but "Please help me" is what they are all saying in one way or another. Nor is any single case report "typical," although in time patterns emerge, procedures are standardized, statistical results become predictable. But if scientific reports may be summarized and conclusions drawn, most patients have singular points of view regarding their experiences. An anecdotal narrative by one may be a little like the proverbial brick thrown through a window that went straight up—unlikely to happen exactly that way again and therefore not statistically significant, but a hell of a case report.

One such account written by a Scottish obstetrician, Dr. Ian Donald, and entitled "At the Receiving End," was published in a 1976 issue of the *Scottish Medical Journal.* It may be scarcely typical of any patient anywhere else, but Donald's conclusion has been echoed, in one way or another, by a remarkably large number of patients who have had cardiac surgery.

Exactly 4 weeks ago to the day, in fact as I write, to the very hour, I was lying on the operating table with my thorax retracted open with a mid-sternal split from suprasternal notch to xiphisternum, my heart stopped, my life sustained on cardio-pulmonary bypass and my brain, for what it is worth, additionally protected by hypothermia.

Actually it was my third heart operation. The previous mitral valve replacement with a homograft had lasted miraculously since 1969. On that occasion, under pressure from my surgical colleagues, I had written up an account of the experience anonymously in the *Lancet.* At that time members of the team who had operated on me had rather reluctantly agreed to the script, but, in fact the effect was so comforting to so many terrified patients about to undergo a similar ordeal that this time I felt a second edition was necessary.

There has been marked improvement in management over the years. I told my precious surgeon that either he had become more slick or I had grown tougher. He modestly denied the former suggestion and rudely rejoined that my alleged toughness was due to pickling in Scotland's national drink, a frivolous allegation which could only be partially sustained. Somehow everything seemed just that bit better and easier this time, although I am still in pain and the memory of the ordeal, for such it certainly is, is vividly fresh in my mind.

I am now totally convinced, as never before, that the more a patient knows what to expect, and the more he understands what the doctors are trying to do, the better. Patients must not be lied to and must be given every opportunity to face and stand up to the truth, as I was.

. . . What really terrified me was the possibility of some major neurological disaster. This fear had been reinforced enormously just a few days earlier by reading a leading article in the *Lancet* on "Brain Damage after Open Heart Surgery." I was very frank about this on arrival in hospital and in discussing the outlook with my anaesthetists, one of whom had anaesthetized me on 2 previous occasions. I detected a momentary shadow of anger on her face, because I let slip some such phrase as "If I get away with it yet again." It was quite clear that she was not going to let me slip through her fingers. My surgeon, too, was very frank with me and, sitting on my bed, very patiently acquainted me with the odds.

The fantastic speed of my recovery compared even with last time must be attributed, I think, to the *ever-increasingly meticulous attention to detail,* including, let us not forget, all the technical and back-up services which are only available in so-called centers of excellence, a term very richly deserved.

[In contrast to earlier days] I was particularly impressed with the slick performance of angiocardiography and catheter measurements which were completed in less than half the time of six and a half years ago. The same symptoms of racing heat were as before, but this time I knew what to expect. They watched me like a cat and by midnight, when obviously all was well, I was getting very fed up with having my blood pressure taken every quarter of an hour, just as I was dozing off, and my toes being scrutinized for defects of circulation.

The operation was obviously hugely successful. Every carefully laid channel of espionage confirmed that fact. It lasted about six hours because, after all, it was the "third time in" but it appears I was not as badly "stuck up" as was feared. I had discussed with both cardiologist and surgeon what type of valve was to be inserted in place of my worn-out mitral homograft. I had heard tell of the Bjork-Shiley valve which I understood was covered with fur and might prove quieter but, as it was, the largest size and latest pattern of Starr-Edwards valve was chosen, partly because of the sheer size of the hole that had to be plugged and, as my surgeon had already explained, he did not wish to have to operate on me yet again.

As expected I came to my senses briefly in the Intensive Care

Unit. Somewhere there was the most almighty pain and evidently I had not registered the anaesthetist's customary remark that it was "all over." I got the strange idea in my head that this was only a half-time interval and that there was worse to come. Consciousness was however quickly blotted out by the addition of more papaveretum to one of the innumerable tubes with which I bristled. As before, mechanical ventilation in the presence of the effects of relaxant drugs was not terrifying. The endotracheal tube, of course, was hateful but I was pleased to observe that there was no gauze bandaging wrapped around it now, which I had found so intolerable last time. Thereafter followed interludes of consciousness and my morale improved with the removal of each successive piece of tubing and I became less and less like a porcupine. From time to time the anaesthetist warned me that I was going to be "sucked out." I was incapable of coughing and curiously did not mind, but was interested to observe from the noises that I was not exactly drowning in my own secretions.

Now followed a period of total frustration at being unable to communicate. Clearly the paralyzing drugs had worn off. Every attempt I made to speak, of course, was frustrated by the tube in my larynx and I was told repeatedly "not to fight the ventilator." At last somebody realized that I wished to say something and a pad was brought to me. I was interested to see if I would be able to write at all in view of the anticipated intention tremor following an anaesthetic of this duration. I wanted to ask if everything was finished but gave up the attempt and finally contrived a note of thanks which it took them some time to decipher. I well remember the laughter which greeted the final translation. I was propped up for portable chest X-ray films and to my delight and no doubt thanks to being a non-smoker I was extubated. I felt very sceptical about this but found that although I was perfectly aware of the removal of each drain I did not experience the agony which I well remembered after my first valvotomy operation.

Presently my dentures were produced and their reinsertion in my mouth evoked such merriment from one of the nurses that I can hear her silvery laughter in my ears to this day. She explained that I looked "so different." I thought thankfully how different I would have felt had it been the other way round. To my great delight, after 30 hours and accompanied by my wife and two of my daughters, I was wheeled back to the ward, in what I felt was a blaze of triumph.

The clarity of my thought processes at this time was very obvious and my wife assured me that I did not at any time talk nonsense. In fact I was trying to engage one of the surgical team in argument on the merits of electronic self-steering gears on yachts, he being a keen yatchsman and I just having bought one. Clearly it was time for more sedation and there now followed the painful period of recovery.

The through-put in this Cardio-Thoracic Unit staggered me. Commonly two cases such as mine were done in a day. There were a lot of us having this kind of surgery and there developed among us all a wondrous fellow feeling reminiscent of my days in the Royal Air Force during the war. We came from all walks of life and all sorts of backgrounds and a great number of different places. They knew I was both a doctor and a professor of gynaecology, but did not hold that against me. . . . Our concern whenever one of our number was rather longer in the Intensive Care Unit than expected was very genuine and the welcome which greeted his eventual return was mingled with great relief. Every one of us came back alive which was an improvement on my experience of several years ago and the legend grew up that in this particular Intensive Care Unit they just would not let you die even if you wanted to.

The experience is sufficiently recent for me to recognize the paramount importance of psychosomatic sequelae following surgery of maximum severity and I fear that we as surgeons are possibly not sufficiently aware of this feature of recovery. In obstetrics of course the phenomenon of "fourth day puerperal blues" is well known and it is always my practice to warn my patients that they are liable to be overwhelmed with temporary depression and possibly crying at this time. . . . Following surgery there is likely to be a period of reactive depression, although this may occur a few days later. It is not necessarily related to pain or discomfort but is in marked contrast to the initial euphoria which follows the realization that one has survived.

[Dr. Donald had three episodes when he "definitely decompensated in the psychosomatic sense," each with an apparently different trigger mechanism. The first was a frightful nightmare which sent him out of bed in a state of unreasoning terror and confusion as to reality. The second episode occurred about ten days after the operation when the normal extreme constipation from drugs had caused him to strain unavailingly at stool. This increased the tick-

ing noise from his prosthetic valve and he panicked. The third episode occurred eighteen days postoperatively in the house of his
brother-in-law, a chest physician. Everyone had gone out.]

Quite suddenly I realized that I was alone in the house. Panic
seized me. My "tachycardia" seemed totally unreasonable and in
no time I was shaking like a jelly, wondering what had gone wrong
and recalling horrid stories of prosthetic valves jamming and precipitating acute failure when provoked by an intolerable bout of
tachycardia. I imagined a fearful 30-mile ambulance drive back to
the hospital for further intensive care. Darkness was descending
and in a desperate way I recognized three alternatives: firstly to
take a double whiskey, secondly to stuff myself with dicoxin, and
thirdly to drink ice-cold water and sit in front of the window
breathing in the wintry night air. Fortunately I chose the last alternative and turned up to its loudest the third act of Bizet's *Carmen*
to distract me. I had to remind myself that I had no dyspnoea and
no anginal pain and simply could not explain my terror. At last I
heard my brother-in-law's footsteps and could hardly tell him what
had happened because of the involuntary twitching of my lips.
What is interesting is that although I could perfectly easily have
taken my pulse I was too terrified to do even that. My brother-in-
law simply examined me and told me firmly there was nothing
wrong and thereafter I fell asleep. I felt thoroughly ashamed of
myself and we agreed that my wife must never know or she would
be afraid to go out of the house again. The episode serves to demonstrate how vulnerable in the psychiatric sense is the patient who
has already endured a great deal. I suppose this is part of the basis
of brainwashing behind the Iron Curtain. . . .

Soon after dismissal from the hospital I was visited by 3 very
bright little children, aged 8, 6 and 4 years. In no time I was identified because of my ticking valve with the crocodile in J. M. Bar-
rie's *Peter Pan*. The 8-year-old, who was determined to be a nurse
and who, in her own mind at least, had already achieved the necessary diplomas, explained that my heart had stopped so that the
doctors could mend it. The 6-year-old thereupon pronounced that
I must have been dead and started to inquire what heaven was
like. Evasive replies filled her with suspicion and clearly she
wanted to know on what grounds I had been kicked out. With a
look of horrified accusation on her face she asked if I had been
caught smoking. The 4-year-old, however, remained confused and

dissatisfied with the crocodile part of the story because, as he observed, I had not yet "gone off." In these days of outrages I am not sure he meant as an alarm or a bomb.

In retrospect, I must admit that, daunting though it has been, I have been through a tremendous spiritual experience. This account is offered in homage and gratitude for all the skill and kindness which have been shown to me in the fabulous Cardio-Thoracic Unit. For most of my life I have thought it fun to be ALIVE and now I am more sure of it than ever!

Both of these "documents" emphasize the individuality of each patient and the importance of the psychological and emotional elements in their "cases." Harken did not think that these elements could be overstressed. Dehumanization and fragmentation of care had to be overcome by the physician and the surgeon closest to the patient, in his opinion, especially in a field as technically complex as cardiac surgery. "The poor patient," he said, "comes in with a complicated heart disease. He's met by a specialist in internal medicine who taps, looks, and listens, and writes on a chart without ever really becoming acquainted with the patient. Then he's sent for such procedures as echocardiography, electrocardiography, phonocardiography, and those specialists do their thing, getting acquainted with his electrical impulses, but not with him. Then a team of specialists, with nothing more than a nodding acquaintance, catheterize him, study his hemodynamics and so forth, and they all assemble in a conference room without the patient present and decide what the patient needs. On the basis of those records and cinefluoroscopic studies and lab findings, the surgeon knows that so-and-so in room number such-and-such needs a certain procedure and that he is scheduled for an operation. The surgeon may only visit the patient to have him sign the informed consent form and then operate, turning post-op care over to somebody else. So the patient has seen a whole lot of different doctors and never gets it straight who is performing what function. This is dehumanization, depersonalization, and fragmentation created by the requirements of the fancy, complex maneuver conducted."

Some surgeons, certainly Harken and Lillehei, insisted on continuity for their patients. They saw them, and their families, before the operation and afterward, monitored their care, and took pains to allow for their individual quirks and needs. Harken's follow-up of his patients often continued for years and years. His "hot line" was always open, and as many as six secretaries at a time labored to keep up with his extensive correspondence, which included communication with patients, their cardiologists, their primary care physicians, their closest of kin. At the end of one long arc of correspondence with and about Mildred Shetterly, operated on in 1957, deceased in 1968, is a letter from her husband, C. Russell Shetterly. Enclosed with it is a copy of another letter Mr. Shetterly sent to the Mount Auburn Hospital in Boston from his home in Denver, Colorado, with a large check as a contribution toward a new heart-lung machine for the hospital in memory of his well-beloved wife "to whom Dr. Harken gave eleven years of life and happiness which she would not have had."

The Shetterly file is a large one. Mrs. Shetterly addressed her surgeon as "Dear Dr. Harken, my Wizard of Oz," and wrote in detail, as he assured her he wanted her to do, of her fears and reverses and of her pleasure in periods of renewed vigor and enjoyment of life. He answered "Dear Mildred," proffering emotional support as well as medical advice. He and her referring cardiologist, Dr. George Robb, well known for his early work in angiography, corresponded regularly about the lady whom Harken referred to as "our wonderful Mildred Shetterly." Her Boston cardiologist and Harken exchanged reports as well.

These warm friendships with his patients usually began in crisis. Of continuing communication, Harken would say, "It's good for the patients, it makes me feel good, and it makes long-term follow-up possible." The relationship ended only with the death of the patient. Ups and downs, good and bad events, including deterioration in the condition of the patient due to his heart disease, were all part of the extended picture.

When one grateful patient, a psychiatrist, congratulated Harken on his "consumer service policy" and expressed the wish that his Cadillac dealer was as conscientious, Harken was insulted by the comparison. That particular patient, in view of his profession, should have had more insight. In fact, whenever Harken thought about it he became more indignant. It made no sense to cure a patient's heart if the patient did not find it out! It was no good equipping them for a good, full life if they were not zestful to live it, given positive motivation! Such motivation was a powerful healing force, especially in the cardiac field where too often in the past patients without surgery had been carefully trained to limit themselves, to restrict their lives. It was *ridiculous* to have a patient with a "cardiac neurosis" and not correct the neurosis when the heart disease was corrected. ("Rather like changing the motor in a car from fifty to two hundred horsepower and not letting the owner know that he could now proceed at normal speed with it," said Harken, using a motor car comparison himself.)

Harken was willing to motivate his patients by any means he could. He even risked the ridicule of his colleagues by whispering in patients' ears in the recovery room that they were better, better, better—hoping that such subliminal suggestions might help. Psychiatrists assured him that planting the idea they were better in this state did help.

Some of the physicians responsible for Harken's patients resented their continued tie with a surgeon. Others were very grateful. These were apt to be the ones who cared most keenly about the so-called behavioral determinants in recovery, which had so much to do with their patients' "social outcome" after heart operations.

Research studies concerning the factors that helped or hindered recovery and rehabilitation after open-heart surgery were being undertaken at many medical teaching centers. The largest one, by a group of doctors from Columbia University, concluded that physical restoration was reached in the majority of cases, and that the primary barrier to full recovery of function was psychological for about one third of the cases. With over seventy thousand patients a year undergoing bypass surgery by 1978, there was a pressing need to know more.

Boston University Medical Center was given a grant to study the effect of major cardiac surgery on patients and their families in both the short and long terms. The university's research team was headed by C. David Jenkins, Ph.D., with Stephen J. Zyzanski, Ph.D., of the Department of Behavioral Epidemiology, and assisted by Drs. Michael D. Klein and Babette A. Stanton. Dwight E. Harken was named special surgical consultant.

In 1978 three members of the university team met with Harken to discuss some of their preliminary findings. Nine hundred and fifty-one major heart surgery patients had answered questionnaires concerning their recoveries, and medical, psychosocial, and work outcomes; 724 had had coronary bypass surgery, 149 mitral, and 78 aortic valve replacement. Summarized by computer, on the basis of patient answers, the results:

As to psychological adjustments: 44% said they were better; 40% just the same; 16% worse than they had been prior to their operations.

As to social adjustments: 31% reported themselves improved; 63% the same; 6% worse.

Of those employed before surgery, 65% returned to work after an average of 4 months.

During an average of four years after surgery, 52% were hospitalized one or more times; 11% of the males and 19% of the female coronary bypass patients reported myocardial infarction.

The team concluded

Those who were female, forced to retire, and Type A (with aggressive-competitive characteristics considered to render an individual more prone to heart disease) had significantly poorer medical outcomes. Even when seven major medical variables as well as age and time since surgery were controlled statistically, psychosocial outcomes were clearly worse in those same three groups.

In summary, far more patients reported heart surgery had improved their life situation rather than made it worse, and psychosocial and medical variables were independently associated with overall recovery.

That early sampling was by no means considered definitive. There was also the fallacy of lumping open-heart patient groups without a closer look at the composition. A multitude of factors in recovery indicated the need for much more thorough follow-through. The whole study was not scheduled for completion until

1980. Already the team had spent many months preparing questions that would provide patient profiles and better data for judging variables. Personal studies of individual patients before and after their operations would be undertaken. The conversation at the team's meeting with Harken was to consider preliminary results from the first questionnaire. During the informal exploratory discussion the team surprised the surgeon in one instance.

The surprise for Harken was a fear uncovered among the patients that he had not anticipated in his thorough briefings nor become aware of postoperatively. A good many patients confessed, in answer to the question about fears, that they were terrified that their incisions would fall open or wires in their chests break loose. "All surgeons should know this!" exclaimed Harken. "It really hadn't occurred to me. When you think of it, it is difficult to warn patients about things that haven't and couldn't occur—especially when the surgeon hasn't an inkling that the dear people would worry about it!"

Considering the group who reported themselves as "distinctly dissatisfied" with the results of their operations, researcher Babette Stanton pointed out that the majority were females who had coronary bypass surgery. Harken, often foresighted about the problems and needs in heart surgery, said he was already aware of this and thought he might have an explanation that was physiologic rather than psychologic. Women, he said, often suffered angina pain from "small-vessel disease"—disease in the extensions of the artery too small to be visualized; it is uncommon among males. This poorly understood disease could be terribly disabling and sometimes produce symptoms of classical angina without showing any coronary disease by angiography. If one of these females did also show some obstruction in the coronary vessels and independently the classical symptoms of angina, it would be entirely reasonable to conclude that coronary bypass surgery was indicated. But if the woman had "small-vessel disease," bypassing the coincidental obstruction revealed by angiograms would not relieve her symptoms or her pain. The symptoms had not been caused by the disease for which the surgeon operated. Also coronary artery spasm might be a confusing factor.

This could explain, he said, why, in their cases, conscientious, competent surgery provided no relief, and dissatisfaction was inevitable. Nobody had studied enough of these people to test this thesis. Perhaps further scrutiny of the little understood and possibly misnamed small-vessel disease syndrome could reduce the incidence of these failures? Drs. Jenkins, Zyzanski, and Stanton were fascinated by this contribution, but quickly returned to their primary concern, which was psychological sequelae

Many psychiatrists had reported a number of patients coming to them after heart surgery, complaining they had suffered personality changes or disturbing mental symptoms. Harken said he himself had worried a lot because so many patients in his early experience seemed "just not as bright as they had been." A good many executives, for instance, did not seem as effective when they returned to their demanding jobs. Were they less alert? Were they going back too soon? Was the altered postoperative performance the result of a change in the patient or was colleague concern a factor in reducing confidence? Was the alteration transient? Were the doctors not allowing enough time for rehabilitation?

Increased myopia (nearsightedness) was noticeable, but this occurred after any very great stress and was transient. (He had measured this on himself after his near-fatal airplane crash and again after an unusually traumatic operation for diaphragmatic hiatus hernia. His nearsightedness had increased by over one-half a diopter after each of these major trauma episodes, but had recovered to prestress state at six months. Routinely he warned his patients not to spend money on new glasses if they had, as they commonly did, "eye problems," until eight months had passed.)

As for strokes and other damage to body or brain, there was no doubt that bubble oxygenators did deliver some bubbles and bits of debris through the blood. The degree of the damage depended on how large the bubbles or debris were. So many variables were involved: low flow of blood at normal body temperatures had proved to cause more changes than high flow at low temperatures. And only recently had the mixed blessing of

membrane oxygenators been available to eliminate bubbles—
membrane oxygenators were much more expensive and complex
but more physiologic.

Certainly in the early days of open-heart surgery postcardi-
otomy delirium and long-term neurologic complications were frequent. Strokes were conspicuous, but other changes were more
subtle and often went unnoticed at the time. ("We see what we
look for and we look for what we know!") Possibly there were
personality changes. These could follow obvious strokes or lesser
strokes that did not produce other obvious neurological deficits.

Surgeons had been pretty quiet about the possibilities because minute changes were hard to see and more difficult to
quantify. And, "Sure," Harken said, "patients in those days had
little choice if they wanted to live at all and the last thing they
needed to worry about was damage to their poor old brains!" Now
there was a new question coming up: Was the fact that all blood
flow by bypass had hitherto been nonpulsatile responsible in any
way for neurological complications?

"The Almighty worked out a system for circulating blood in a
pulsatile pattern," said Harken. "It might make a lot of difference
to the brain whether blood flow is pulsatile or not." His son,
Alden Harken, cardiac surgeon at the Pennsylvania Medical
School, thought it probably made no difference, but his opinion
was based on a study of leg muscles. "There's a recent study that
suggests that when patients are on bypass with steady flow they
essentially put out water from their kidneys, and when this flow is
pulsatile they put out something like urine."

"Whew!" commented Dr. Jenkins. Zyzanski and Stanton
drew in their breaths.

"However," said Harken, "the guys using pulsatile delivery
are also using high flows and much more sophisticated cardiopulmonary bypass. The returns aren't in on pulsatile flow."

As serious investigators, the four people present at this
meeting paused to enjoy an antiphonal diatribe against slipshod
and inadequate methods used to arrive at "stupid" conclusions.
The recent VA study of coronary bypass was a case in point.
Doubtless some operations had been unnecessarily performed. "If
some don't prove to be unnecessary, the chances are you aren't

doing enough," said surgeon Harken. "It can be easy to ignore serious indications and fail to do what you should. A further study compared the VA patients after coronary bypass surgery with private groups, and the private patients returned to work three to one compared with the veterans!"

Another article in the *New England Journal of Medicine* questioned the surgery on the basis of a follow-up of just twenty-two cases. Public suspicion was fostered by Richard Knox, a Boston *Globe* investigative reporter, who picked up the article and came, said Jenkins, "to a remarkable conclusion that this revascularization surgery did not eliminate occlusive disease in other parts of the heart system and so bypass patients might continue to have pain."

"No," said Harken, "and it doesn't eliminate prior brain damage or anything wrong with the adjacent nonvascularized muscles or the legs or what may be wrong with the neighbors either!"

If the studies had been scrutinized with care as to specifics they would not have been misleading or have added, through the media, fuel to antimedical/antisurgical bias.

The VA study did conclude correctly that the results of medical treatment were similar to VA surgical results, at thirty-six months, in stable angina, leaving out common trunk coronary artery lesions and patients with triple vessel coronary disease, et cetera. Even then, at thirty-six months, the VA surgery patients had closed the gap and come equal to the medical survivors, and were gaining steadily. Therefore "medical treatment equaled surgery? What kind of science was that?" asked Harken. The effect on the public of conclusions that *unnecessary surgery was being performed* could be tragically misleading. And some physicians might superficially infer that "bypass surgery may improve quality of life, but it has not been proved that it lengthens life," and therefore is "unnecessary."

In preparing their next study, Zyzanski and his team tried to come up with a more scientific and broad-based sampling of heart surgical patients. In fourteen centers where randomized comparisons with those who had medical treatment had been projected, many patients refused the luck of the draw, opting for surgery.

"There comes a time," said Harken, "when the question of randomizing something that is clearly beneficial becomes very questionable. If you had had randomized mitral valve surgery during the last ten years, it would have been immoral!"

Zyzanski regarded his high stack of computer printout sheets and said, "If you look at what we have so far, and cluster depression, anxiety, social adjustment, mood, current well-being, et cetera, you see that for the valves there has been a dramatic change for the better. They perceive the change. Mitrals more than aortics feel improvement. The aortics don't see so well that they are better."

"The aortics are the ones who might well have dropped dead without the operation," Harken reminded him. "The indications for aortic valve replacement may become urgent long before the patient perceives limitation, and Sudden Death may preclude any suffering at all! In contrast, take a woman with mitral stenosis. She will always recall her distress at sex, or her husband's departure, or her inability to climb the stairs. One sees the figures, and then one must look to their meaning. You can prove by tests and the cinematic mapping of the larger coronary arteries that patients had the 'widowmaker.' They might have dropped dead without having had memorable inconvenience, but they may feel no better after surgery. Others forget the recurrent angina that took them to the hospital; it's the person with mitral stenosis who seldom forgets his or her previous trouble."

"Speaking of those with job loss," said Zyzanski, "a sizable percentage feel they were forced to retire because of prejudice, because the insurance carriers would not permit such people to go back to work, and even refused the patients' waivers of responsibility in the event of heart-related disabilities. In a few cases taken to workmen's compensation boards, they got favorable decisions, but for rheumatic and coronary artery diseased—*no way!*"

"Maybe the most important thing you uncover will be the factors of length and quality of life versus cost," commented Harken. "Is it more expensive to have this surgery or not to have it? Do they come back to the hospitals as much after surgery? Or is it just cheaper to let them die! Dr. Collins' Peter Bent Brigham study supported the premise that it was cheaper in the long run to have surgery, but it seems pretty good sport to question such a study if it is made by surgeons."

"So far," said Zyzanski, "the valves feel they have lots more energy, more time out of bed, a dramatic difference. Not like the coronary bypasses, who found not much change, and 10 to 12 percent felt worse. We've questioned over a thousand people so far and two hundred of them sailed through four years post-op without any complications at all. Among the various complications, medical, emotional, social, the women certainly average worse than the men. You get a percentage of both males and females who do not do well, although their surgery is a success and recovery excellent. They just can't cope. We want to find out if you can identify them before surgery. Know that for sure a year later, no matter how well mended, they will still moan the blues. Who are they?"

Included in the overall research design was this question and many others. The next step was to enlist twelve hundred to fifteen hundred patients as volunteers for a study that would begin in the weeks preceding their major heart surgery. Nurses and trained research workers would be used to collect information. In-depth patient interviews would be conducted before and after surgery.

The preliminary study by questionnaire had been a limited one. For the most part the questionnaire had been sent through the cooperation of Mended Hearts, Inc., to a random sampling of over a thousand of their active members. That was the readiest resource for reaching postoperative open-heart surgery patients, and an astonishing 81 percent had carefully filled out the forms; but *were* they typical? People who joined Mended Hearts, Inc., might not represent the average heart surgery patient.

Typical or not, membership in the club was a way of reinforcing the morale of those who had had heart surgery. That was health giving, or at least health aiding, and in some cases actually life saving. In the interplay of factors that added quality of life to those surviving serious health impairment, transient or permanent, Harken had always rated the emotional, environmental, and psychological elements high on the scale of medical importance.

The Boston University Medical Center's preliminary study was carried out in 1977. Questionnaires were sent to a random selection of roughly 25 percent of the active members in each of ninety-five chapters of Mended Hearts, Inc., in cities all over the United States and ranging through Canada and as far away as Haifa, Trinidad, Buenos Aires, and Santiago de Chile.

Active members had had major cardiac surgery; those with only pacemakers were eligible for associate membership, as were family members and interested parties. But only active members were entitled to wear the club logo in the form of pin, pendant, tie clasp, or lapel button. This was a bright red valentine heart, gold trimmed. A graceful symbolic suture line was stitched across the heart, which was topped with a symbolic gold flame representing the club motto: "It's Great to Be Alive . . . and to Help Others."

After 1967 Mended Hearts' active membership list grew to be 75 percent male and 25 percent female, reversing the percentages of earlier years. Coronary artery bypass surgery accounted for 73 percent of that membership, mitral valve surgery 14 percent, aortic valve surgery 8 percent, congenital repairs 3 percent, and 2 percent had undergone the Vineberg procedure of coronary artery bypass. Six times as many men as women had had coronary artery bypass, twice as many men as women had had aortic valve repair. Women had three times as much mitral valve surgery. This was comparable to figures for the United States as a whole.

Over 98 percent of Mended Hearts' members were white. Three-quarters were between the ages of fifty and fifty-nine; only 3½ percent were under forty and only 4½ percent were over seventy. Averages indicated first major heart symptoms at age forty-nine, surgery at fifty-three; the age of those responding to the questionnaire averaged fifty-seven. Most members came from middle or upper social strata. Their average of education was well above the national level. Family income averaged $15,000 in the year prior to surgery and 88 percent of those who answered the questionnaire were married.

The study's results indicated that the economic impact of the operations had not been drastic. In an average of four years since the surgical episode, family income had gone up for 47 percent. About half of the rest indicated little or no change. Among those whose income decreased, some suffered considerable hardship, periods of financial crisis, depletion of savings, debts. In spite of that, 77 percent reported no decline in their standard of living since surgery, and housing remained the same for 81 percent.

In the social and emotional area, results were surprisingly upbeat. Changes in marital status were very little higher than for the population as a whole, but there was a difference between the two sexes. Only 3 percent of the males had a change; 11 percent of the females. Nearly two-thirds of the members questioned said their relationships with spouses, children, employers, co-workers, and friends remained the same. Among the remaining third, the majority felt that those relationships had improved rather than deteriorated.

Many reported that, by comparison with the years before their operations, they took more pleasure in life, worried less, were not as tense or depressed. Female patients who had undergone mitral valve surgery were the most positive as to improvement; female coronary bypass patients the most negative.

Perhaps most pleasing to their surgeons would be the rating on a scale of one to six as to whether the patients were pleased with their surgery. A thumping 75 percent picked the "extremely pleased" response and only 2 percent the "extremely displeased." Asked if they would undergo their operations again, considering them in retrospect, 63 percent gave an unqualified "yes"; 5 percent said "no." Male valve patients, both aortic and mitral, were the most affirmative; female coronary bypass patients the least.

It will be interesting in 1980 to find out whether a broader sampling in the continuing study reinforces these, on the whole, optimistic conclusions. The findings for the small number of non-members included in this preliminary survey were similar. But it must be kept in mind that all the answers on the effects of surgery were estimated only by the patients themselves, and that the overwhelming majority of them had joined Mended Hearts.

Veterans of many kinds of experience have joined clubs or groups, and often there has seemed to be a considerable difference between them and the people who do not join such organizations: this is certainly true among war veterans. Until recently those who shared the same illness, living through related life-and-death experiences because of this, rarely organized publicly. Perhaps this was because while war was regarded as honorable, illness was seen as somehow private, even shameful. Now organizations for self-help and help-to-others who have suffered specific afflictions are becoming ubiquitous. Of these, Alcoholics Anonymous is undoubtedly the best known; Recovery, Inc., founded in 1937 by former nervous and mental patients, perhaps the least publicized. Mended Hearts was initiated in 1951 by four patients of Harken's at the Peter Bent Brigham Hospital and was derisively often called, during its first years, "the Dwight Harken fan club."

Doris Silliman, Mended Hearts' founder and first president, came to Harken for surgery at a time when every cardiac operation was a newsworthy event. Bea Murray, newly appointed as the Peter Bent Brigham Hospital's first public relations officer, was warned to play down the exciting new and risky cardiac surgery. Not everyone agreed that such surgery was justified, and any vulgar, distorted public image of the Peter Bent Brigham as a guinea pig institution rather than as an important research center and a house of healing must be corrected. Her job was to see that accurate reports informed the public, but some of his colleagues thought Harken was too flamboyant and the press far too interested in what he was doing.

Mrs. Murray's first encounter with Dr. Harken filled her with alarm. He was leading his entourage of students and visiting doctors in a headlong rush through the corridors. Timidly she approached him, mindful of his reputation for high temper, to approve a mild release. He took it, scanned it, and approved it except for one unpardonable journalistic sin: she had misspelled his name. "*KE*n not k*I*n," he said and rushed on, leaving her shaken. She tried to keep out of his sight—until she ran into an inconsolable Harken just after he had lost a patient. "That was a different man," she would say, "and after that I trailed him around like a little puppy." Taking it upon herself to visit his patients on the hospital's "Bridge B," she called this her "heart beat" and on this beat she met Doris Silliman.

Bea Murray never expected to see Mrs. Silliman alive after her surgery; she had a very poor chance for survival. Among the physicians and her friends, only her surgeon clung to his bulldog belief that she would wake up after the operation. Doris Silliman did wake up and, said Bea Murray, "she was so surprised to be alive she was really on Cloud 9, almost psychotically happy." Most heart surgery patients do experience hours of euphoria immediately or soon after regaining consciousness, but they are usually followed by a much more alarming equivalent of the post-delivery mother's "fourth-day weeps." Harken always warned patients and their families that patients could slump into depression and even a paranoid state. Doris Silliman sailed through her recovery in an uninterrupted manic and joyful state of mind.

She conceived the idea of a club named Mended Hearts with the motto: "It's Great to Be Alive." There were three other Harken heart patients from the Massachusetts area on Bridge B and she enthusiastically enlisted them as a "bridge foursome" and the nucleus of her club. Her sense of organization and ultimate purpose were vague, but it seemed to her "I had heart surgery, too," constituted a unique bond.

Bea Murray, sub rosa, helped the four to turn the idea into a real organization, to draw up a charter and a program. Harken suggested adding "and to Help Others" to the motto, extending the purpose from self-congratulation in the direction of sensible charity. A program to visit preoperative patients, encouraging them by the example of their own restored health, was proposed. Bea Murray arranged for these willing amateurs to get the training that would make them acceptable and useful in hospitals.

Initially the club was widely considered "a naïve and unprofessional movement" of New England ladies, but it began to grow. As patients came in from all over the world to the Peter Bent Brigham, they were recruited at the club's headquarters, and by 1975 membership spanned the globe and members from chest and heart centers everywhere had joined chapters. By this time Harken had retired discreetly into the background so that other prominent physicians and surgeons would join him on the

Board of Advisors. Programs were formalized and members who volunteered as "visitors" were accredited following training by other members and by medical personnel. Armed with licenses to do so, they took their own joy in "It's Great to Be Alive" into hospitals, serving it like nourishing soup to patients suffering the fears and uncertainties of contemplating or recovering from cardiac operations.

From the beginning, active members put their best hearts forward. To celebrate the club's first decade, Mary Richardson, with the first successful implanted ball valve inside her heart, danced with a male member of Mended Hearts. Two patients who possessed five artificial valves between them were photographed as they greeted each other. One was national secretary of the club, the other the Boston chapter president.

The men boasted of the most athletic among survivors. Truck driver Roland Cyre, from Melrose, Massachusetts, had gone back to work after his valve surgery. He rolled 350-pound oil drums and juggled 53-pound cases to load the giant trailer truck he was driving 140 miles a day. Ruben Harris and Charles Langrock bicycled thirty miles in a cyclethon held on Long Island to raise money for the Nassau County Heart Fund. Seth Goodwin, active member and president of the Denver chapter of Mended Hearts, spoke at a dinner meeting; he had been golfing all day, he said, and added, "And I was skiing at Loveland Basin yesterday!"

By the time of its twenty-fourth annual convention in the Bicentennial year 1976, visiting and reassuring patients and participating in public appeals for money to forward heart research were only two of the club's purposes. They helped the Red Cross to recruit blood donors. They took it upon themselves to aid patients with such things as postoperative housing and information about procuring needed drugs at the lowest prices. They provided their membership lists for informational research programs such as the ones Columbia and Boston universities undertook.

Although as an organization Mended Hearts avoided controversy, members backed efforts being made to persuade insurance companies to cover heart patients. A club blood credit bank was extended so that heart sufferers anywhere, especially over-

seas, could borrow from them the eight pints often required prior
to operations.

Jokes accumulated equating Mended Hearts with Lonely
Hearts because so many marriages took place among members.
There were even "children of Mended Hearts." Dwight Harken
is still known affectionately as the club's "father," although he
did not take a prominent part in the field of coronary bypass
surgery, which was followed by an immediate increase in membership and a change in the ratio of men to women.

Harken believed that people who had survived, whole, such
an experience were better people for it, and so did Mended
Hearts' members. The positive was deliberately stressed. There
was a rigid club rule that members were not to gather for discussion of misery, pain, or the unpleasant details of their surgery. No
competitive boasting about endurance was permitted, only competition, restricted by honesty, as to the rapidity with which they
had recovered.

Most of them agreed that whatever their trials, whatever
coin it cost them in money, psychological, or social problems, it
had been worth it.

Nevertheless, before contemplating the future of cardiac
surgery, there are questions to ask. Increased knowledge opens
up new vistas of ignorance. Power to improve is power to abuse.
These truisms apply as much to medicine as to any other area of
authority.

15.

The Time Has Come to Ask Questions

The time has come to ask questions to which there are no historical answers, only consensus and various opinions. I will do what most of us do in the field of medicine and ask "my" doctor. That possessive "my" before the professional title, an indication of peculiar trust and confidence, has been in use, I suspect, since human beings first refused to accept their physical fate the way animals do and confided their ailments to specialists in healing, from witch doctors to M.D.s.

"My" doctor, as is obvious in this book, is Dwight Harken. His opinions are those of a world-recognized authority, prophet, reformer, teacher, and preacher, not only in his field but in the broadest aspects of medicine. He is opinionated, but one of his guiding principles is a quotation from Francis Peabody, a great and kindly Boston physician who died in 1926: "The secret of caring for the patient is caring for the patient." He does not think of patients as compartmentalized ailing bodies.

That principle has actually been jeopardized by solutions for heart disease. Solutions inevitably lead to problems created by the solutions. Three words, adapted from the Greeks, whose physicians added science to the art of healing, cover the syndromes patients may suffer following medical treatment: *iatrogenic*, "caused by the physician"; *nosocomial*, "from the house or hospital" where patients are treated; *monocigenic*, "derived from or due to money," the cost of care. These syndromes are as ancient as they are current. In 1969 Harken had asked classics scholar Mrs. Laurence Ellis and Professor Lowell Edmunds of Harvard for a word suitable for a brand-new syndrome: the constellation of adverse factors that had developed from treatment in intensive care units (ICUs). By the late 1960s these (and subsequently coronary care units, CCUs) were standard in most hospitals. They enabled patients to survive surgical and other trauma that had previously been routinely fatal. They were marvels in terms of machine care. But *periotogenic*, "genesis in things about," was the word he adopted to cover the syndrome that could result from their use.

My first question would be about ICUs, which represented to me the ultimate in modern medicine's tendency to dehumanize patients. Patients, often stoic about other aspects of major surgery, seem to react with extraordinary distress to their memories of time spent in them. I had learned through Nurse Edith Heideman, chief of nurses at the Henry Ford Hospital in Detroit, that the first ICU in the world had been the one she and D.E.H. established in 1951 at the Peter Bent Brigham Hospital. (The earliest mention she could find of a similar unit appeared in the *Index Medicus* for 1955. At that time the idea was postulated as a "radical invention.")

On April 9, 1971, Nurse Heideman had written to Dr. Harken:

> Twenty years ago we determined that fresh postoperative patients did not receive optimum care for their smooth recovery in an open ward. We recognized that the equipment and facilities would have to be first rate, the nursing staff more educated, more willing to accept responsibility, and (not least of all) we had to convince the skeptics that we needed a greater number of nurses for patients in this area than in the rest of the hospital.
>
> Dr. Harken, you and I were present at the birth of this baby, and I feel very strongly that we must take some responsibility in guiding it back in the right direction. I have no quarrel with instrumentation per se, but *only* if it used as an adjunct in the service and support of the patient, rather than having the patient

regarded as a terminal designed to supply the data requested. Doctors and nurses forget quite often that patients are people!

Has not our idea, which was to give superior care and attention to each patient *as an individual*, been so subverted that it is now evidenced only by the wavering of monitoring gauges and the mechanical recording of fluid balance, cardiac function and blood gas and electrolyte status? Was it part of our objective to threaten a patient's sanity by creating for him a day with 24 glaring fluorescent hours? Did we plan to overwhelm him with banks of instruments that click, blink or beep with (or without) the slightest provocation? Whatever happened to our concept of privacy? Cutdowns and arterial taps, cardiac resuscitation and defibrillation—to name a few—are scarcely the entertainment one would prescribe for a recent postoperative patient! In our eagerness to embrace new technical advances, some of the basic principles of environmental control seem to have been kicked aside. I do not say that this is "unfortunate"—I state flatly that it is *criminal*. Patients may retain the psychic scars acquired in ICUs for many years—often for life.

I have patients coming back five years later for another operation more afraid of returning to the ICU than of death itself!

Harken replied to her that he was already on the attack. Wherever he could, he had been speaking about it to audiences of people concerned with health care, particularly hospital administrators. He would remind them that originally the ICUs had to be given space in hospitals already crowded. Surgeons who wanted them had to wrest storerooms from the cleaning services and to convince administrators, many of whom considered such units "just another example of the cardiothoracic staff crowding others out," to give them even that much space. Even after the value of ICUs had been conclusively proven, the units were largely relegated to windowless corners in hospitals. As the techniques and devices employed in intensive care were steadily elaborated, the balance of emphasis had gone from patient care to machine care for patients.

Question: What about your periotogenic syndrome, resulting from ICUs, Dr. Harken?

Answer: Well, first you have to cure the disease and then you have to cure the cure!

Following are notes from one of D.E.H.'s lectures on the subject, using his capitals and emphases:

DEHUMANIZATION and SENSORY DEPRIVATION and SENSORY OVERLOAD are components of *periotogenic* disease, common to ICUs. They come when a person's diurnal and circadian rhythms [sense of day and night, sun and moon] are upset, from timelessness, noise sustained around the clock at intolerable decibel levels, continuous "daytime" light and never-ending activity.

The patient, in varying degrees of pain, is also suffering from physical restraint, encumbered as he is by intravenous feeding lines, monitor lines, oral and rectal sensing devices, external and even internal electrodes, chest tubes, nasogastric and urinary catheters. He is frightened and exhausted and has awakened to feel like GULLIVER immobilized by the Lilliputians while he slept. He may literally PANIC.

This psychological and emotional "future shock" in a scientific environment is DEHUMANIZING, a major factor in monitoring and machine care. It has resulted physiologically and psychologically in an enormously complicated and little understood physio-patho-psycho metabolic reaction, embracing all systems, to the point of paranoia, agitation, and even delirium. It frequently reverts the exhausted, terrified, disoriented patient to the infantile state emotionally.

There are other possible periotogenic manifestations in ICUs, which should be suggested *not* for their probability but because awareness of possibility reduces the likelihood of occurrence. In the past there have even been a few deaths by electrocution following equipment failure or misuse. The more and better the equipment, the more need for expert biomedical engineers and technicians for proper maintenance. Some patients have even undergone cruel and violent "resuscitation," inappropriately instituted because an electrode slipped off an arm and the flat electrocardiogram was interpreted as cardiac arrest. Also required are sophisticated nurses, physicians, and surgeons alert to these possibilities and above all to their patients' needs.

Some answers are obvious. Windows if possible. At least place clocks, calendars, and pictures of outdoor scenes on the walls. Organize the services to allow intervals of REST. DIM the lights, when possible, at night.

If house officers, physical therapists, visiting clergy, cleaning people, and so on do not respect the rest intervals, hang a sign on the patient's bed (in the ICU and everywhere else for that matter) DO NOT DISTURB, F.C.S. ("For Christ's sake!"). GROUP THE TREATMENTS, pay attention to what must be done as opposed to what *could* be done.

And above all, remember what the behavioral sciences teach, that TENDER LOVING CARE is IMPORTANT.

Everyone accepts now that TLC at regular intervals can be life-saving to the infant or child. It is equally important to the terrified, exhausted, pain-racked adult. Frightened, very ill, slightly or over-whelmingly disoriented patients have a tendency to revert to the infantile state. They pull their knees up under their chins, lie on the right side with bent back and bowed head, arms around their knees, and retreat to semiconscious limbo [the *in utero* position].

NEVER permit the urgency of scrutiny and the expertise required to monitor complicated equipment to outstrip human competence and thereby kidnap personal attention from the patient. Embarrassment inhibits too many of the scientific-minded nurse/physician health delivery segment. Above all these patients need UNABASHED AFFECTION, UNABASHED TENDER LOVING CARE.

The answer to DEHUMANIZATION IS REHUMANIZATION!

Question: It seems to me small or community hospitals are often more human. Should cardiac surgery be done only in major centers?

Answer: The answer is no. However, the only medical question to which that monosyllable is sufficient answer may be "Can you cure the common cold?" I must elaborate.

First, I don't know what a "major center" is, and second, there are two advantages to good—I underline *good*—heart surgery in something less than a so-called major center. It takes care of the patient within the readily accessible area, and heart surgery in a hospital makes that hospital better per se. Their ICUs and CCUs are better, their nursing is better, operating rooms, blood banks, laboratories, and X-ray departments—the whole hospital is better for having this type of surgery—*if* it can be done without hurting the patients, that is, with quality and safety.

Whether *good* heart surgery is done depends on reasonable minimum volume—something like three or four major open-heart cardiopulmonary bypass operations a week—by people who get consistently acceptable results and who send the complex congenital problems, the very ill multivalvular or multivascular coronary problems, to special major centers, if and when they are transportable.

I want to lean toward open-heart surgery off the great center areas. There is a rapidly broadening awareness that unstable angina, acute myocardial infarction [damage to the heart muscle secondary to the loss of its blood supply], and cardiogenic shock patients cannot be moved. If these types of patients have such heart attacks where there are no institutions with cardiac surgery backup, they will die.

The terribly important additional factor is that the advantages to the hospital must never be promulgated at the expense of the heart surgery patient. The most prostituted form of this hospital advantage is when the hospital is improved and everything there is improved—except the poor devil who has the heart trouble and needs heart surgery, but gets less than the best.

Question: I know you have had two heart attacks since you turned sixty-six, and that you have been cardioverted, once in a small hospital in Keene, New Hampshire, and once at the Mount Auburn in Boston. Both times you seemed to get very well again, very quickly. Cardioversion and counterpulsation are two of the techniques for dealing with heart attacks with which you were greatly involved. Your first cardioverter is a "character" in this book, but what about counterpulsation?

Answer: I well remember the laboratory brainstorming session where Dr. Stanley Sarnoff spoke about the fresh awareness we had gained of the greater oxygen consumption the heart muscle used when it was doing pressure work versus flow work. This led me to speculate that if a volume of blood could be aspirated from a large leg artery at the instant when the heart ejected blood, the heart would empty against less pressure. This would reduce heart muscle oxygen demand. Conversely, that unit of blood could be returned in diastole, between heartbeats, when the aortic valve is closed, which would increase the coronary blood supply to the heart muscle. Then we created the word "counter-pulsation."

This effect proved to be obtainable by threading a sausage-shaped balloon on a catheter through the femoral [leg] artery into the chest aorta. Inflating it and deflating it created "counterpulsation," and made it possible to reduce the amount of heart muscle death in cardiogenic shock and help patients dying of heart attacks until they could be studied by angiographs and have emergency surgery. There was slow acceptance of the value of counterpulsation, but now it's used worldwide. External forms of noninvasive counterpulsation circulatory assistance may well be one of the greatest technical therapeutic advances on the horizon. It is my conviction that within the decade we shall make more discriminating assessment of myocardial infarctions by bidimensional echocardiograms [a new technique something like radar for studying the heart and many other organs]. Then we can find a place for *external* counterpulsation to reduce the damage of infarctions.

Question: That was a bit of a digression, but while on the subject of treatment, may I ask what you recommend to your own postoperative patients and how well they comply?

Answer: General advice is simple. A patient may exercise to the point of fatigue but not to exhaustion. He should avoid salt and smoking. His doctors should cut back on medications as rapidly as possible.

The primary care physicians can follow one simple rule: Treat a postoperative patient exactly as you would one who had had heart failure without surgery. Liberalize his treatment the same way. If the patient has had coronary artery bypass surgery but has never had heart failure, manage the patient as if he had had a coronary attack. Patients do need certain medications that are basic and important, overcomplicated at first, to be decomplicated in the months following surgery.

The problem is that patients and their families tend to overcomplicate or undercomply. A patient may continue his medication without consulting his doctor for years or decide to eliminate his own medications. The primary care physician, for his part, may either overprotect his patient or be so alarmed at carrying a postoperative heart patient that he undertreats him. There's no mystery, really: don't overdo or underdo. Careful compliance on the part of patients is the problem and underlines the need for good doctor-patient relationships.

Question: Is it true that in heart surgery the high-risk patient gets a bad deal these days?

Answer: That's a difficult if not unanswerable question. It takes a surgeon of enormous stature to take on the terminal, extremely bad-risk patient. The surgeon's reputation is wounded by high mortality records that are inevitably associated with such risks. The cardiac surgical record of his hospital may be inappropriately damaged. Not only that, but the surgeon is almost inevitably misunderstood by those of the medical service of the hospital, the administration, and the trustees. The whole geographic area may suffer.

It's a delicate balance and one of the areas where public relations and courage on the part of the surgeon and critical, accurate insight by the physicians are vastly important. Sometimes the equation is impossible.

[*Note:* D.E.H. never refused his old patients who needed reoperation—and often multiple valve replacement increased the risk greatly—if there was hope to give them more years of good life. Also, as a senior surgeon in the field, he had long been expected to assume other surgeons' bad risks.]

Question: I presume it would be difficult for a patient to sue for omission, that is, refusal to operate? So that brings up the iatrogenic diseases, those created by the physician or surgeon, and the general question of malpractice.

Answer: Abuse of a perfectly legitimate method of protection for the public has brought about a malpractice crisis! Hospitals alone pay $2 *billion* a year for insurance. This is intolerable. It adds $5 per day per patient to hospital costs. Furthermore the unconscionable malpractice insurance rates for physicians and surgeons, especially in high-risk surgical areas, are conditioning the way they practice, where they practice, and indeed whether they can continue to practice.

The crisis has come about because of the litigation-mindedness of our people, stimulated by lawyers operating on the contingency system, and supported by a climate of consumerism and the prevalent attitude that "the world owes me a living." The enormous expense of defending against plaintiff action, be it absurd or legitimate, coupled with the unrealistic amounts granted for damages, has led to these runaway insurance rates. Frequently there are out-of-court settlements even when there is no justification *whatsoever* for the award. Even the most frivolous actions have become profitable because insurance companies find quick settlement cheaper than defense. Profitable chiefly for the lawyers, because when the dollar for indemnity is broken down, we find that after court costs, the cost of the contingency lawyer, et cetera, the plaintiff, the patient or his family, can be left with less than 30 percent of the award.

Question: Is anything being done about it? Can anything be done about it?

Answer: Yes, and it is absolutely essential to work out a system that protects the patient yet protects the physician against unjustified suits and unrealistic judgments.

Former Attorney General Griffin Bell has indicated that some twenty states have adopted measures to cope with the malpractice crisis. The tribunal system as it operates now in Massachusetts appeals to me. In this state malpractice complaints are screened by a tribunal before proceeding to trial. The tribunal consists of a judge, with a physician and an attorney whom he selects from carefully chosen panels. That three-man tribunal reviews the plaintiff's grievance and the defense by the physicians and hospital. The tribunal does not decide for or against the charge of malpractice, but simply whether or not there is a basis for further inquiry. If the tribunal finds that the charge is frivolous or without justification, the suit is generally and rightly dropped. About 50 percent have been so judged. Conversely if the tribunal finds that there is basis for further inquiry and additional scrutiny, an out-of-court settlement is often concluded, avoiding the expensive trial system. Should the plaintiff wish to, he may have his lawyer continue the action, whatever the tribunal decides, but the lawyer is obliged to post bond covering defense expenses if the trial goes against his client. As a consequence of this system, malpractice insurance rates in

Massachusetts have not increased during the past three years. Rates are still too high and judgments still often unreasonable, but the tribunal system constitutes progress. The FTC [Federal Trade Commission] is considering a national tribunal system.

The most common complaint in malpractice suits is that the doctor did not explain that there was risk! Litigious patients seem to recall that they were told there was absolutely no risk involved, even though I suspect *no* reputable doctor *ever* said that about any major procedure.

Question: What about informed consent to surgery? Isn't that the best protection for the surgeon?

Answer: Well, it's a mixed bag. When shrouded in legalese and with every conceivable accident or possible complication paraded before the patient, he may well elect *not* to have a much needed procedure. Is it good medicine to scare a patient away from what's good for him?

Once one of my hospitals gave me a consent form that required the most awful description of real and remotely possible complications. The patient and I were to initial each paragraph after reading. My patient, a lawyer, asked me how long we had been using this form. I said it was just being introduced.

"Would it help," asked my attorney patient, "if I indicated to your board of trustees that I'm bringing an action against them for cruel and unnecessary aggravation of a pre-existing anxiety?"

That form was withdrawn. In fact, currently many well-run, fine institutions feel that on balance it is better not to have these forms and painful rituals at all. The more complex the form, the more devastating to the patient, and none of the forms offer any reasonable advantage in court. It may well be better to depend on the patient-physician relationship and do away with consent forms.

Question: Now what about possibly faulty devices in this age of machine care and prostheses? Do you approve of the legislation to protect the public?

Answer: Of course I want to protect the public! The public must be protected at any reasonable cost.

However, let us beware of the fact that protection, while preventing errors of *commission*, may be so restrictive as to cause errors of *omission*. For a decade or so it was obvious that some sort of protective legislation about devices was going to be passed. The Supreme Court decision on the Difco and Amph cases [manufacturers of a laboratory device and a knot-tying instrument involving tissue ligatures] declared that devices were, in fact, drugs. You can imagine the consternation within the Food and Drug Administration when told that devices were their responsibility, as well as drugs. The FDA was already overwhelmed with the burden of the world of pharmaceuticals. This meant, *reductio ad absurdum*, that thermometers, bedpans, hospital beds, you name it, were now "drugs." The conscientious FDA people all but decompensated.

In 1968 and 1969 some of us began working with FDA and legislators on reasonable legislation. Surgeons Arthur Beall of Baylor, Gerald Rainer of Denver, Congressman Paul Rogers of Florida, and I, with many FDA people and others, hammered out the Device Act of 1976. That helped to order the chaos; it called for classification of devices into three groups. When the device involves matters of life and death, it requires premarket clearance. A second group requires only good manufacturing practice and registration. The third group can be accepted as safe and effective without the foregoing complications.

If some of our colleagues think that the Device Act of 1976 is a horror, they can have no idea how difficult it was to get as realistic a law as we have. As I have said so many times, "A device is safe when it is safer than the disease it corrects and is the best available." At any rate, we must live with the 1976 act and can only pray that the FDA uses great common sense in its enforcement. This means, particularly, enforcement consistent with the intent of the act.

Question: Is the "strict liability" law involved with the Device Act?

Answer: Well, not really. The Device Act is only indirectly involved in malpractice, but the strict liability concept is a real horror that the public should, indeed must, know about. It could completely kill off innovation and the manufacture of very important devices.

"Strict liability" means that the manufacturer of a medical instrument or device must guarantee it not only against malfunction but also against misuse. I have asked, if I put in a valve upside down, would that mean the manufacturer could be held responsible and have to pay damages to the plaintiff? The answer was yes. The presumption was that such damages paid by the manufacturer would then be passed on in added costs to subsequent purchasers/users. The absurdity of the concept is immediately apparent. If carried to its ultimate conclusion, as manufacturers added the cost of damages to the cost to subsequent users, think of the cost of a baseball and a baseball bat! Under such a concept, $500 for the ball and $1,000 for the bat.

This law could well put device makers out of business. For devices with known hazards, such as prosthetic valves, many manufacturers have already left the field and others are trying to get out of it. So the fate and future of valves is uncertain and gloomy. It doesn't seem to matter that perhaps 300,000 people are enjoying longer and better lives because of valves.

Remark: You are frightening me!

Retort: I call this the "scared age" as distinct from the "golden age" of heart surgery. Consumerism has certainly grossly handicapped or even eliminated experimentation and innovation where "absolute safety"—a chimera—cannot be guaranteed.

For example, at one time I had a valve which I was sure would be better than existing valves. In addition to excellent function and long wear it would perhaps avoid the need for anticoagulation. It was never manufactured because I was told that I should place the new valves in a hundred calves and follow them for two years before trying them in humans. How many operations is that to obtain a hundred survivors in calves? What a capital venture in animal husbandry it would require and, at two operations a week, many years and a large farm. And in the end there would be no real assurance that the coagulation factors in calves are like those in humans with heart, lung, and liver problems. It is this sort of silly "safety and security" that spawns phony defensive research and discourages serious inventive research.

Remark: But there must be protective laws.

Reply: Of course! I urge such laws as the national standardization of parts for devices and the release of drugs in standard measurements, so that patients can afford and follow their therapy more cheaply and easily. Such protective legislation would be genuinely in the public interest.

But even the best laws, no matter how carefully written in consultation with the best experts in the field, still must be administered sensibly. Sensible regulations and sensible interpretation might free us from fear in the "scared age" and lead to another golden age of creative innovation, saving more lives than could ever be saved by excessive caution.

After all, Bill Bigelow, the Canadian pioneer in cardiac surgery and research, said that if cardiac surgery was something of an American invention, perhaps that was because research and experimentation were so much part of the American scene at the time! If that freedom is too much curtailed in the United States, new procedures, devices, and drugs may have to come from other countries.

I can only quote Juvenal: *Quis custodiet ipsos custodes—* Who will protect us from our protectors?

Question: We, the public, have been badly scared by media stories of unnecessary operations. Will you speak to that?

Answer: I could fill volumes. I suffer from the same ambivalence that you do. Of course, unnecessary operations are performed. I cannot defend overaggressive surgeons or venal, evil men.

There are *good* and *bad* unnecessary operations. Just as there are good and bad statistics. If that sounds crazy, let me tackle the question of bad-good mortality statistics.

When some clinics present a large series of patients with, for example, valve disease, with very few or no deaths, we must wonder if they are excluding those very sick patients—the bad risks—who should be given a chance but, in the aggregate, would make the figures look less good.

I am reminded of the late great Dr. John Homans, one of my heroes at the Brigham. When one of his colleagues boasted a phenomenally low mortality rate with a certain type of abdominal surgery, Dr. Homans exclaimed with his characteristic lisp, wry smile, and twinkle in his eye, "You ought to be ashamed of yourself—you aren't trying hard enough!" He meant, of course, that his colleague was rejecting needy patients who might have enjoyed some salvage and were being denied the chance to live. That is a way to attain good statistics, so good that they reflect a selfish selection of patients. When I was a young man training in general surgery it was considered bad practice to have no normal appendices in one's pathology reports. If all the specimens were reported as diseased, it meant that the surgeon was not being liberal enough in his indications for removal in patients with suspicious acute abdomens.

We must be a little cautious about some of the publicized announcements about "unnecessary surgery" where series of operations from suspect fields of surgery and conducted in atypical geographic areas are extrapolated for our whole country. I don't say these things to defend bad or venal surgeons, rather to indicate that some of the dramatic news may not be what it appears to be.

Medical reporting demands extra care and checking. Otherwise it can raise hopes about a "breakthrough"—sometimes claimed by overenthusiastic medical sources—that might be a long way from being ready or available to the public. And one horror story about a small series of faulty valves and faulty pacemakers was leaked to the press before surgeons could inform their patients. It scared hell out of the thousands and thousands who had perfectly good devices that they depended on. My own switchboard lit up like a Christmas tree with calls from all over the world, although I had never used these particular devices. It isn't good for heart patients to be frightened out of their wits. But I must not be overdefensive of surgery. It comes down to the fact that *good* surgeons and physicians make good selections of candidates and bad ones make bad selections.

Question: What about second opinions as a safeguard?

Answer: Second opinions are fine if they constitute added thinking of high quality. When a second opinion is less than excellent, the patient might as well have flipped a coin or asked the first three people who got on the bus. Multiples of zero are still zero, and a bad opinion is worse than zero. So, yes, get second opinions *if* they are good opinions, and if two good opinions differ, get a third.

The assumption prevails that if a second opinion does not agree that surgery is necessary, an "unnecessary operation" has been avoided. Obviously the second opinion could be right or wrong, or there might be a choice of two methods for handling the problem. In some instances there is no good choice, and choosing the lesser of two evils is very difficult. Or there could be a situation where surgery is elective and the patient chooses a definitive surgical solution in preference to prolonged medical management, or vice versa. Which is right or wrong? Does the surgical choice mean that it is an "unnecessary operation"?

Sometimes a second opinion is really not a second opinion. When a primary care physician seeks consultation from a specialist, that is not a second opinion. It is a request for advice. And if that advice, that *consulting* opinion, is medical rather than surgical, the decision may or may not favor surgery and may be wrong in either event.

In the case of heart surgery, the so-called second opinion is almost uniformly built into the system. I do not believe I have ever performed a major heart operation without the concurrence of my regular, independent medical colleagues. Fortunately they have been men of whose company I can boast, Drs. Burwell, Ellis, Forwand, Gorlin, Samuel Levine, Sprague, and Paul Dudley White. In addition to my consultations with them, there were always preoperative conference presentations and discussion of all but emergency operations. That is second opinion at its best— more than second opinion.

Question: Now to costs, of such concern to us all. Hospital costs are the major monocigenic disease of the present, and they are getting worse. How can we cut costs and still get good care?

Answer: I'm glad you didn't lump all costs. Physician cost escalation, bad as it is, is a relatively minor area. Most of the escalation of health care cost is in hospital cost.

Now, a neighbor of mine is the chairman of the board and driving force in one of our country's largest corporations. He says he could run a more efficient company if the unions allowed him to pay every third employee to *stay at home*! Hospitals, of all "companies," should learn from that. Personnel constitutes some 60 percent of the cost. It is the obvious place to tighten up. There are a vast number of 250-bed hospitals with more than a thousand employees. If that increased the quality of care, we *might* justify the attitude "better medicine no matter what the cost"—but it does not, although further expansion might absorb the unemployed like a blotter.

Cut redundancy, inefficiency, top-heavy administration, maintenance, and ancillary services and you might end up with hospitals delivering better care and making profits instead of accumulating deficits.

Miss Marguerite Brooks at the General Hospital in Moline, Illinois, did just that. She built and equipped a multimillion-dollar hospital out of profits. She accepted no government aid and had no public fund raising. When I said, "You must have had to make exorbitant charges," she answered, "Oh, yes, indeed, the regular Blue Cross insurance rates!" Before making major purchases, she consulted doctors, engineers, and others. She lived with the nurses and did not allow nursing supervision, maintenance, and administrative hierarchies to expand and proliferate. She made a great hospital profitable.

Now bed utilization committees generally help to correct the malignant tendency to keep patients in the hospital when the costs are borne by third-party carriers, that is, insurance. However, very often the extended care of minimally ill patients is of low cost to the hospital—"the well patient is no effort." Even the senile people awaiting transfer to our abysmally inadequate nursing home facilities are of low patient cost to the individual hospital, but they represent a disgraceful augmentation of the national cost of health care.

One area where I have long sought reform is in the tendency of physicians, particularly young people in training, to write orders for procedures with no consideration of costs. New diagnostic or therapeutic modes are often ordered, simply added to existing tests rather than substituted for the older, outdated modes that they replace or even render obsolete. I favor a plan that would require the physician ordering medications or minor procedures costing over $10 to enter the cost after the order. If it is more than $25, he would be obliged to specify in his progress note what actions a positive or negative test would evoke. If there is no alteration in active/positive versus negative, the test or study should not be made. This may sound like more paperwork, but it would not only reduce costs by enhancing cost consciousness, but also bring about more critical clinical thinking.

There is also the horrible matter of "defensive orders"—ordering every conceivable study as protective armor in the event of malpractice action. This, coupled with defensive consultations, adds significantly to costs.

Many discussions of cost cutting indict new devices, new instrumentation, as causes of unnecessary escalation in costs. Never mind the minor impact of the $10 billion annual cost of devices within the more than $180 billion annual cost of health care. Indeed, equipment may be the best place to spend money. Where there is the finest equipment, you will see the highest morale and the greatest efficiency in life saving, pride in the work, and competence in the doing.

Diminish the effect of litigation, and reverse the operation of Parkinson's Law, Peter's Principle, and Murphy's Law in our hospitals! Peter's Principle, you know, promotes people to the level of their own incompetence. Parkinson's Law triangulates and increases administration, adding to costs, and Murphy's Law says that if an accident can happen, it will. Nature favors the hidden flaw, and Mother Nature is a bitch.

That sounds obvious, doesn't it? Now let me ask you a question. What is the basic way to cut all medical costs?

Question: Prevention?

Answer: Of course! Prevention. We surgeons want prevention or medicine to take over from us. For example, surgery has only a *small* impact on the overall problem of death from heart disease—although it has a big impact on the person involved, the individual whom it cures or helps when there is no other way.

On the general subject of prevention and on the future of cardiac treatment, Harken had his own strong opinions, but wanted to call in colleagues. So in this one-to-one question-and-answer session I asked for his thinking on only one more subject: the burning, controversial one of euthanasia. I knew this was a tough issue for all doctors because they are committed to saving lives. Harken was committed even more than many, but he was also vehement about the quality of life as part of any judgment he must make on treatment for a patient. Keeping someone alive as a vegetable with no further awareness of his own being or in unrelievable pain was not part of his creed. So I asked him, "What about our right to die? Or not to be kept living in intolerable, irreversible conditions?"

His answer was a letter he showed me that he had written to Lewis J. Amster, clinical editor of *Modern Medicine*, in 1978:

Dear Editor Amster:

The discussions of euthanasia are so endlessly repeated that the more significant the comments they evoke, the more hackneyed they seem. Perhaps we can assume the obvious and push beyond the "active versus the passive" (euthanasia versus dysthanasia to the sophisticates), Papal omission of "extraordinary life support," "no tranfusion for the pain-racked cancer-riddled patient," and "pulling out the plug."

The time has come to ask questions that plague one who has dealt with these problems for several decades. Yes, one whose "pain-racked and cancer-riddled" patients have suffered minimally; one who has been shocked by the too frequent looseness defining "brain death." Indeed one who has had patients sent simultaneously as recipient and donor for heart transplantation, and having decided against this give and take, has then seen the proffered donor (a twenty-eight-year-old mother) leave the hospital healthy and intact along with the intended recipient rehabilitated by three artificial valves. Two grateful, useful people versus two dead.

Now for some questions and one suggestion.

What distinction is drawn between euthanasia and dysthanasia? I am not always certain which is which, and furthermore, I do not make a moral distinction. Of course, there are examples at opposite poles, e.g. allowing that pain-racked, cancer-riddled unfortunate to pass on quietly without cardiopulmonary resuscitation versus blowing him to bits with a shot gun. Here discussion of the extremes is silly *but* consider that same patient to whom one gives enough morphine to relieve his pain, even though such doses will lead to pneumonia and blessed death! Is that euthanasia or dysthanasia? Have we followed the Papal edict and "used no extraordinary means to prolong" or have we given the fatal injection . . . and indeed is there an ethical distinction? Yes, there are arguable but hardly moral differences.

Would a balanced committee, e.g. theologian, lawyer, psychiatrist, physician and family member, be helpful in deciding about the pain-racked, or the brain dead? For the "pain-racked hopelessly ill" the decision may hinge on the condition *"hopeless."* "Hopeless" varies with the medical competence. Both the *diagnosis* and *treatment* relate to local professional quality. Just so does the decision of the balanced committee. Therefore, I seriously question the validity of the committee, for I can assure the public that where the diagnosis of the hopeless is adequate, there also the care of the borderline is best, *and* in that very center, *there is no need* for committee action on euthanasia. I believe that *now* unencumbered by committee deliberation, family emotional torture and painful patient delay, the decisions are more accurate and quietly appropriately promulgated than would be possible by committee action. And, God have mercy on committee action if predicated on lesser standards of diagnosis, treatment or loose definition of brain death. (Those standards of the definition of brain death exist, let all physicians adhere to them absolutely!)

What, then, do we do about these balanced committees? We give serious thought as to where in the above circumstances the committee is really a safeguard as opposed to a potential source of confusion or delay.

Are there areas that do need new consideration, possibly committee action? Yes, for an essentially different but related area. Here the committee may serve a purpose. Though estimates vary there are thought to be upwards of 300,000 people in nursing homes who have lost their brain function so that they know not who they are, where they are, cannot feed themselves nor care for their personal toilet. The diagnosis and prognosis of these vegetative, nonindividual, metabolizing nonpeople can be established with certainty. In those situations does not food and fluid by attendant, feeding tube or intravenous become "extraordinary means of life support"? While we may find it easier to discontinue intravenous or feeding tube, is that different than interrupting the attendant's offering of food and fluid by spoon and drinking tube?

In short, I hope that I have suggested areas where public deliberations are possibly both unnecessary and counterproductive. At the same time, let us address ourselves to an enormous existing problem . . . and one that is growing.

Thanks for including me.

Sincerely,
Dwight E. Harken, M.D.

16.

The Now and Future Heart

Three doctors joined Dwight Harken in his study at his house in Cambridge, Massachusetts. They gave of their overburdened time because he asked them to, to talk informally about the present and future of heart disease. Each one was a world-recognized expert in his particular field.

Lewis Dexter, immediate past chief of cardiology at the Peter Bent Brigham Hospital and Harvard Professor of Medicine (emeritus) was the first man to assess the function of the heart's left ventricle by extending catheterization to the study of capillary pressure in the lungs. Now called "wedge pressure," this was considered one of the great contributions to hemodynamics since it provided a method of studying the function and failure of the left ventricle. Tall, quiet of voice, in his late sixties, Dexter's was primarily the clinical approach through the mind of the investigator.

George Blackburn, the youngest luminary, was Associate Professor of Surgery at Harvard, director of Nutritional Support Services at the New England Deaconess Hospital, and chief of the Nutrition-Metabolism Cancer Research Laboratory there. Dark and dynamic, his international reputation was as an authority on nutrition in health and disease, embracing body factors relating to arteriosclerosis, obesity, and wound healing. His was essentially the epidemiological approach.

Bernard Lown, with Barouh Berkovits, invented the cardioverter, and was well known for his clinical work and laboratory experimentation. An authority on arrythmias, he was Professor of Cardiology in Public Health at Harvard, with two laboratories there and a practice at the Peter Bent Brigham Hospital. A naturalized American citizen, his speech faintly reflected his boyhood in Lithuania, the country from which he had emigrated, to graduate from Johns Hopkins and go on to his remarkable career in Boston. Stocky and vivacious, he had an approach that might be called broadside.

It was as if four generals, wearing sixteen stars, had gathered to discuss strategy, weaponry, and progress in a destructive, continuing war. Their mutual optimism about our increasing defense capability offered the hope that at least our children's children might triumph over cardiovascular disease, the number one enemy of health and reasonable longevity.

That enemy accounted for 997,766 deaths in the United States alone during 1978, according to the American Heart Association's statistics. Nevertheless 1978 was the second year in which the total had dropped slightly, indicating at least the beginning of a downward curve in the number of casualties. Each man there had made contributions to public education about prevention, to which they credited the drop. Each man there was prepared to express his current thoughts on the subject that consumed them all.

The floor was given first to Lewis Dexter. He tackled atherosclerosis, the endemic disease that has beset mankind since the beginning of medical history. "Hardening of the arteries" is not only an almost inevitable result of age, but can affect children.

Dexter: There seems to be real progress in the very basic field of finding out just what an atherosclerotic plaque is, how it develops, and some of the factors that influence it. For instance, the atherosclerotic plaque on a coronary artery, or on any artery, starts as a little fat streak and begins to build up in one place. Call that a lesion on the way to becoming a plaque. It becomes a plaque and finally gets bigger and bigger and occludes the artery.

A lot of evidence indicates that the process starts on the endothelium [cells forming the inner lining of blood vessels] in defects—really holes or abrasions—perhaps produced by such forces as high blood pressure. The blood flow may attack where an artery branches, causing eddy currents at these favorite, especially vulnerable places for plaque formation. Then heaven only knows what other factors come into play, such as lack of oxygen. If there is a break in the inner lining, platelets come along to seal over that little defect. In doing so they release all sorts of substances, many of which have not yet been defined. It's difficult chemistry. We know the substances are there, but the biochemists haven't been able to isolate many of them. Yet. Progress has been slow, but new methods are making my hopes higher. Basic researchers now know the *action* of these substances—they make cells in that inner lining proliferate.

The lipids—the fatty stuff in the blood—go through and are attracted to the vessel cells. The cells start to grow in that area. As the cell fills and swells with cholesterol, that is the beginning of atherosclerosis. All sorts of enzymes in this process influence the way the cell handles the cholesterol. For instance, the high-density lipoproteins [HDLs] carry cholesterol away. People who happen to have a high level of HDLs have greater protection against atherosclerosis, and people who have a lot of low-density lipoproteins [LDLs] do get it, or tend to get it.

Now as far as I can see, nobody has the foggiest notion how to raise the level of high-density lipoproteins, but there is a lot of research going on at the basic biochemical and cellular level. This makes me fairly confident that it is only a matter of time until the basic disease process gets under control and surgery will no longer be necessary.

I'm awfully grateful for surgery at this point. I'm sending people to surgery all the time, but I don't think it's the fundamental approach to this problem. However, and note well, it is of prime importance to these people suffering from coronary artery and other vascular diseases that are surgically correctable—such as I had! [Dexter had had an abdominal aortic aneurysm replaced surgically seven years before.]

We need to know much more about the underlying causes of atherosclerosis, but in the meantime we can assess the value and ultimate place of surgery.

Harken immediately contributed his view of a development in angioplasty (plastic surgery performed upon arteries), which he felt would alter the picture in the future.

Harken: I think we are on the verge of one of the most important quantum jumps forward in heart surgery. I have just reviewed a large series of patients at the Lenox Hill Hospital in New York. A catheter was threaded from the arm down the aorta and out into the first and second order of coronary arteries. Then, having localized the obstruction with a combination of angiography, fluoroscopy, and catheterization, a little balloon on the catheter was introduced into the obstruction and inflated, thus dilating and opening the obstruction.

Surgeons have said you can't do that—you will break open those little vessels or you will send a shower of cementlike bits downstream and you will have more occlusions. Wallsh, a brilliant surgeon at Lenox Hill, and others have demonstrated in autopsy that when one breaks open the atherosclerotic vessel, the intima [inner lining of the artery] cracks longitudinally. It does *not* rupture circumferentially, which would, of course, be dangerous because the lining might then peel off and go downstream or flap in the bloodstream and obstruct it. So they *can* use the little balloon at the end of the catheter—which was originated by Grundzig, supported by Senning, in Zurich, Switzerland, who demonstrated it to Dr. Stertzer of Lenox Hill. This procedure eliminates, in many instances, the need for open-chest coronary bypass surgery. It also adds a whole new dimension to open-heart coronary bypass surgery as beautifully extended by Dr. Wallsh. Since the vessels do break open longitudinally, the bloodstream keeps the lumen [passageway] open. Angioplasty is here and extensions of it are part of our future. The medical people will make great advances in this field, and the surgeons can jump on the bandwagon and use this technique at the time of surgery. Small-vessel disease has defeated medicine and surgery in the past, but now small-vessel obstructions can be treated way out at the periphery where vessels are too small for bypass surgery. Even three-vessel disease with many minuscule peripheral obstructions can be dilated by the surgeon at the operating table.

Wallsh takes out a big plaque or goes into the coronary artery just beyond it. Then, before anastomosing [connecting] the saphenous vein to it, he takes a string of plastic thinner in diameter than the lead in a pencil and pushes it clear around the apex of the heart thus dilating the tiny little vessels. Interestingly enough, instead of plugging up those tiny little vessels, blood comes back, which indicates vessel communication with other coronary arteries. So angioplasty as done in the catheter laboratory might eliminate a lot of surgery, and angioplasty combined with coronary bypass surgery could extend effective surgery!

Sudden Death, that is death by unheralded cardiac circulatory arrest, was the single biggest killer in 1978; of the 997,766 deaths from cardiovascular disease, 646,073 were by Sudden Death. Approximately 60 percent of those victims died outside the hospital, and 60 percent of that 60 percent had seen a doctor within sixty days of their demise. This had been Bernard Lown's preoccupation since 1959.

Lown: As we sit here, one person is dying of Sudden Death every minute! Some people say why worry about that way of dying? It's a beautiful way to go. But it afflicts men in a ratio of four to one, and accounts for the great disproportion of females to males in our country today, and furthermore the peak of its occurrence, the median time, is age fifty-nine. Sudden Death cuts down people in their prime. That is tragic. This cardiovascular mortality is four times as important as death from cancer. It must be prevented, but the level of priorities in our research establishments does not reflect this. I feel like Cato who stood up every day in the Roman Forum and said *Delenda est Carthago,* Carthage must be destroyed or it will be the undoing of Rome!

In 1959 it was clear that sudden cardiac death was most likely due to arrhythmia, but it was uncertain whether it was due to asystole [no beat] or ventricular fibrillation, that chaotic, multiple sort of twittering that is ineffective in propelling blood. Lack of interest in the problems reflects something wrong with the medical profession, to speak very frankly.

The medical profession is disease oriented and hospital based, and Sudden Death occurs most often outside the hospital and generally instantaneously. In the early sixties I thought that Sudden Death was due to a heart attack, by coronary artery occlusion, so after a big hassle we got a coronary care unit at the Peter Bent Brigham, one of the first, to study heart attacks. What rapidly became clear was that people who died suddenly had *not* generally had a heart attack in the form of coronary occlusion. That was an important finding. Everybody had presupposed that dying suddenly was a catastrophic event involving an occlusion of a coronary artery. However, pathologists began to point out that Sudden Death victims generally did *not* have fresh coronary occlusions. Death was often unwitnessed, so the time could not be determined precisely, but it certainly occurred within an hour of the first symptoms and was often instantaneous.

So—aha!—you may have an injury or death of the myocardium, the heart muscle, so-called myocardial infarction without coronary occlusion. If the supply of blood is already inadequate, excessive stress may make the supply so inadequate to the demand that there is death, although there is no obvious sign of tissue damage. So the supposition became that myocardial ischemia [deficiency of blood] was the villain, but it was too early to establish a connection with arrhythmia.

Then something else happened. People who "died" from Sudden Death were beginning to be resuscitated. If they had suffered a heart attack by coronary occlusion they would have shown significant changes in the electrocardiograms, in enzymes, or whatever. They did not, so now there is a chorus of people around the world saying, "What the heck happened?" To some of us the conclusion is clear: Sudden Death could be an electrical accident Like for example, if the switch is turned off, the light goes out That doesn't mean the wiring is bad or the bulb burned out. The switch was shut off. This happens to some people and not to others, and if it is due to some electrical instability in the heart, as we vaguely conjectured, we must recognize it ahead of time and do something.

We formulated the hypothesis that certain skips in the heartbeat, so-called VPBs [ventricular premature beats], could be indicators of electrical instability in patients who have heart disease. So we might do something to protect them from Sudden Death. This early speculation opened up a whole new activity—monitoring. Patients starting carrying little boxes, the size of a tape recorder, to monitor what was happening over twenty-four-hour periods. Manufacturing such equipment got to be big business—and business often determines the direction of equipment for medicine.

It became clear that the number of premature beats, among other factors, was a function of age—the older the person, the more likely he was to have them. Ninety percent of people who have coronary disease have VPBs anyway, so it is not a good warning of impending Sudden Death, although further studies showed that *some* people who have VPBs are at higher risk. This is a conundrum. It became our view that not merely the presence of VPBs but the type—certain attributes, certain frequencies—made people with such VPBs three- or fourfold times at higher risk. This proved to be the case.

So we introduced exercise testing to expose arrythmias in a controlled environment. We have just now demonstrated that people who are at risk from Sudden Death can be protected if they are identified. In the last three years we've had about 110 patients who have had recurrent Sudden Death and were fortunate enough to be shocked, [defibrillated] out of this type of ventricular action.

We know a lot. We can treat people who have recurrent episodes by selecting a program that protects them. We think we know how. A majority of those we have treated have not had recurrences, but the difficult problem is how to identify them before the cardiac arrest. And the protection program now is very costly in terms of time. We keep the patients in the hospital three weeks, test them with diverse drugs, and meantime we ask the important questions: If they have electrical instability of the heart, and there is every reason to believe they've had it for years, why are they alive at all? Why does Sudden Death happen when it happens? What is the trigger?

We make a hypothesis: Of the transient risk factors that change the excitability of the electrophysiology of the heart, the key one is in the brain. We started a series of fascinating animal experiments to study Sudden Death in dogs.

I am amused to relate it all so easily, after all the work, suffering, false starts, and cul de sacs. We want to study the psychologic factors, but when a dog drops dead and we resuscitate him, he is through. The experience is too formidably traumatic. So we counterfeit Sudden Death. We know it is Sudden Death, but the dog doesn't—that's complicated. We settle on a stimulus at a certain part of the vulnerable period of the cardiac cycle [as identified by the great twentieth-century physiologist Wiggers], increasing susceptibility to Sudden Death short of the point where the dog would die.

We take the dog and put him in a cage in a room where everybody is nice to him. Then we suspend him in a sling with his feet barely touching the ground, a stressful situation. If human beings have no escape, it's terribly stressful; the same is true with animals. The dog stays quietly, seems passive, but there is no escape. We use noise and light and give the dog only one small electric shock. We repeat this for three days and then no more. The dog is returned to the cage. His heart is normal. Put him back in the sling and the dog's threshold, his susceptibility to lethal arrhythmias, increases precipitously. We have demonstrated that the dog, with no heart disease, has become exquisitely susceptible to Sudden Death just by putting him in that sling.

So now we occlude his coronary artery and release it while the dog is in the cage. Nothing happens. We occlude it and release it in the sling. Consistently, the dogs drop dead. We are in the midst of modeling a problem that demonstrates the importance of psychologic stress. Nothing happens to the dog for weeks, but memory traces about the sling are there permanently and modify his response characteristics to an environment he interprets as stressful. The blood-circulating hormones, like epinepherine, are markedly increased. This indicates stress.

We are now dealing with the brain. It has been found that if you increase serotonin [a mediator of nerve activity in the brain] there is a diminution in sympathetic nerve impulses to the heart, and stress is reduced. To increase the serotonin, we give the dog an essential amino acid, tryptophan, which enters the brain and is the precursor of serotonin, and also enters the body and provokes the production of serotonin. We have to block the conversion of serotonin, which is rapidly metabolized, so that the maximum amount accumulates specifically in the brain to protect the dog.

We ask ourselves about other factors and recently have investigated melatonin, produced in the pineal gland, which the ancients regarded as the seat of the soul. It modulates the organism's diurnal responses and is produced when you sleep with your eyes closed. More melatonin apparently lessens sympathetic nervous activity to the heart, we thought, and this is the case. It has become very exciting. We are searching for means to prevent the factors that lead to Sudden Death.

The neurophysiologists, neuroendocrinologists, and nutritionists have found, in the last few years, that one can modify brain chemistry by diet. In the future physicians need to pay more attention to such relations.

If research proves that we can protect patients at risk, what is the next problem? At present we can identify but a small subset of patients who die suddenly, namely those who have had coronary heart attacks, but they constitute only one-third of those who die suddenly. We cannot screen the entire population, catheterize them all, subject millions to coronary angiography, and repeat the process every few years. So, first, screen and identify those at risk. Second, once they are identified, learn how to interdict the trigger. Third, learn how to modify electrophysiologic instability. I think the scientific community is on the verge of solving these screening problems and developing the prophylactic methods. Then we shall be able to contain sudden and accidental death!

Dr. George Blackburn, acknowledged by those present to be the expert on the general subject of prevention, which absorbed them all, reviewed the subject of risk factors and public education.

Blackburn: Epidemiologically, we have identified and tried to educate everybody about six primary and secondary factors. I think we can make a frontal attack on all six because they dovetail—on the big three: hypertension, high cholesterol, and smoking, and on obesity, stress, and lack of exercise. The effort to diet leads to exercise, the person who exercises has the best stress control, eating less and weight reduction make him feel so good he doesn't need to smoke, et cetera, et cetera. It's a longitudinal study; you make a measurement, subjectively and objectively, and watch people progress through your behavior chain, and, lo and behold, educational programs do work. There is less smoking, less overweight, more exercise, better diet, and, fingers crossed, time will show a further diminution of the incidence of heart attacks.

Let's take up the fundamentals. Some of the factors have been confused because high- and low-density lipoproteins have not been separated in the studies and the meaning of cholesterol has been too loosely assessed. When the difference in lipoproteins—high density (HDL), the "good guys," versus low-density lipoproteins (LDL), the "bad guys"—began to be appreciated, we were getting someplace. These factors make still more sense when assessed against the backdrop of high cholesterol (evil) versus low cholesterol (good) factors.

One of the first studies Dr. Paul Dudley White used to illustrate the advantages in diet and exercise were the findings in autopsies of Canadian children under ten years old killed in accidents. Those children had already begun to show coronary artery disease. It is interesting to note that studies of children in Brooklyn, New York, and the Ashkenazim in Israel showed similar findings. The groups had similar dietary styles. The Yemenites, with Semitic backgrounds similar to the Ashkenazim, but who were wandering, walking, nomadic goat milk drinkers, showed no such incidence of coronary artery disease in childhood.

One of the first major comparisons of plasma lipids, separating alpha or high-density lipoproteins from beta or low-density lipoproteins in racial groups, showed no differences in HDLs—the same in Cape Cod or Cape Town, but slightly higher among the Bantus. Subsequent studies by Ansell Keyes and others in the 1950s and 1960s did not usually separate the alpha and beta lipoproteins, but cholesterol averages for Japanese living in Los Angeles were higher than for those in Japan. Eskimo men on the west coast of Greenland have higher cholesterol than the Danes, and mainland adolescents have lower cholesterol than the New Zealanders of European origin, et cetera, but the factor of the influence of HDLs, the good kind, within the groups has to be worked out.

To pursue HDL—high density, high hope—a little further, we note that HDLs are higher in female children, still higher in female adolescents and young women. Thus females have more protection than males until menopause. Estrogen, the female hormone, raises HDLs, and androgen, the male sex hormone, lowers HDLs. Within limits, alcohol and exercise raise HDLs. The female versus male advantage persists until age sixty, when the estrogens go down and the androgens begin to match up and close the gap.

I believe intuitively that we will get control. There is enough evidence. You don't need any more of it to decide about smoking, for instance. Dwight, you have more perspective on this. Can you say whether people will grab responsibility that really works, day in and day out?

The conference was thus opened for general discussion. It returned again and again to prevention through the education of physicians, patients, and the general public about all aspects of heart disease. All four men were dedicated to this purpose. Among other public projects he had embraced, Harken's strong, activist approach had been an important factor in sweeping cigarette advertisements from the airways. Blackburn was on his way to Washington to preach the epidemiological approach to diet. Lown had a program of lectures on Sudden Death.

Harken: Citing risk factors with shotgun indictments is like a return to the days when they decided malaria was due to living in swampy areas. Certainly it was a big risk factor to live in swampy marsh areas. If you moved people away, they had less malaria. But it's a hell of a lot more direct to kill the anopheles mosquito that's carrying the plasmodia. Now there are some thirty-five million Americans who have definite high blood pressure and are at risk for stroke, renal failure, and heart failure. The National Heart, Lung, and Blood Institute says another five million have borderline high blood pressure. Here is a fruitful area for attack. We have effective treatment *now* for these people. But even though diagnosis and treatment are available and awareness is high, continued long-term compliance with treatment is low!

Dexter: Well, my confreres will forgive me if I say most of the agents that we have used to control blood pressure have been terrible. They do lower blood pressure and allow people to live longer, but they all have had side effects. There are, however, new medications—transfer enzyme blockers—right at this moment, and 80 percent of hypersensitive patients tested on them benefit without significant side effects. It is too soon to say it's the sort of answer the field is waiting for, but hypertension *can* be essentially eradicated. How about a substance you could put in your shredded wheat? I think this is just around the corner. I'm not sure.

Harken: Peeking around the corner, that shredded wheat additive might obviate the big problem of compliance—patients who just don't continue medication. Maybe we'll get perfect compliance when we have a slow-release pellet that can be planted under the skin or in a muscle and last for months or years, eliminating strokes from hypertension, as well as related kidney failure, and overworked hearts. Medication is a small price to pay for insurance against death or worse!

Dexter: No question, hypertension is one of the greatest, call it the worst, of the constellation of risk factors.

Blackburn: Let's see. We've got the genetic thing, and that's very powerful. You can smoke a lot of cigarettes and eat a lot of eggs if you were born right. But if your ticket is punched by heredity, nothing can save you, and up until menopause the females can laugh while the men are falling over dead in their forties and fifties. Work on smoking first. Then we have exercise, which, independent of diet, will raise the good type HDLs. Brisk walking twenty minutes every other day will do it, according to a Harvard alumni study. It doesn't have to be masochistic running or jogging. The more you do, the more intensely you have to work to burn up the calories, so it needn't be tough. Control obesity, and that is a tremendous way to reduce dying. Alcohol is interesting. A little is probably good and seems to stimulate the right kind of lipoproteins (HDLs).

Dexter: Most people who drink don't have anything wrong with their hearts, but there are certain people who develop real heart muscle disease as the result of either moderate or heavy drinking. If you know the cause, you can stop it, whatever it is.

Harken: I like to drink, and as far as I can determine, for me, the alcohol factor is mostly calories. I went to a meeting where Dr. George Burch, Professor and Chairman of the Department of Medicine at Tulane Medical School, made the claim that anyone who had an ounce of alcohol a day was an alcoholic. I looked out at the audience and said, by the one-ounce standard, all alcoholics raise your hands—almost everyone in the audience did.

Blackburn: Well, we know that exceeding two drinks, 120 calories a day, is without merit. And we know that lowering cholesterol a little bit, plus lowering the saturated fat in our diets, has resulted in a plateauing of the incidence of heart disease, and it has even gone down. Cross-sectional epidemiological studies have indicted cholesterol.

Then Blackburn added as another note of cheer, "One heart disease has fallen off the chart at the Center for Disease Control in childhood morbidity. New cases of rheumatic heart disease are really down."

Harken paused to boast of his father's observation of the con-

nection between childhood joint pains, fever, tonsillir streptococcal infections, a certain kind of myocarditis, and death. A remarkable deduction for a small-town country doctor to make and
publish at the turn of the century.

Harken: I take a long-term conservative view about eliminating all heart disease because we are dealing with many different diseases. The great plague of heart disease is not like the
white plague [tuberculosis], not quite like diabetes, not quite like
cholera. It's a whole bag of different diseases. Basic science may
identify subsets and we may find specific cures within these subsets. There would be my optimism. The causal relationship of
rheumatic fever to myocarditis is not altogether clear, but it is
certainly dramatically correlated. People who do not have this
particular identifiable streptococcus in their throats, as far as we
know, never get that kind of myocarditis—and this one kind of
bacteria almost always remains sensitive to penicillin. So penicillin prophylaxis has changed the incidence of rheumatic fever in
this country.

Dexter: The incidence of *chronic* rheumatic heart disease
has declined, impressively. Acute rheumatic fever has all but dis-
appeared from the American scene. We are seeing less myocarditis, and chronic rheumatic heart disease has decreased to the
point that it is now rarely seen in pregnancy whereas it used to be
the leading heart disease in that age group.

Harken: If you markedly reduce active rheumatic carditis,
you will suppress a chronic disease. After all, most chronic diseases were acute once! Let's discuss, *pro bono publico,* that terrifying set of facts trying to tell us something about the enormous
number of people who died of Sudden Death after having been to
see a doctor within the past two months. How does the primary
care physician, 90 percent of whose patients merely come to him
with the "blahs," separate the "blahs" from those with a real risk
of heart failure?

Lown (reacting to Sudden Death like a firehorse alerted by
the sirens; no matter how many warnings people had had, those
with known risks were liable to die unexpectedly anyway): Cardiopulmonary resuscitation [CPR] salvages many more than the

CCU. "Instantly" is the critical intervention factor. If death by heart stoppage occurs, the stopwatch starts—three minutes, none or minimal brain damage; five minutes, more; six to ten minutes and brain damage is probably irreversible. You may resuscitate the heart and end up with a vegetable. The object is to reach the victim instantly. *Everybody*, I say, should learn to do CPR. I've always been amused because you cannot graduate from Harvard College unless you can swim fifty yards; how could a Christian-oriented university, dedicated to serving man, teach you to save yourself but not your fellow man? Nobody should graduate from Harvard until they know CPR. It would be nice to know that you might save my life or I might save yours. That would create a greater togetherness in society at a time when centrifugal forces are working to tear people asunder. You would look on your fellow man as your potential savior.

All of them commended a program in Seattle, organized by former Peter Bent Brighamite Dr. Leonard Cobb, that had trained 125,000 people in CPR at a cost of $1.75 per person, an investment the whole United States could afford. Dr. Mark Vasu had followed Cobb by introducing such a program in Michigan. People who did get to CCUs in time were effectively monitored and saved if Sudden Death occurred. Harken asked Lown about a study in Great Britain that had turned up plausible statistics indicating that CCU care for patients with myocardial infarctions was less effective than good home care.

Harken: Perhaps you feel you are biased in favor of CCUs, Bernie?

Lown: Certainly I'm biased. He who says he has no bias is biased. I'm biased and I was very active in the sixties traveling the length and breadth of America preaching for coronary care units. Let's look objectively at the arguments of the British centers. The most recent is from Nottingham University by John Hampton. He concluded that there is no advantage in treating people in CCUs rather than at home. I think the British are reaching that conclusion through economic necessity—*their* bias.

Care in a CCU is very costly—the sophistry of the human mind is always enchanting. You can make a virtue of necessity.

Remember that doctors can generally, within two or three hours of a heart attack from coronary occlusion, come to a relatively sound conclusion as to who is likely to survive and who is not. They can, with some degree of safety, keep some at home and take those with early lung congestion or those with a lot of arrythmias into hospital CCUs. With such proper triage they have already separated out the worst from the best. This is possible in Britain where there is a national health care system; the United States doesn't have such a delivery of health care, which reaches out to home care with nurses, ambulance attendants, and doctors making critical judgments early. Even so, if you look closely at their figures, you may find that comparatively hundreds treated in the hospital have no deaths, while those treated at home have one or two deaths. We have more people in the United States, and even if we did intelligent triage and took out most of the at-risk and left behind the lesser risks among whom there would be this subtle, small mortality, it would multiply out to maybe twenty thousand deaths, and that's a lot of deaths. The British say that that small but real mortality doesn't pay. That's a matter of profound value judgment, pivoting on the unanswerable question of what a life is worth to society.

Lown went on to attack developments in CCUs as Harken had for both ICUs and CCUs.

Lown: When a person is trained in a special skill, he makes an effort to use that skill, which can result in excess. A psychiatrist once said, "If you're trained only in how to use a hammer, you will look at everyone as if they were nails." The number of invasive procedures in some CCUs has become so excessive, so flagrant, and so inhuman that I'm frequently apprehensive about walking through the very units I helped to develop. Now you have a lot of house staff with much less supervision. Techniques do enable more precise diagnosis, but the rate of change in technology is so rapid that older doctors abdicate and the young assert their revenge against age by saying "You older guys don't know about technetium 99 or two-dimensional echocardiography," or what have you. So the older man's judgment, skill, experience, greater knowledge, are not sought. That is what is so impressive about the Chinese and their respect for older people. We shouldn't romanticize it, because it can become the tyranny of age, but this should not be substituted for the opposite.

Harken: It's apparent to me that many of our older physicians have not always disciplined themselves enough in continuing education. "Repetition of error is not experience."

Lown: We, the American people, have been sold a bill of goods—that medicine is a science. Medicine partakes of science, but medicine is an art and the greater the doctor, the greater the artistry. When I'm brooding about the philosophy of medicine, healing, and the care of the sick, I think the physicists—the Einsteins, the Bohrs, and the Bornes—are way ahead of us. They recognized the uncertainty of knowledge, the fact that the observer influences the observed. It was, I believe, T. S. Eliot who said, "Where is the wisdom we lost in knowledge? Where is the knowledge we lost in information?" Philosophically the physician is still in the middle of the nineteenth century. Technically he is brilliant, but philosophically he is a moron. He regards the human apparatus, the human being, as machinery. The modern physicist has introduced the quark as some ultimate particle. They talk of "virtuous" quarks—"strange" quarks, "charmed" quarks. They aren't crazy. They have comprehended the elements of subjectivity and uncertainty that are inherent in our perception of reality.

Blackburn: I'm bothered by judgments of therapies based only on longevity. I strongly believe that the quality of life must be in the equation. People say that is such a soft science, but there are techniques for objectively measuring the quality of life. Are you confined to bed? Can you get your own clothes off? Go to work? Enjoy retirement?

Harken: Do you *think* you are better? I accept the value of the charisma of the surgeon or the placebo effect of an operation; if the patients are clearly a lot happier, that is a cardinal plus.

Blackburn: It's the total package. I'm a great believer in the placebo. You have to regard the whole aura of the phenomenon of care. In surgery, there is the intense encounter and then emotional catharsis, and on the other side of it you feel better for whatever reason. For instance, in the field of diet, we are in constant competition with the health stores and they just beat the pants off us because they are really slick with, so to speak, placebo medicine.

Harken: I'd like somebody to study the positive metabolic effect of motivation, the healing effect of believing. I know I see older people give up, return to the fetal position, and quit. And then somebody comes along and pats them on the head and gives them TLC and they start to eat and feel better. I know how to deliver it and that it works, but I don't know how to measure it.

Blackburn: We're talking about the Latin meaning of placebo, to *please.* It started with witch doctors who gave little potions or totems, and those Egyptian physicians who wrote commands on little pieces of white writing material that were get-better contracts. Very powerful communication.

Lown: We, biologists and physicians, have lost not only wisdom but knowledge in the deluge of information. We must begin to perceive the whole human being and put Humpty-Dumpty together again. Put the brain back into the equation; a psychologic dimension needs to be restored. The greatest development in medicine will be when the doctor integrates modern science with the legacy of what medicine is all about, an empathy for the whole human being!

Blackburn: We all have visions of immortality, that disaster will strike the folks next door, not us. Take the risk factors we recite so glibly. We know there is a stress factor and that people with Type A [combative, competitive] personalities tend to get stressed. A lot of people were shocked to discover that our GIs killed in action, young, well-nourished, supernourished individuals, had rather substantial degrees of already irreversible atherosclerosis. Diet was blamed, but now a lot of people are recognizing the importance of stress. You are in combat, running the risk of being killed in action; the stress catecholamines are involved. We don't know the rate at which you can develop atherosclerosis, but perhaps prolonged stress has a lot to do with it.

It is remarkable how well Bernie's stress experiments with the dog fit into all this. It's a serious question whether you can re-make your personality, but you can revise your lifestyle. Planning can do a lot to control stress for Type A's. You can organize your life so that you don't make yourself so vulnerable to stress. People with too many irons in the fire let their Type A personalities take control of them. Behavior modification! People didn't really listen to what B. F. Skinner taught us about the science of behavior. It was converted into Freudian encounter stuff. You were supposed to get with a group of people and tell them what you really thought and that sort of thing. It was counterproductive. Stress-ful. Some people even committed suicide or did other terrible things. Then we got through that, and developed some sort of simplistic plan for an orderly life. Now it's education, adult educa-tion: lectures, workshops, homework, implementation. Who is the great therapist and long-term help? Me! It's each one of us! We are our own best physicians, benefiting from education by professional people in the field. Atherosclerosis will be around unless we, as individuals, definitely take responsibility. You can't get vaccinated against it; you can't buy a treatment. You've got to do it yourself! We might well have it in our power to put athero-sclerosis into oblivion by three generations of behavior modifica-tion.

The four professional men then began speculating about medical contributions in the future. Dexter dreamed of a whole host of new drugs. There were already new ones that reduced the afterload (resistance against which the heart works) and were ben-eficial in aiding patients in refractory stages of heart failure. Lown was excited about work being done by neurophysiologists, neuroendrocrinologists, and nutritionists on modifying brain chemistry that might bring solutions at the cellular level. Harken, ever a pragmatist as well as a theorist, spoke of stapling that was replacing stitching in surgery, and better still of tissue glues to replace the traditional one stitch at a time, as well as other refinements and advances in surgery.

"The holdup," said Dexter, "is partly grant money for research. Basic science is, after all, basic. It must have more extensive support."

"Well," said Blackburn, "there are a thousand and one projects, all of which make sense, to fill those little gaps of knowledge by methodology. Some methods now not even in existence. I look at the research that has gone on and is continuing to go on and where it is headed, and I take a rather optimistic view. There will be an understanding, for instance, of the pathogenesis of atherosclerosis and knowledge of how to control it; if there could be ways of getting high HDL levels for everybody, creating a disposal system for cholesterol, you could probably eliminate this plague."

"Meantime," said Dexter, as the others took their leave, "thank God for surgery!"

When the two old friends, Dexter and Harken, who had worked together so many years, were alone, Dexter said, "Dwight, you may not approve of what I say now, but it would appear to me that in about five or ten years if any of us have anything wrong with our hearts, we will just go to the surgeon and get a new heart. You would think U.S. industry would be able to make a plastic material that would not damage or clot blood, effective valves and lasting implantable power sources. They've come close, haven't they?"

"The main problem," said Harken, "is the energy source for an artificial heart. Nuclear sources are currently too hot to implant without shielding that is excessively heavy."

Dexter said, "I recall that you could put enough atomic energy on the head of a pin to drive the *Queen Mary* across the Atlantic. I don't see the problem. Atomic energy pacemakers are in use now."

"The difference is that a pacemaker requires only a billionth of the energy needed to run a heart," said Harken, "and even the nuclear pacemakers are so heavy people don't like them. If you could get nuclear power to run a heart, you probably couldn't get the patient to carry it. Probably the physicists can and will solve the shielding/weight problem, but they must spend more time on nuclear power and waste, which is equally important.

Perhaps when basic science eradicates the waste-disposal problem, a usable power source for artificial hearts will follow."

The artificial heart might be a commonplace in the future, but what had happened in their lifetimes, Drs. Harken and Dexter agreed, was far more important. The human heart, which could never be surpassed in the performance of its function, had proved to be reparable and revivable. It *could* be restored by medical men. It *could* be protected by intelligent people, to serve them well throughout their lives. It *could* be mended! That seemed to them worth all they and their professional colleagues had done to make this so.

Dwight Harken, born in 1910 in Osceola, Iowa, Harvard College class of 1931, retired as an operating surgeon, mused after the others were gone. Even in a contemplative late-night mood, he sat within an almost tangible field of energy. Two heart attacks and white hair had not visibly aged him, although he complained of reduced vigor. Resignation was no part of his nature and he damned the word "impossible." Because of failing eyesight, he had relinquished surgical activity with sufficient grace, but refused to temper his heavy schedule otherwise.

He spoke of heart surgery as a continuum, a stream of activity with neither segments nor interruptions. Now the course of that stream would be altered as responsibility was transferred from the pioneers to the next generation, the torch handed on. "The transfer of the torch," he remarked, "is noted largely by those giving it up!"

By evolution, not revolution, many new things would happen. The now and future leaders must define what they want to know and build an orderly set of steps to learn it. Solid building blocks were things known, facilities extant. When these are marshalled, it is often remarkable how close the future becomes. No one can ever say, "Everything is known; there are no fields for me to conquer."

He recalled his class reports as a Harvard College alumnus. For his twentieth reunion, in 1951, he had written: "Many types of operations combine to promise that heart surgery, the youngest of the surgical specialties, will become, if good fortune stays with us another five years, a full-scale department of surgery." Five years later, for his twenty-fifth reunion, he reported: "Heart surgery *is* a full-fledged field of surgery. All valves, walls, and partitions have been attacked by blind [closed] techniques. We are struggling to reduce the need for heart function during surgery by lowering body temperatures [hypothermia] and with mechanical substitutes for the heart and lungs, so that we can open the heart and operate under direct vision. Heart surgery, the reality, is more fantastic than were the dreams."

He then went on, in that 1956 report, to project what he expected to be able to write for his fiftieth reunion in 1981: "I reflect [he fantasized] on my crude operations in 1954 and 1955 under lowered body temperature and how machines afforded direct vision. Now, as a spectator, I record how Alden Harken [his son, in 1956 aged sixteen] went on to medical school and later replaced a diseased heart with a good one, or how he substituted a simple, dependable little self-activating plastic machine that became infiltrated with and incorporated into the recipient's tissues. Perhaps [his prophecy ended], Alden didn't go to medical school and do all this. Never mind, someone else will."

Alden Harken did go to medical school and was doing his own remarkable heart surgery in 1979 as a professor of surgery at the University of Pennsylvania. Part of his father's prophecy had already come true.

As if for his son as well as all the younger men in his profession, Harken warned that change is a witches' brew of good and bad from which progress must be distilled; that forces had altered the course and speed of heart surgery's continuum. They must now contend with all the facets of protectionism, laws to cover the fear men had of what was imperfectly understood, the temptation to say no to innovation. They had to be concerned with the overwhelming amount there was to be known, with time too short for learning it all and heads too small to contain it. That would force them, he thought, to question more and more the future of the Gutenberg system of learning from the printed page, and to look to electronic storage and retrieval. The whole matter of teaching, learning, and communication was a field for fresh research.

The younger surgeons could rejoice in basic science and the

new ways of looking at diseased heart muscle and valves: as vulnerable at the intracellular level, the energy source, and the enzyme and electrolyte levels. These methods would lend precision to their surgical timing and action and to therapy. Their work now would of necessity be in groups. They would lean heavily on their colleagues, which would multiply the exhilaration of success and dilute the pain of failure. They were lighting the way to prevention.

Prevention was the ultimate goal of the professional; prevention, which would eliminate the need for his profession.

Harken ended his musing that night with the words of Sir Isaac Newton. It was a sentence he had often quoted in lectures and discussions with his contemporaries to honor the great historical figures of the past, from Galen the Greek, to William Harvey, to the immediate predecessors of his own generation, Souttar, Churchill, Cutler, Tudor Edwards, and so many others. "Remember," he said, "we see so far because we stand on the shoulders of giants!"

Appendix

The Heart and How It Works

The heart weighs well under a pound and is only a little larger than the fist, but it is a powerful, long-working, hard-working organ. Its job is to pump blood to the lungs and to all the body tissues.

The heart is a hollow organ. Its tough, muscular wall (myocardium) is surrounded by a fiberlike bag (pericardium) and is lined by a thin, strong membrane (endocardium). A wall (septum) divides the heart cavity down the middle into a "right heart" and a "left heart." Each side of the heart is divided again into an upper chamber (called an atrium or auricle) and a lower chamber (ventricle). Valves regulate the flow of blood through the heart and to the pulmonary artery and the aorta.

The heart is really a double pump. One pump (the right heart) receives blood that has just come from the body after delivering nutrients and oxygen to the body tissues. It pumps this dark, bluish red blood to the lungs where the blood gets rid of a waste gas (carbon dioxide) and picks up a fresh supply of oxygen, which turns it a bright red again. The second pump (the left heart) receives this "reconditioned" blood from the lungs and pumps it out through the great trunk-artery (aorta) to be distributed by smaller arteries to all parts of the body.

Before the heart muscle will contract, it must receive an electrical impulse. Normally, this impulse comes from the natural pacemaker, a center of specialized muscle tissue. As long as these impulses are sent regularly, the heart pumps at a steady pace. But if something interferes with the electrical impulses, the natural pacemaker cannot do its job. The heart then pumps too quickly or too slowly or irregularly. This means not enough blood—carrying oxygen and nourishment—gets to the body cells.

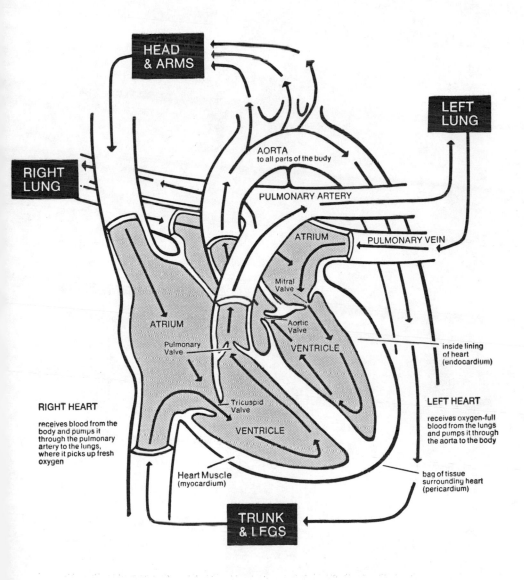

HEAD & ARMS

RIGHT LUNG

LEFT LUNG

AORTA
to all parts of the body

PULMONARY ARTERY

ATRIUM

PULMONARY VEIN

ATRIUM

Mitral Valve

Aortic Valve

Pulmonary Valve

VENTRICLE

inside lining of heart (endocardium)

RIGHT HEART

receives blood from the body and pumps it through the pulmonary artery to the lungs, where it picks up fresh oxygen

Tricuspid Valve

VENTRICLE

LEFT HEART

receives oxygen-full blood from the lungs and pumps it through the aorta to the body

Heart Muscle (myocardium)

bag of tissue surrounding heart (pericardium)

TRUNK & LEGS

Glossary

adhesion–A band or fiber. Abnormal bands that bind the organs to one another.

analgesic–Pain-relieving medication.

anastomosis–The joining together of two or more hollow organs.

anemia–Insufficiency of red blood cells, either in quality or quantity.

anesthesia–Loss of sensation, usually produced in order to permit painless surgical operation.

aneurysm–An abnormal condition characterized by the dilation of the wall of an artery.

angina pectoris–Pain in the chest, sometimes radiating to the left arm, generally due to obstructive disease of the coronary arteries, which reduces the oxygen supplied to the heart muscle.

angiocardiography–X-ray visualization of the chambers of the heart and the large blood vessels entering or leaving the heart.

angiography–X-ray of blood vessels after injection of a radiopaque substance to show their outlines.

anomaly–A deviation from the normal, such as a congenital deformity.

anoxia–Inadequate oxygen supply, with consequent disturbances in body functions.

anticoagulant–A substance that prevents blood from clotting.

anticubical–In front of elbow.

aorta–The large artery originating from the left ventricle of the heart. Its branches carry blood to all parts of the body.

apex–The summit of an organ, as the apex of the lung.

arrhythmia–Lack of rhythm, applied especially to irregularities of heart-beat.

arteriosclerosis–Hardening of the arteries.

artery–A vessel carrying oxygenated blood from the heart.

atherosclerosis–Hardening of the inner lining (intima) of arteries.

auricle–The upper chamber of the heart, which receives blood from the veins. The atrium.

bacterial endocarditis–An infection of the valves of the heart, usually attacking valves already damaged by rheumatic fever or congenital disease.

bicuspid–Two cusps; the bicuspid valve is of the heart.

biopsy–The surgical removal of tissue in order to determine the exact diagnosis.

cannulation–To put a catheter or tube into a vein or artery.

carcinoma–Cancer derived from lining cells of organs.

cardiopulmonary bypass–Bypassing the heart and lungs.

cardiotomy–Opening of the heart.

cardiovascular–Relating to the heart and blood vessels.

cardioverter–Machine for converting irregular heart rhythms into regular rhythms.

carditis–Inflammation of the heart.

catheterization–As applied to the heart, refers to the passage of a catheter (tube) via an artery or vein into the great vessels and chambers of the heart to measure pressures, flow, and to inject radiopaque substances for angiographic X-ray study.

cholesterol–A chemical compound of animal oils and fats.

chordae tendineae–Strands of tissue attached to the papillary muscles of the ventricles of the heart and extending to the valves, which are located in between the atria and the ventricles.

cineangiography–The taking of moving pictures to show the passage of an opaque dye through blood vessels.

coarctation of the aorta–A narrowing of the passageway of the aorta, due to contriction of the walls of the vessel.

collagen–Connective tissue, such as that in the walls of the arteries.

commissure–The tissues that bind together opposite but corresponding parts.

commissurotomy–An operation upon the heart in which a deformed heart valve is cut so as to permit a more normal flow of blood.

communis–In common with or participating in.

coronary arteries–Arteries supplying the heart muscle.

coronary occlusion–Closure (thrombosis) of a coronary artery.

cyanotic Bluish color due to insufficient oxygen in the bloodstream.

diastole–The period between beats when the heart fills with blood, the opposite of systole.

digitalis–A drug helpful in treating heart ailments, particularly those in which the heart muscle is weak.

dyspnea–Shortness of breath.

echocardiography–An ultrasound reflection technique, such as radar, to image organ and fluid structure throughout the body. Especially useful in visualizing tissue density and motion patterns of the heart walls and valves.

edema–Excessive accumulation of fluid in the tissues, thus causing swelling, seen in certain cases of poor heart function.

electrocardiogram–The recording of the electrical impulses of the heart.

electrolytes–Substances that can, when in solution, convey an electrical impulse.

embolism–The obstruction of an artery by an embolus, usually a piece of clotted blood that breaks away from one part of the circulatory system and travels to another.

empyema–The presence of pus in a cavity, as in the chest (pleural) cavity.

endocardium–The membrane lining of the chambers of the heart.

epithelium–The tissue cells composing the skin surface; also the cells lining all the passages of the hollow organs of the respiratory, digestive, and urinary systems.

esophagogastrectomy–A surgical operation in which a new communication is fashioned between the esophagus (food pipe) and the stomach.

exsanguinate–The loss of huge quantities of blood.

extrasystole–An extra heartbeat occurring before its normal time (commonly referred to as a "skipped beat").

femoral artery–The main artery supplying the thigh and leg.

fibrillation–An irregular heart action due to abnormal spread of impulses from one portion of the heart to another.

fluoroscopy–X-raying a part of the body and recording the rays on a fluorescent screen, in order to view various organs in motion.

gastrointestinal–Relating to the stomach and intestines.

hemodynamics–The study of blood flow, volume, and pressure.

His, bundle of–Conduction system in the heart.

homeostasis–Stability of all body functions at normal levels.

homograft–A graft of tissue taken from the body of another person.
hypertension–High blood pressure.
hypertrophy–Increase in the size of an organ.
hypothermia–A lower than normal body temperature.
infarct, infarction–An area of tissue deprived of its blood supply because of a clot within the artery; the infarcted area usually undergoes degeneration and is replaced by scar tissue.
interatrial septal defect–Hole or defect in the partition of the atria.
intercostal–Between the ribs.
interventricular–Between the two ventricles of the heart.
ischemia–Lack of blood supply to an organ or organ part due to a spasm or shutting down of the artery that supplies it.
ligation–Tying off of blood vessels or other structures during the performance of an operation.
lobectomy–An operation for the removal of a diseased lobe (one portion) of a lung.
lumen–The passageway inside a hollow organ or structure, such as the lumen of an artery.
mammary artery–One of two paired arteries on either side of the breastbone (sternum).
mediastinum–The space beneath the breastbone containing the heart, aorta, vena cava, trachea, esophagus, and other vessels and nerves.
metabolism–The process by which foods are transformed into basic elements that can be utilized by the body for energy or growth.
midaxillary–Middle of the armpit.
mitral stenosis–Constriction or narrowing of the mitral valve of the heart.
myocardial infarction–Damage of heart muscle secondary to the loss of its blood supply, as in coronary thrombosis.
myocardium–Heart muscle.
norepinephrine–Hormone from body of adrenal gland that combats low blood pressure.
palpation–The act of feeling some organ or part of the body in order to make a diagnosis.
palpitation–Feeling one's own heartbeat, usually associated with excessively forceful "pounding" heart action.
patent ductus arteriosus–Open connection between the pulmonary artery and aorta (to bypass lungs while fetus is in the womb).
perfuse–To flood or inject fluid into or through an organ or structure of the body in order to permeate it.
pericardium–The sheath of tissue encasing the heart.

phenobarbital–One of the barbiturates, useful in calming the nerves and inducing sleep.

pleura–The membrane lining the chest cavity and covering the lungs.

pneumonectomy–Removal of a lung, surgically.

pneumothorax–Air in the pleural (chest) cavity surrounding the lung.

prednisone–A cortisone preparation.

premature ventricular contraction–Early abnormal contraction of the heart.

prosthesis–An artificial part.

pulmonic stenosis–Obstruction of the pulmonary valve or artery.

regurgitation–A backward flow.

resection–Surgical removal or excision.

resuscitation–The revival of a patient who appears to be dead, or almost dead.

saphenous vein–A vein in the leg (expendable for use in pulmonary bypass).

sclerosis–Hardening of tissues, with deposit of fibrous tissues to replace the original structure, as sclerosis of the walls of the arteries.

septal defect–An abnormal opening between a right and left chamber of the heart; atrial defects occur between the two auricles, ventricular ones between the two ventricles.

septum–A partition between two structures or cavities.

shunt–A bypass, an alternate route. A shunt operation is one in which blood is detoured so that it alters its course; it is performed to bypass clotted (thrombosed) vessels.

stenosis–Constriction or narrowing of a passageway or opening.

sternum–The breastbone in the front of the chest.

subclavian–Beneath the clavicle (collarbone).

subcutaneous–Underneath the skin.

suture–To stitch surgically.

syncope–Fainting.

systole–The phase of the heartbeat during which the heart contracts and expels the contained blood.

tachycardia–Rapid heartbeat (more than 100 beats per minute).

tamponade–Stopping a discharge or flow of blood.

therapeutic–Healing.

thoracic–Referring to the chest.

thoracoplasty–An operation upon the chest wall in which several ribs are removed.

thoracotomy–A surgical incision into the chest cavity, performed either for diagnostic purposes or to carry out treatment.

thrill–A vibration felt by the physician's examining hand when placed upon a heart in which there is a murmur, or over a blood vessel containing an aneurysm.

thrombosis–Formation of a blood clot.

trachea–The windpipe.

tricuspid–Having three cusps, as the tricuspid valve of the heart.

tryptophan–An essential amino acid, needed for growth in infants and protein metabolism in adults.

valvuloplasty–An operation to relieve constriction and to reconstruct a valve, as for mitral stenosis.

valvulotome–Instrument for cutting valves.

valvulotomy–Opening of a valve, as contrasted with valvuloplasty (repair) and valvulectomy (removal).

vascular system–Blood vessel system.

vena cava inferior–The large vein in the abdomen that transports blood back to the heart from structures and organs located below the diaphragm.

vena cava superior–The large vein above the heart that transports blood from the head, neck, and upper body and extremities.

xenografts–Grafts between two animals of different species, as rat to mouse or baboon to man.

Acknowledgments

The medical people who permitted me to tape interviews with them were, for the most part, still active professionally. Their schedules were strenuous. Nevertheless, in response to Dr. Harken's requests and mine, they found time for me and talked freely. In no instance was I refused an interview, although when I was in Palo Alto, California, Dr. Norman Shumway was unable to keep his appointment with me. However, his associate, Dr. Donald Harrison, came to his office as the sun rose so that I could interview him before his first appointment in a very busy day.

With all my heart, I thank those interviewed:

In Boston, Massachusetts: Drs. Laurence B. Ellis; Lewis Dexter; Leroy D. Vandam; Francis D. Moore; Paul Zoll; George Cahill; Leona Norman (Zarsky); J. Hartwell Harrison; David Rutstein; Bernard Lown; George Blackburn; Jorge Albertal from Buenos Aires, Argentina; Rowan Nicks from Sydney, Australia; Kenji Honda from Fukushima, Japan; Mariano Alimurung from Manila, Philippines; Peter Alivizetos from Athens, Greece.

In New York City: Drs. Lawrence E. Hinkle; Roy H. Clauss; Henry I. Russek; Robert S. Litwak.

In Detroit, Michigan: Drs. Conrad Lam; E. Grey Diamond from Kansas City, Missouri; Arthur Beall from Houston, Texas; Lord Russell C. Brock from London, England; Charles P. Bailey from Philadelphia and New York; Charles DuBost from Paris, France; Helen Taussig from Baltimore, Maryland.

In Minneapolis, Minnesota: Drs. Owen Wangensteen; C. Walton Lillehei; Richard L. Varco.

In Palo Alto, California: Dr. Donald C. Harrison.

In Toronto, Canada: Dr. Marjorie Davis.

The following doctors sent me long, helpful letters: Drs. Ernesto Castro Farinas, Madrid, Spain; Norman R. Barrett, London, England; D'Arcy Sutherland, Adelaide, Australia; Poul Ottosen, Aarhus, Denmark; Erich Wagner, Giessen, Germany; June Howqua, Melbourne, Australia; Juro Wada, Sapporo, Japan.

Also for interviews I am indebted to: Nurse Edna Duncan, Boston, Massachusetts; and Nurse Edith Heideman, Detroit, Michigan.

For permission to tape a conference with Dr. Harken at Boston University in Boston, Massachusetts, I thank Drs. C. David Jenkins, Babette A. Stanton, Michael Klein, Stephen J. Zyzanski, and thank them for the research material with which they provided me.

William D. Nelligan, Executive Director of the American College of Cardiology, granted me an interview in Boston.

Several patients gave me records and wrote or talked to me about Dr. Harken, among them Leland E. Evans, Holden, Massachusetts. I thank most particularly Melvin Meyers, Cincinnati, Ohio, the husband of patient Georgette Meyers, and Russell Shetterly, Denver, Colorado, the husband of patient Mildred Shetterly, for making records and correspondence on their wives' cases available to me.

In the field of public relations, every effort to contribute to this book was made by Bea Murray (Chapman), Peakes Island, Maine; Edward Bernays, Cambridge, Massachusetts; T. Van Pelt, the University of Virginia Hospital; and Spiro Andreopoulous, the Stanford University Medical Center.

And special thanks to the loving members of Dwight Harken's family who opened their memory books: Anne Hood Harken; Dr. Alden Hood Harken and his wife, Dr. Laurel Harken; Ridgway M. Hall, Jr., and his wife, Anne Louise Harken Hall.

In addition to the interviews and letters, the following sources supplied important information. In many instances material was generously provided for my use by authors, editors, and public relations departments.

"The Growth of Cardiac Surgery: Historical Notes" by Robert S. Litwak, M.D., in the Cardiovascular Clinics Series: Cardiac Surgery 1,

Cardiovascular Clinics, Vol. 3, No. 2; *The History of Thoracic Surgery* by Richard H. Meade, M.D. (Springfield, Ill.: Charles C. Thomas, 1961); and *The Risk Takers* by Hugh McLeave (London: Frederick Muller Ltd., 1962) provided essential general and historical information on developments in thoracic surgery. *Pages in the History of Chest Surgery* by Rudolf Nissen, M.D., and Roger H. L. Wilson, M.B., B.Chir. (Springfield, Ill.: Charles C. Thomas, 1960) contained reprints of historical documents as well.

Patients by Jurgen Thorwald (New York: Harcourt Brace, 1972) contained fascinating portraits of various patients.

Report on the Second Henry Ford Hospital International Symposium on Cardiac Surgery, edited by Julio C. Davila, M.D. (New York: Appleton Century Crofts, 1971), provided information on that event.

On the history and development of anesthesia, *Introduction to Anesthesia: The Principles of Safe Practice,* 4th ed., by Robert D. Dripps, M.D., James E. Eckendoff, M.D., and Leroy D. Vandam, M.D. (Philadelphia: W. B. Saunders Co., 1972), and the articles "Anesthesia" by Leroy D. Vandam, M.D. (*Annual Review of Pharmacology,* Vol. 6, 1966) and "The Origins of Professionalism in Anesthesia" by Leroy D. Vandam (*Anesthesiology,* Vol. 38, No. 3), proved valuable. "Medical Progress, Hypothermia" by Leroy D. Vandam and Thomas K. Burknap (*New England Journal of Medicine,* September 10 and 17, 1959) provided information on that particular development.

The history of the medical use of electricity is covered in the November–December 1975 issue of *Medical Instrumentation,* Vol. 9, No. 6. Especially useful were "Historical Notes on Electroresuscitation" by David Charles Schecter and "A Survey of the History of Electrical Stimulation for Pain to 1900" by Dennis Stillings.

For material on Drs. Michael DeBakey and Denton Cooley, *Hearts: Of Surgeons & Transplants, Miracles & Disasters Along the Cardiac Frontier* by Thomas Thompson (New York: Saturday Review Press, 1971) was invaluable. Dr. Christiaan Barnard told his own story through the first transplant in his book *One Life* (by Christiaan Barnard with Curtis Bill Pepper, New York: Macmillan, 1969).

Heart Surgery Founders Group

Alley, Ralph D., M.D.
Albany, New York
1. Organization man, contributing to communications within the specialty of thoracic and cardiovascular surgery.
2. First successful resection traumatic aortic arch aneurysm using external shunts (1953).
3. Exemplary teacher and clinician who has built strong national and international bridges of professional and social exchange.

Austen, W. Gerald, M.D.
Boston, Massachusetts
1. Collaborator with Kantrowitz and Buckley in intra-aortic balloon circulatory assistance.
2. First repair of patient in shock from acute ruptured papillary muscle from myocardial infarction (1963). This was a forerunner of emergency coronary surgery in early infarction or unstable angina.
3. With Buckley, Daggett, Mundth, Laver and MGH Group in combining metabolic, pharmacologic, mechanical, and technical support for critically ill heart surgery patients.
4. Especially effective in teaching students and developing cardiac surgeons.
5. Past president American Heart Association (1977–78)

Bahnson, Henry T., M.D.
Pittsburgh, Pennsylvania
1. Innovator of operations for aortic aneurysms.
2. Collaborator under Blalock in surgery of congenital and acquired heart disease.
3. Teacher and organizer.
4. Introduced monocusp aortic valve to palliate aortic heart disease.

Bailey, Charles P., M.D.
New York, New York
1. Co-founder of modern cardiac surgery.
2. Developed "commissurotomy" for mitral stenosis.
3. Creator of many closed operations for congenital and acquired cardiac disease.
4. Collaborated with Bolton, Likoff, Glover, Nichols, Neptune, Morse, O'Neil, and many other early cardiac physicians and surgeons.
5. Clarified and applied many physiologic principles for clinical use collaborating with Zimmerman, Hirose, and others.
6. Edited massive first "position paper," a textbook on cardiac surgery. The state of the art at that time.
7. Innovator in valve reconstruction and coronary artery surgery.
8. Helped demonstrate heart surgery as a practical therapy to an unwilling world, while evoking both frivolous and responsible controversy over patient, personal, and public relations.

Barnard, Christiaan N., M.D.
Cape Town, South Africa
1. Performed first heart transplant using Shumway Technique (1967), and has continued these efforts.
2. Conducted other assisted circulation procedures by tandem homografted hearts.
3. Worked with new heart valves.

Barratt-Boyes, Sir Brian G., F.R.C.S., K.B.E., Chm.
Auckland, New Zealand
1. Brilliant developer and standardizer of aortic valve homograft technique.
2. Promulgator/developer of deep hypothermia technique.
3. Innovator of surgical connection of congenital defects.

Beall, Arthur C., Jr., M.D.
Houston, Texas
1. First successful emergency pulmonary embolectomy using total cardiopulmonary bypass.
2. First successful emergency operation for traumatic aortic valve insufficiency.
3. Prosthetic valve developer.
4. Fostered medical, engineering, industrial, and government communication via The Association for the Advancement of Medical Instrumentation of which he is a past president.
5. Past president of the American College of Chest Physicians.
6. Advisor to the government and private sectors regarding device safety legislation.

Beck, Claude S., M.D.
Cleveland, Ohio
1. Proponent of collateralization of coronary circulation by vascular adhesions similar in principle to procedures of O'Shaughnessy, Lezius, and Harken.
2. Reversed coronary venous flow by arterial shunt.
3. Pioneer in open-chest cardiac resuscitation.
4. Co-worker in Cutler and Levine's mitral valvulectomy (1923).
5. Articulated Beck's Triad (constrictive pericarditis and cardiac tamponade).

Berkovits, Barouh, F.A.C.C.
Wellesley, Massachusetts
1. Developer of direct-current defibrillator, tested by Lefemine.
2. Engineered cardioverter, tested and used by Lown.
3. Engineer-designer of demand pacemaker with Zaroff and Harken.
4. Designer of atrioventricular sequential pacemaker.

Bigelow, W. G., M.D.
Toronto, Canada
1. Studied and applied clinically extensive observations of microcirculation, deriving source material from anatomist Knisely. Presented material (1949) and continued in collaboration with Drs. Harrison and Heimbecker.
2. Developer of biologic valves.
3. Pioneer investigator in hypothermia hibernation.

316 | Heart Surgery Founders Group

4. Collaborated with Callaghan and Hopps in early pacemaker work with two-point focal electrode to excite SA node. The selfless sharing of information with Zoll is a tribute to them and a model to the scientific world.
5. Clinician, teacher, investigator, and organizer by whose conduct a laudable standard is established.

Billroth, Professor Christian Albert Theodor
Zurich and Vienna

Great abdominal and general surgeon, but also classical obstructionist and nihilist who is best characterized by his own words: "Any surgeon who would attempt an operation on the heart should lose the respect of his colleagues." (Circa 1875)

Björk, Viking O., M.D.
Stockholm, Sweden
1. Developed direct percutaneous left-heart catheterization and angiography.
2. Investigator of biomaterials and artificial intima.
3. Developer of a disc-oxygenator (1947) with Crafoord and engineer Anderson.
4. Pioneer in patient monitoring, intensive care, and innovator of involved mechanical devices.
5. Inventor of prosthetic heart valves.

Blalock, Alfred, M.D.
Baltimore, Maryland
1. Physiologist/surgeon, innovator, and teacher.
2. With Burwell, studied and corrected constrictive pericarditis.
3. Studied the thymus and its effect on circulation, including myasthenia gravis and shock, specifically and in general.
4. Developer, with medical pediatric cardiologist Taussig, of subclavian-to-pulmonary artery shunt for congenital cyanotic heart disease.
5. Conducted fundamental studies on the nature and treatment of shock.
6. As teachers and investigators many have been credited in this report; however, to name a few of those surgeons whose lives he influenced leaves him without peer: Bahnson, Cooley, Gott, Hanlon, Longmire, Maloney, McGoon, Morrow, Muller, Sabiston, Scott, Spencer.

Brewer, Lyman, M.D.
Los Angeles, California
1. Clinician, teacher, and leader in national and international scientific organizations.
2. His clinical work has simplified and standardized techniques to extend the service of both thoracic and cardiac surgery.
3. World War II pioneer in "Wet Lung in War Casualties," the treatment of which by intermittent positive pressure oxygen improved the care of severely compromised cardiopulmonary function (1944).
4. Introduced elective cardiac arrest to control hemorrhage of heart wounds (1965).
5. Explored the nature of spinal cord injuries following correction of coarctation of the aorta. This had clinical and medico-legal significance.
6. Chairman of National Thoracic Surgery Manpower Study to improve thoracic surgery (1970–1974).

Brock, Lord Russell
London, England
1. Closed mitral valvulotomy, closed pulmonary valvulotomy, and closed pulmonic infundibular resection (1948).
2. Percutaneous left ventricular puncture to assess aortic obstruction.
3. Description of functional obstruction of left ventricular outflow tract (1955).

Brunton, Sir Thomas Lauder
London, England
Experimental pharmacologist and surgeon who in 1902 drew attention again to English cardiologist Samway's suggestion that notching of the stenotic mitral valve should constitute a palliative compromise through insufficiency. He suggested extensive experimental preparation, which he had too little time to conduct himself . . . but suggested that others carry on the project. For not doing the work himself and "suggesting that others carry on with a dangerous operation," he was ruthlessly criticized for both his concept and principles.

Carpentier, Alain J.
Paris, France
1. Assessed behavior of biologic valves with various methods of preparation and use.
2. Developed and evaluated techniques of tricuspid valve repair.

Carrel, Alexis, M.D.
Lyon, France
1. Devised practical techniques for arterial anastomoses (1905).
2. Visualized artificial hearts and created (with Lindbergh) perfusion pumps.
3. Conceived of open-heart surgery by caval occlusion.
4. Planned (experimentally) heart valve surgery and correction of localized coronary artery disease (1910).
5. Described methods for future resections of aortic aneurysms.
6. Predicted and experimentally practiced organ transplantation and was aware of problems of "biologic relationship between tissues."
7. First American Nobel Laureate in Medicine and Physiology (1912).

Castaneda, Aldo R., M.D.
Boston, Massachusetts
1. Extensive laboratory work with the Minneapolis group on the effect of cardiopulmonary bypass on formed blood elements and the use of cardiopulmonary bypass for combined heart-lung autotransplantation in primates, leading to long-term survival of animals after heart-lung transplantation.
2. Applied his laboratory work to the correction of complicated general lesions in the first few months of life, particularly using deep hypothermia and circulatory arrest.

Cooley, Denton A., M.D.
Houston, Texas
1. One of heart surgery's most brilliant technical surgeons.
2. Aggressive developer of improved techniques for relieving congenital and acquired heart disease.
3. Proponent of ischemic arrest for open-heart surgery.
4. Extended the use/availability of the bubble oxygenator in the disposable plastic form as developed by Gott.

Crafoord, Clarence, M.D.
Stockholm, Sweden
1. Developer of ventilators and respirator equipment techniques predicated on early work of Sauerbruch, Giertz, and others.
2. Student of thromboembolic diseases.
3. Colleague and friend of Erik Jorps, who determined chemical formula of heparin and introduced it in its pure form. With the

physiologist Howell, he was the first to point out anticoagulant effect of substance he called "heparing."
4. Co-developer with Björk, Senning, and engineer Anderson of heart/lung machines.
5. Second successful open-heart operation, removal of myxoma of left auricle.
6. Pioneer thoracic surgeon—coarctation of aorta, lobectomy, pneumonectomy, et cetera.

Cutler, Elliott Carr, M.D.
Boston, Massachusetts
1. Initiated valvulotomy for mitral stenosis with Samuel A. Levine as collaborating cardiologist. This was a brave but disappointing adventure.
2. Perhaps one of the last surgeons to believe that the great surgeons should be competent in all areas (a standard that he very nearly attained).
3. Gave Harken his valve instruments. Made Harken Consultant in Thoracic Surgery, ETO, World War II, and stimulated renaissance in modern heart surgery by supporting Harken's removal of shell fragments from the heart.

Davila, Julio C., M.D.
Warsaw, Wisconsin
1. Performed first operation which corrected mitral regurgitation by annular constriction, proven by hemodynamics and cinematography.
2. Built first mechanical pulse-duplicator in America for study of cardiac valve mechanics.
3. Various original observations on valvular function and on role of left ventricle in valvular disease.
4. Elucidated mechanisms of thrombosis in valvular prosthesis in relation to healing and to altered-flow patterns.
5. Confirmed validity of radiographic methods for measurement of left ventricular volume by comparison with an original method. Edited a symposium on measurement of LV volume which helped to open up the area of clinical measurement of left ventricle performance.
6. Experimented in early refinements of cardiopulmonary bypass (with cooling and with plasma dilution), in development of thermodilution for measurement of cardiac output in clinical setting, in the study of biomaterials, and in applying various instrumental methods for physi-

ologic measurement in valvular disease (i.e., first to measure, directly, transmitral valve flow).
7. Organized Second Henry Ford Hospital International Symposium on Cardiac Surgery (1975) and edited its proceedings.

Day, Hughes, M.D.
Kansas City, Kansas
Founder and developer of Coronary Care Units.

DeBakey, Michael E., M.D.
Houston, Texas
1. Developer of roller pump used on John Gibbon's machine and other heart/lung machines.
2. Developer of Dacron artificial arteries and biomaterials for cardiac implantation.
3. Developer of effective surgical methods for treating of a wide spectrum of aneurysms of the aorta and major arteries (1952 and later).
4. First successful carotid endarterectomy (1953).
5. Early observer of arterial disease as localized and segmental in a substantial number of instances, thus permitting rational treatment, including bypass.
6. Developer of left ventricular bypass for circulatory assistance.
7. First aortocoronary saphenous vein bypass with long-term survival performed on his service by Edward Garrett in 1964.
8. Pioneer developer of mechanical hearts.
9. Champion of cardiovascular causes, *pro bono publico*.

Dennis, Clarence, M.D.
Setauket, New York
1. First to use pump-oxygenator to carry out circulation during open-heart operations (two patients, April 1951—neither survived).
2. Studied reduction of oxygen utilization by left-heart bypass (1963).
3. First to use mechanical pump support for chronic heart failure (1955) and myocardial infarction with shock (1958).
4. Experimented with caged-ball heart valves (1957).
5. External counterpulsation with Senning and Wesolowski (1963).
6. Physiologic and metabolic studies assessing cerebral ischemia, embolism, and bleeding.

Dewall, Richard A., M.D.
Dayton, Ohio
Pioneer developer of first clinically useful bubble oxygenator, subsequently modified to the Bentley disposable oxygenator.

Dodrill, F. Dewey, M.D.
Detroit, Michigan
1. Performed first open-heart surgery using right and left bypass successfully with the patient's lung as the oxygenator. First used left bypass for mitral stenosis.
2. Started experimental work (1949) with mechanical help from General Motors' Research Laboratories.

DuBost, Charles, M.D.
Paris, France
1. First resection and restoration of continuity in aoritic abdominal aneurysm (1951).
2. Innovator of instruments and techniques.
3. Co-developer with A. Carpentier of glutaraldehyde-preserved heterografts for mitral and aortic replacement.
4. Endocardiectomy for fibrous constrictive endocarditis.
5. Developer of isotopic pacemaker.

Edwards, Jesse F., M.D.
St. Paul, Minnesota
Made and continues to make correlations of morbid pathology and physiology to give a new order of understanding of the heart as a surgical goal.

Effler, Donald B., M.D.
Syracuse, New York
1. Crusader for the treatment of ischemic heart disease; pioneer heart surgeon.
2. His own epitaph: "The S.O.B. had enough talent to do a given operation well and was smart enough to reduce it to its simplest form."

Elkin, Daniel C., M.D.
Atlanta, Georgia
Pioneer in repairing wounds of the heart (1941 and later).

Favaloro, René G., M.D.
Buenos Aires, Argentina
1. Developed bilateral internal mammary artery implant as an extension of the Vineberg operation through midline incision (1966). Combined this form of revascularization with aneurysmectomy.
2. Saphenous vein grafts first as interposition and bypass, then aortocoronary saphenous vein bypass (1967).
3. Saphenous vein bypass in acute coronary insufficiency in impending and actual infarction (1968).
4. Leader in the development of aortocoronary artery bypass surgery.

Gerbode, Frank L., M.D.
San Francisco, California
1. Developer with Bramson and Osborn of clinically successful membrane oxygenator.
2. Developer of operations dealing with complicated endocardial cushion defects.
3. Developer with Osborn and IBM of computerized monitoring for critically ill cardiopulmonary patients.
4. Teacher and organizer of national and international mechanisms of communication.
5. Established, with Osborn, a very important private research institute, The Institutes of Medical Science.

Gibbon, John H., Jr., M.D.
Philadelphia, Pennsylvania
1. Developer of IBM heart-lung machine in collaboration with his wife, Mary.
2. First successful open-heart operation using complete cardiopulmonary bypass closing atrial septal defect (1953).

Glenn, William W. L., M.D.
New Haven, Connecticut
1. Developer of techniques for correcting congenital and acquired heart disease, including division of patent ductus arteriosus, mitral stenosis, and diverticulum approach to the chambers of the heart and great vessels.
2. Introduced use of elective electrical ventricular fibrillation.
3. Developer of artificial heart and techniques of right-heart bypass.
4. Developed operation to bypass the right ventricle and carry out pulmonary valvulotomy.

5. Developer of artificial cardiac pacemakers.
6. Author, investigator, clinician, and teacher.
7. Past president American Heart Association.

Glover, Robert P., M.D.
Philadelphia, Pennsylvania
1. Collaborator with C. P. Bailey, in performance of first modern mitral valve operation (commissurotomy). The patient was admitted, and operated on, on his service at Episcopal Hospital in Philadelphia.
2. He had the gift of simplifying scientific and medical information which made him one of the most effective proponents and popularizers of cardiac surgery (mitral commissurotomy), in particular among the general medical public and the laity.
3. He performed the first resection of a postinfarction aneurysm of the left ventricle (1953). His patient died 10 days after from massive G.I. bleeding secondary to stress gastric ulcer. The ventricular incision was clean and healing well.
4. He was among the most active founders of the American College of Cardiology and one of its first presidents.
5. He died at the peak of his career, of cancer of the colon. His studies of the lymphatic spread of this tumor, while a trainee at the Mayo Clinic, are recognized as a classic investigation.

Gorlin, Richard, M.D.
New York, New York
1. Cardiac physiologist and clinician.
2. Developed with his engineer father the formula for calculating effective valve orifices. The constant in the formula derived from the assumption that Harken's digital estimate was correct. This assumption served remarkably, as Harken's estimate was within 0.1 cm^2 in 12 of 13 autopsy specimens. Subsequent prospective estimates in hundreds of patients solidly confirmed the validity of "the Gorlin Formula."
3. Promulgator and innovator of many physiologic measurements and their clinical correlation.

Gott, Vincent L., M.D.
Baltimore, Maryland
1. Developer of thrombus-resistant heparinized surfaces for use in heart valves (1963).

2. Collaborated with Weirich and Lillehei in developing transthoracic myocardial tracing systems (1957).
3. Co-developer with Dewall of bubble oxygenator (1957) and modified it to disposable oxygenator as used by Cooley.
4. Developer of biomaterials as vessels and shunts.

Grondin, Pierre, M.D.
Montreal, Quebec, Canada
1. Aggressive in early heart transplant activity.
2. Prime assessor of prognosis in coronary artery disease by repeat angiograms.
3. Leader in Heart Institute.

Gross, Robert E., M.D.
Boston, Massachusetts
1. Closure of patent ductus arteriosus (1938) as suggested by John Munro (1907).
2. Resection of coarctation of aorta in collaboration with Hufnagel (1945).
3. Developer of numerous techniques dealing with congenital cardiovascular anomalies.
4. Teacher, investigator, author, early leader in developing field of general pediatric surgery, as well as pediatric cardiac surgery.

Harken, Dwight E., M.D.
Cambridge, Massachusetts
1. First consistently successful elective intracardiac surgery (removal of shell fragments from the heart) (1944–1945).
2. Shared in the development of mitral valvuloplasty for mitral stenosis (1948).
3. Developed technique for closed aortic valvuloplasty. Developer of heart valves, heart-lung machines, instruments, and surgical techniques for acquired and congenital heart disease.
4. First successful human implantation of caged-ball valve in normal anatomic site (1960).
5. Developer with Clauss and Birtwell of counterpulsation as a mechanism of reducing pressure work and increasing coronary perfusion.
6. Placed first totally implantable demand pacemaker (1966), developed by Berkovits and tested with Zaroff, Zuckerman, and Matloff.
7. Tested with Lefemine the efficacy and safety of Berkovits' direct current defibrillator in the laboratory, and applied its first clinical use.

8. Collaborator with Beall and others in developing The Association for the Advancement of Medical Instrumentation as a forum for medicine, engineering, industry, and government. Past president and editor of the official organ, *Medical Instrumentation,* of that association.
9. Established the first designated Intensive Care Unit with Nurse Edith Heideman at Peter Bent Brigham Hospital (1951). Nurse Heideman is now a director of nursing at the Henry Ford Hospital in Detroit.
10. Past president American College of Cardiology, chairman Heart House campaign.

Heimbecker, Raymond O., M.D.
London, Canada
1. In vivo microcirculation research in collaboration with Bigelow from 1949, with special emphasis on microaggregation in shock.
2. Homograft valve placement in thoracic aorta with Murray in 1955, and the first clinical homograft mitral valve replacement in March 1962, following laboratory studies of their function and fate from 1959.
3. Early development of extracorporeal circulation with special emphasis on hypothermia and temperature control by heat-exchanger devices.
4. Experimental studies of acute myocardial ischemia and the effects of acute and chronic resection.
5. President of the First World Congress for Microcirculation, Toronto (June 1975).

Hufnagel, Charles A., M.D.
Washington, D.C.
1. Developer of plastics for blood contact implants, blood vessels, heart valves, extracorporeal instrumentation, and artificial kidneys.
2. Ball-valve concept and ball valve used in the descending aorta for aortic insufficiency.
3. Pioneer in low-profile mitral valves.
4. First clinical use of cloth-type prosthesis for vascular replacement. Introduced autogenation of prostheses.
5. Internal and external shunts for general use including the correction of coarctation of the aorta.
6. Pioneered modern homografting and vessel preservation by rapid freezing.
7. Developed ethylene oxide tissue sterilization.

8. Multiple-point fixation for holding arteries or prostheses without necrosis.
9. Local hypothermia for myocardial protection.

Jude, James R., M.D.
Miami, Florida
1. Developer with Knickerbocker and Kouwenhoven of external manual systole. This was of extreme importance of and in itself, but also substantially because it stopped the epidemic of open thoracotomy and manual systole.
2. External manual systole was important particularly in the Intensive Care Unit, and it led to the development of Coronary Care Units by Hughes Day, M.D., who in turn discovered that external manual compression systole itself was not important if arrhythmias were controlled.
3. External manual systole was carried to the scene of Sudden Death by public and rescue squad education. There is an increasing national urgency for cardiopulmonary resuscitation training.

Kantrowitz, Adrian, M.D.
Detroit, Michigan
1. Demonstrated that augmentation of diastolic aortic pressure could increase coronary blood flow (1953).
2. First human implantation of permanent left ventricular assist device (1967).
3. Early developer of cardiac pacemakers.
4. Second human heart transplant after extensive laboratory procedures. He was totally unaware of Barnard's preparation for a similar procedure, leading to its performance three days previously (1967).
5. First successful use of balloon counterpulsation pump in humans (1967).

Kay, Earle B., M.D.
Cleveland, Ohio
1. Developer of numerous closed-heart operations (1946–1956).
2. Developed operation for transposition of great vessels (1955).
3. Developed with Cross the rotating-disc pump oxygenator parallel to and independent of the work of Lillehei (1955) with a bubble oxygenator and Kirklin with a screen oxygenator (1955). Began open-heart surgery with the disc oxygenator (1956).

4. Pioneer in myocardial protection by metabolic and perfusion techniques.
5. Developed heart valves simultaneously and independently of work by Harken and Muller (1960).
6. Developer of tricuspid stent annuloplasty for tricuspid and mitral valve insufficiency subsequently applied by Blondeau, DuBost, and Carpentier.
7. Worked with biologic heart valves and developed with Suzuki an early low-profile mitral valve with essentially physiologic function.
8. One of the most versatile clinical surgeons in myocardial revascularization, cardiopulmonary instrumentation, and valve surgery. Worked with retroperfusion of coronary sinus systems.

Kay, Jerome Harold, M.D.
Los Angeles, California
1. Student of cardiac arrest and its management by "external" massage (i.e., external manual systole) and external defibrillation.
2. Developer of instruments, heart-lung machines, and heart valves.
3. Strong advocate of valve repair rather than replacement, if possible.

Kirklin, John W., M.D.
Birmingham, Alabama
1. Improved Gibbon's screen oxygenator for wide and practical use.
2. Leader in computerization of monitoring and treatment of critically ill patients.
3. Pioneer in biologic valve replacement (particularly homografts).
4. Possessed of a unique ability to simplify and apply new surgical techniques.
5. Master of harvesting, distilling, and presenting in usable form multifaceted experimental and clinical material.

Kolff, Willem J., Ph.D., M.D.
Salt Lake City, Utah
1. Pioneer in development of artificial organs, particularly the kidney during World War II and the heart (1957).
2. Developed with Moulopoulos and Topaz the intra-aortic balloon for counterpulsation (1961).
3. He continues as a pacesetter in the field of artificial organs.

Lam, Conrad R., M.D.
Detroit, Michigan
1. Pioneer of many surgical techniques for correcting congenital and acquired heart disease, including induced cardiac (potassium chloride acetylcholine) arrest, correction of pulmonic stenosis, homograft valves, and vessels.
2. Physiologic studies involving mechanism of death from intracardiac air and its reversibility—with T. Gahagan.
3. Pioneered the use of newly purified heparin (1939).
4. Organizer, teacher, and international surgical ambassador.

Landsteiner, K., M.D.
Vienna, Austria
1. Discovered that "human blood contained isoagglutinins capable of agglutinating other human blood."
2. Divided human blood into types (1900).
3. His work clarified by Moss and Jansky (independently), DeCastle/Sturli, Hektoen, and Ottenberg.
4. Infinite refinement continues to be required by heart surgery.

Lev, Maurice, M.D.
Chicago, Illinois
1. Gave Maude Abbott's morbid pathology of congenital heart disease a renaissance in kinetic pathology as a sound foundation for corrective surgery.
2. His instruction of Harken made the right-sided correction of left ventricular septal resection for IHSS practical.
3. His own epitaph: "The guy who saved a few kids from heart block."

Lillehei, C. Walton, M.D.
St. Paul, Minnesota
1. Creator and innovator of perhaps more techniques and concepts than any other living heart surgeon.
2. Open-heart surgery by "extracorporeal oxygenation" achieved by cross circulation of a father to his infant in intractable heart failure (1954).
3. Collaborated with Dewall in development and use of bubble oxygenator (1955).
4. Plastic disposable-bag bubble oxygenator developed (1957).
5. Introduced hemodilution and moderate hypothermia techniques for open-heart surgery.

6. Developed simple disposable membrane oxygenator with Lande (1967).
7. Inventor of heart valves.
8. Made possible the extension of the opportunities afforded him by Wangensteen to his own illustrious disciples, including Shumway, Gott, Barnard, and others.

Litwak, Robert S., M.D.
New York, New York
1. Early investigator of intracardiac homografts.
2. With Gadboys evolved the concept of and some understanding of homologous transfusion reactions. This and subsequent work supported hemodilution techniques for open-heart surgery.
3. Developed left ventricular circulatory assist system that can support the heart action in critically ill patients and be discontinued without reopening the chest.
4. Leader as heart surgeon, teacher, speaker, and editor.

Lower, Richard R., M.D.
Richmond, Virginia
Pioneer in cardiac transplantation and investigator of rejection modes.

McGoon, Dwight C., M.D.
Rochester, Minnesota
1. Pacesetter for surgical procedures to correct complex congenital heart disease.
2. Sponsor of professional bridges of communication, national and international.

Magill, Sir Ivan Whiteside
London, England
Opened opportunities for thoracic and heart surgery with intratracheal anesthesia.

Magovern, George J., M.D.
Pittsburgh, Pennsylvania
1. Early advocate of central venous pressure monitoring in the postoperative patient as a rough guide to blood volume replacement.
2. Developer in 1961 of the sutureless technique of fixation for aortic and mitral ball-valve prostheses. His collaboration with engineer and instrument designer Harry Cromie was central to this success.

3. Developer of various ingenious valvuloplastic techniques and sutureless vascular anastomotic procedures.

Malm, James R., M.D.
New York, New York
1. Remarkable ability to consolidate the contributions of innovators into
   first-class surgical programs.
2. Demonstrated the reproducibility and low mortality in the correction
   of tetralogy of Fallot and developed infant cardiac surgery in several
   areas.
3. With others, including Kirklin, has given solid evaluation of homografts, their potential, and limitations of some sterilization and preservation techniques.

Meredino, K. Alvin, M.D.
Riyadh, Saudi Arabia
1. Investigator in laboratory and clinical use of behavior of biologic
   valves.
2. Ingenious developer of plastic techniques for acquired valvular insufficiency and atrioplastic procedures to correct congenital transposition of the great vessels.
3. Excellent organizer of symposia and educational efforts that have
   furthered heart surgery.
4. Carries the torch of American surgery to new areas of unique opportunity.

Morrow, A. Glenn, M.D.
Bethesda, Maryland
1. Left-heart catheterizations by transbronchial technique based on Alli-
   son's concept.
2. First direct-vision valvotomy under general hypothermia for congenital aortic stenosis.
3. First successful complete replacement of mitral valve with flexible
   material simulating normal mitral valve in collaboration with Nina
   Braunwald. This was March 11, 1960, one day after Harken's first
   successful caged-ball aortic valve replacement below the coronary
   ostia.
4. Investigator of biomaterials for patches and valve cover.
5. Basic studies of hypertrophic subaortic stenosis, its mechanism, diagnosis, and surgical correction.
6. Contributed to the concept of porcine heterografts on flexible stent,
   first implantation (1970).

7. Indubitably the only surgeon to have made exhaustive hemodynamic and angiographic studies of the complex circulation of the American alligator. (The important purpose of this study remains obscure.)
8. Contributed to the unique climate in the National Heart and Lung Institute that has improved diagnostic and surgical techniques for correcting congenital and acquired heart disease.
9. Creative teacher of a host of second-generation heart surgeons.

Muller, W. Harry, Jr., M.D.
Charlottesville, Virginia
1. Developed pulmonary vascular changes in experimental animals secondary to pulmonary hypertension.
2. Developed pulmonary banding operation, with F. Damman.
3. First operation for total anomalous venous return.
4. First use of complete aortic valve replacement with bicuspid prosthetic valve.
5. Definitive repair of Marfan's syndrome by resecting ascending aortic aneurysm and repair of aortic valve.
6. Definitive repair of dissecting aneurysm with pump oxygenator.
7. Teacher and organization leader.

Murray, D. W. Gordon, M.D., F.R.C.S. (C), F.R.C.S. (E)
Toronto, Canada
1. Innovative and technical genius whose vast contributions are multifocal and only sporadically exposed.
2. Early use of heparin to prevent pulmonary emboli.
3. First human homograft valves (inserted in descending aorta). Used homograft veins and showed that they arterialized.
4. Tried subclavian coronary artery anastomosis in dogs (1940s).
5. Tried fascia lata for valve replacement.
6. Produced first artificial kidney in America (second in the world).

Mustard, W. T., F.R.C.S.
Toronto, Canada
Ingenious and courageous pioneer in the surgical correction of transposition of the great vessels.

Nadas, Alexander S., M.D.
Boston, Massachusetts
1. Clinical and physiologic correlation leading to the establishment of the specialty of Pediatric Cardiology.

2. First comprehensive textbook in Pediatric Cardiology.
3. Medical collaborator with surgeon Robert E. Gross in developmental phases of open and closed cardiac and great-vessel operations.

O'Shaughnessy, Lawrence, F.R.C.S.
Newcastle-on-Tyne, England
1. Used omentum and irritant paste to cause revascularization via vascular adhesions (1933) (relates to no. 4).
2. Suggested valvotomy for congenital pulmonary valve stenosis.
3. Died in his own casualty-clearing hospital of tension pneumothorax in the Dunkirk retreat, World War II.
4. Aware of Thorel's case (1903) of patient who died of carcinoma of the lung, but who had "adhesive pericarditis" and complete obliteration of the main coronary arteries.

Paget, Sir Stephen
London, England
Leading surgeon of his time who serves as a lesson to us all not to decide what others will be incapable of attaining. His classical dour prediction of 1896 was: "The heart alone of all viscera has reached the limits set by nature to surgery. No new method and no new technique can overcome the natural obstacles surrounding a wound of the heart." (Ludwig Rehn of Frankfurt succeeded in 1896.)

Potts, Willis J., M.D.
Chicago, Illinois
1. Brilliant pediatric surgeon.
2. Developer of pulmonary artery/aortic shunt for cyanotic congenital heart disease.

Rehn, Ludwig, M.D.
Frankfurt, Germany
Successfully sutured a stab wound of the heart in 1896. A great victory of a "doer" over the "doubter" Paget. (The doubters always have a statistical advantage.)

Roe, Benson B., M.D.
San Francisco, California
1. Pioneered use of elective ventricular fibrillation.
2. Utilized left atrial pressures after open-heart surgery to reduce the mortality of the low-output syndrome.

3. Promulgator of the disposable bubble oxygenator.
4. Developer and refiner of techniques for congenital anomalies, including Ebstein's anomaly.
5. His only cardiac transplant is alive and well six years after operation.

Ross, Donald N., F.R.C.S.
London, England
1. Described sinus venosus congenital defect.
2. Was the man who introduced aortic homograft valves and autograft aortic valve replacement into clinical use.
3. Performed the "Rastelli operation," right ventricular outflow tract reconstruction with valve conduit before Rastelli (1966).
4. Educator, investigator, and clinician.

Sabiston, David C., Jr., M.D.
Durham, North Carolina
1. Extended understanding of physiology of the myocardium and coronary circulation as it relates to myocardial contraction and collateral/revascularization.
2. Augmented surgical management of congenital and acquired coronary circulation.
3. Studied the diagnosis and nature of pulmonary embolism.
4. Explored fluid fluorocarbon as an oxygen conduit in experimental extracorporeal circulation and as a blood substitute.
5. Added clarity to physiopathology of myocardial infarction.
6. Performed early aortocoronary artery bypass (probably first in a human—patient lived 3 days) (1962). Published with beautiful illustrations (1974).
7. Structured the management of dissecting aneurysms.
8. Related aortocoronary bypass grafts to myocardial contractility.
9. Editor important surgical textbook.

Sakakibara, Shigeru, M.D.
Tokyo, Japan
1. Developed a cardioscope for use before open-heart surgery was available.
2. Devised competent and ingenious oxygenators and has combined them with hypothermia (1956 and later, originally with Dr. Konno).
3. Developed many ingenious operations in the laboratory, then clinically, for congenital heart disease (with Dr. Arai).
4. Computerization of diagnosis and care (with Dr. Imai).

5. Founded Heart Institute of Japan.
6. Developed transvascular myocardial biopsy technique.

Sealy, Will C., M.D.
Durham, North Carolina
1. Explained postoperative arteritis and paradoxical hypertension related to coarctation of the aorta and the nature of the hypertension of such coarctation.
2. Pioneered surface cooling with extracorporeal circulation; deep hypothermia and circulatory arrest controlled by extracorporeal circulation; and first heat exchanger (with Ivan Brown and Glenn Young).
3. Mapped atrial internodal conduction paths.
4. Explained disturbance and shunt-flow pathophysiology.
5. First correction W.P.W. dysrhythmia in now 40+ patients.
6. Explained bundle of His and AV node exclusion from atrium in dysrhythmias. The work on arrhythmias, including tachycardia, is a cardinal remaining frontier of cardiac surgery.
7. Studies on hypercapnea, alkalosis, and changes in the internal environment of man related to organ function.

Sellors, Sir T. Holmes, F.R.C.S.
Aylesbury, Bucks, England
Early British surgeon who worked with pulmonary valvotomy, septal defects, and explored the etiology and nature of constrictive pericarditis.

Senning, Ake, M.D.
Zurich, Switzerland
1. Introduced elective fibrillation in heart surgery.
2. Combined efforts in developing heart-lung machine with Crafoord/Björk (1954).
3. Corrected total anomalous venous return (1956).
4. Developed circulatory assist techniques by left-heart bypass (some with Dennis).
5. Correction TGA (1958).
6. First total pacemaker implantation (1958).
7. Strip biologic graft introduced (1958).

Shumway, Norman E., M.D.
Stanford, California
The prime investigator and cardinal man in the field of cardiac transplantation. He, as no other, has forged the multidisciplinary effort.

He now records significant long-term human heart transplant survival.

Sones, Mason, M.D.
Cleveland, Ohio
Fashioned equipment and techniques of angiography as a cornerstone to clarify the diagnosis, prognosis, and results of both medical and surgical treatment of heart disease. His work added the essential precision to the foundations of Steinberg and Raab required to open the field of coronary artery surgery.

Souttar, Sir Henry, F.R.C.S.
London, England
Successfully explored mitral valve digitally via the left atrial appendage (1925). When asked by Harken why he did not repeat the magnificent operation, he replied, "Because I could not get another case . . . the physicians declared it was all nonsense . . . it is of no use to be ahead of one's time."

Spencer, Frank C., M.D.
New York, New York
1. "The Larrey of the Korean War" for his excellent management of arterial injuries in battle casualties.
2. Pioneer in monitoring of patient after open-heart surgery and supporting patients with circulatory assistance guided by appropriate blood gas and electrolyte assay.
3. Technical innovator and designer of instruments, including silastic coronary perfusion cannulae and visual aids.

Starr, Albert, M.D.
Portland, Oregon
1. The most meticulous investigator, innovator, and clinical user of caged-ball valves. His standards of quality control in valve development and follow-up of patients are models for the world.
2. Innovator of surgical techniques in correcting and caring for acquired, and early correction of congenital, defects.
3. Pioneer in the marriage of medicine, biology, and engineering.

Strieder, John W., M.D.
Boston, Massachusetts
Made first attempt to close the patent ductus (1937). Though the patient died, he and his medical collaborators gave clear definition of

the ethical place for risk taking and experimental surgical adventure. This standard has been widely, but unfortunately not universally, followed.

Swan, Henry, M.D.
Denver, Colorado
1. First resection of aneurysm with arterial homograft (1949).
2. First peripheral arterial replacement with homografts.
3. First series of open-heart operations under hypothermia. (Lewis preceded with atrial septal defect closure, and Varco with open correction of pulmonic stenosis without hypothermia.)
4. Continues efforts at identification and synthesis of antimetabolic hormone.

Swan, H. J. C., M.D.
Los Angeles, California
1. A cardiologist and physiologist who views the heart and lungs from the surgical point of view.
2. Gave clinical assessment of left ventricular function currency by the pulmonary artery catheter that bears his name and his coworker's, "Swann-Ganz."
3. Past president of the American College of Cardiology.

Taussig, Helen B., M.D.
Baltimore, Maryland
1. Recognized that cyanotic children often died when the ductus closed. A clinical/autopsy study.
2. Inspired by Gross's closure of patent ductus arteriosus, she sought a surgeon to "build a ductus." Persuaded Blalock to try it in the laboratory, then in humans.
3. Designed an experimental cyanotic model, corrected it in animals, then in man.
4. The collaborator, with Blalock, in surgical legend.
5. Her selection of patients for the Blalock-Taussig operation gave the benefits to the world.

Urschel, Harold C., M.D.
Dallas, Texas
1. Leader among second-generation heart surgeons.
2. Innovator and extender of revascularization procedures.

3. Effective organizer of societies and publications for dissemination of knowledge.
4. Past president American College of Chest Physicians.

Varco, Richard, M.D.
Minneapolis, Minnesota
1. Collaborated in early open-heart surgery with Dennis (1951).
2. Collaborated with Lillehei in cross circulation (1954).
3. Actively pursuing ileal bypass as a metabolic prophylaxis against atherosclerosis.
4. Surgical leader who supported pioneering efforts of his group of leaders in heart surgery.

Vineberg, Arthur, M.D.
Montreal, Canada
1. Creator of Vineberg mammary artery implantation for coronary artery disease (1946). (Continues to date with various additional maneuvers.)
2. His work was based on careful, extensive experimental laboratory research.
3. He addressed a reluctant world until patency was proved by Sones.

Wada, Juro J., M.D.
Tokyo, Japan
1. Bubbled and debubbled venous blood to oxygenate (1953). Those working with him failed to recognize the relevance to cardiopulmonary bypass.
2. Developed pump oxygenator—heart exchange devices.
3. Pioneered tilting-disc hingeless valves.
4. Multitude of regional (Japanese) surgical firsts.
5. Advocate of innovations in Japanese medical education based on the American system.
6. Director of Japanese Heart Institute at Tokyo Women's Medical College.

Waterston, David J., F.R.C.S.
Old Iselworth, England
1. Devised aortopulmonary anastomosis.
2. Outstanding surgeon and teacher.

Wiggers, Carl J., M.D.
Cleveland, Ohio

A cardiac physiologist who linked the laboratory to clinical application for medicine and surgery.

Zerbini, Euriclides DeJesus, M.D.
São Paulo, Brazil

1. Brilliant innovator of surgical techniques and instruments.
2. A multitude of regional first operations and led Brazilian manufacturers to create the equipment not otherwise available from the outside world.
3. Creation of biologic valves (dura mater).
4. Founder of Heart Institute.
5. Leader, modest and creative teacher, clinician.

Zoll, Paul M., M.D.
Boston, Massachusetts

1. Pioneer of external, then implantable cardiac pacemakers.
2. Made precise anatomical studies of coronary arteries in health and disease with Blumgart and Schlessinger.
3. Collaborated with Harken as cardiologist in World War II foreign body work.

Zuhdi, Nazih, M.D.
Oklahoma City, Oklahoma

1. Combined efforts in developing rotating screen oxygenator with Clarence Dennis and Karl Karlson (1953). Collaborated in first mechanical pump support for chronic heart failure (1955).
2. Combined efforts in developing plastic sheet oxygenator, bubble type, with Gott, Dewall, and others (1956).
3. Developer of several heat exchangers and systems, including the double-helical reservoir heart-lung machine.
4. First glutaraldehyde porcine aortic valve in human in America, following Carpentier, and collaborator in evolving the stabilized glutaraldehyde process porcine aortic valve in aortic and mitral positions in humans (with Warren Hancock, manufacturer, 1970).
5. First total prime of a heart-lung machine with 5 percent dextrose in water, hemodilution with moderate hypothermia for open-heart surgery (experimentally and clinically, 1960).

Index

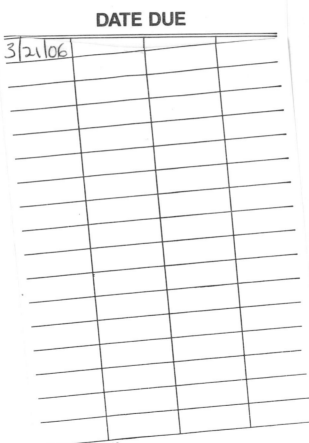

DATE DUE

3/21/06			

Demco, Inc. 38-293